Monographs on Endocrinology

Volume 16

Edited by

F. Gross, Heidelberg · M.M. Grumbach, San Francisco
A. Labhart, Zürich · M.B. Lipsett, Bethesda
T. Mann, Cambridge · L.T. Samuels (†), Salt Lake City
J. Zander, München

J.E.A. McIntosh
R.P. McIntosh

Mathematical Modelling and Computers in Endocrinology

With 73 Figures and 57 Tables

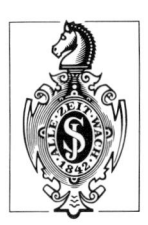

Springer-Verlag
Berlin Heidelberg New York 1980

James E.A. McIntosh M.A., Ph.D. (Cantab.)
Department of Obstetrics and Gynaecology,
University of Adelaide, Adelaide, S.A., Australia

Rosalind P. McIntosh Ph.D. (Cantab.)
Lucy Cavendish College, Cambridge, U.K.

ISBN 3-540-09693-0 Springer-Verlag Berlin Heidelberg New York
ISBN 0-387-09693-0 Springer-Verlag New York Heidelberg Berlin

Library of Congress Cataloging in Publication Data.

McIntosh, James Edward Alister, 1942-. Mathematical modelling and computers in endocrinology. (Monographs on endocrinology; v. 16) Bibliography: p. Includes index. 1. Endocrinology – Mathematical models. 2. Endocrinology – Data processing. 3. Biological models. I. McIntosh, Rosalind Phyllis, 1943- joint author. II. Title
QP187.3.M36M34   591.1′42′028   79-28283

This work is subject to copyright. All rights are reserved, whether the whole or part of the material is concerned, specifically those of translation, reprinting, re-use of illustrations, broadcasting, reproduction by photocopying machine or similar means, and storage in data banks. Under § 54 of the German Copyright Law where copies are made for other than private use, a fee is payable to the publisher, the amount of the fee to be determined by agreement with the publisher.

© Springer-Verlag Berlin, Heidelberg 1980
Printed in Germany

The use of registered names, trademarks, etc. in this publication does not imply, even in the absence of a specific statement, that such names are exempt from the relevant protective laws and regulations and therefore free for general use.

Typesetting, printing and binding: O. Brandstetter, Wiesbaden
2125/3020 – 543210

Preface

The building of conceptual models is an inherent part of our interaction with the world, and the foundation of scientific investigation. Scientists often perform the processes of modelling subconsciously, unaware of the scope and significance of this activity, and the techniques available to assist in the description and testing of their ideas.

Mathematics has three important contributions to make in biological modelling: (1) it provides unambiguous languages for expressing relationships at both qualitative and quantitative levels of observation; (2) it allows effective analysis and prediction of model behaviour, and can thereby organize experimental effort productively; (3) it offers rigorous methods of testing hypotheses by comparing models with experimental data; by providing a means of objectively excluding unsuitable concepts, the development of ideas is given a sound experimental basis.

Many modern mathematical techniques can be exploited only with the aid of computers. These machines not only provide increased speed and accuracy in determining the consequences of model assumptions, but also greatly extend the range of problems which can be explored. The impact of computers in the biological sciences has been widespread and revolutionary, and will continue to be so.

The aim of this book is twofold: we wish to portray to endocrinologists the productive interplay of concepts in biology and mathematics, and at the same time provide illustrative examples and practical information about computing to enable the reader to apply many of the techniques presented to his or her own subject of interest. The approach is descriptive, with the minimum of mathematical nomenclature and equations. Although the formulation of ideas in words rather than in mathematical symbols necessarily entails some loss of precision, the text should thereby be made approachable for the biologically trained reader. It would be pleasing also if mathematicians could perceive here some of the richness, challenge and reward of working with biological systems, difficult and "imperfect" mathematically but "perfect" in their ingenuity of adaptation to biological purpose.

Mathematical modelling is not the answer to all endocrinological problems, but where applied appropriately it offers substantial reward for effort. Some kinds of mathematical modelling can contribute to endocrinological investigations at the descriptive level. Knowledge of endocrine systems is, however, becoming increasingly quantitative and the relevance of mathematical methods suited to more precise measurements is growing rapidly. Mathematics appears to be essential for formulating and testing hypotheses on biological control and organization.

The techniques described in this monograph are completely general—the examples, however, reflect the experience and interests of the authors, many being related to reproductive endocrinology. Computer techniques are given prominence throughout.

The scope of the book is as follows. Chapter 1 discusses in general terms the nature, purposes, advantages and limitations of mathematical modelling, and some of the mathematical and biological concepts involved. Chapter 2 concerns the characteristics and utility of a selection of mathematical techniques appropriate to the formulation of a varied range of biological models; these also are presented generally. Chapter 3 shows how models can be compared with data, and how to determine when a model is adequate, or requires modifying. Computer methods are introduced using two computer programs for comparing models with experiments, and illustrative examples are given of how they are applied. Chapter 4 describes statistical techniques for designing effective experiments, and includes a computer program to control sequential experimentation. Chapters 5 and 6 deal with several subjects of endocrinological interest to which the quantitative computer methods of earlier chapters are applied. Chapter 7 is concerned with rhythmic processes. The first part describes how theories of cyclic processes have begun to be applied in modelling biological rhythms, while the second outlines methods for analysing rhythmic behaviour empirically. Chapter 8 illustrates the mathematical modelling of large endocrinological systems by discussing the use of several approaches described in Chap. 2 in modelling the ovulatory cycle. Chapter 9 contains examples of two kinds of statistical models of great practical usefulness in endocrinology.

Appendix A briefly introduces statistical concepts and tests required in mathematical modelling, while Appendix B provides details of the computer programs referred to above.

While this monograph is the result of an enjoyably co-operative effort, particular responsibility is taken for Chaps. 1, 2, 7 and 8 by R.P.M., and for Chaps. 3–6, 9 and the appendices by J.E.A.M.

The latter is grateful to the Department of Obstetrics and Gynaecology, University of Adelaide, and the Agricultural Research Council's Unit of Reproductive Physiology and Biochemistry, University of Cambridge, for encouraging and supporting his research, and we are appreciative of the generous policies of both Universities in providing free access to excellent computing facilities. R.P.M. thanks the Department of Obstetrics and Gynaecology, University of Adelaide for an honourary Research Associateship.

We welcome this opportunity to express gratitude to our friends and colleagues in Adelaide, Cambridge, Bethesda and elsewhere (and particularly Dr C. Lutwak-Mann, Dr R.F. Seamark, and Mrs B. Godfrey) for helpful discussions, and for kindly reading and commenting upon many sections of the typescript. Mrs Godfrey also assisted in the coding of the computer programs SIMUL and DESIGN. The reviewers made several helpful suggestions and we are grateful to them for their careful reading of the text.

Most of all we happily acknowledge the unfailing inspiration, enthusiasm and encouragement of Cecelia and Thaddeus Mann.

December 1979

J.E.A. McIntosh
R.P. McIntosh

Contents

1		**Modelling in Biology**	1
1.1		The Nature of Scientific Models	2
	1.1.1	Different Kinds of Models	3
	1.1.2	Reductionism in Biology	4
	1.1.3	The Scope of Modelling	5
1.2		Clarity from Complexity	6
	1.2.1	Experimental Frames	7
	1.2.2	Variables and Parameters	7
	1.2.3	Diagrams	9
	1.2.4	Lumping	9
	1.2.5	Hierarchical Levels	10
	1.2.6	Stochastic and Deterministic Behaviours	11
	1.2.7	Problems of Individuality	12
1.3		Experimental Data	13
1.4		Predictions from Models – Simulation	13
1.5		A Model of Complexity Producing Organized Simplicity	14
1.6		Subjectivity in Modelling	17
1.7		Mathematics in Modelling	18
1.8		Computers and Models	20
1.9		Description of Models	22
1.10		Modelling in Perspective	23
1.11		Advantages in Modelling	25
2		**Mathematical Descriptions of Biological Models**	26
2.1		Theoretical Modelling – Analysis of Mechanism	26
	2.1.1	Differentials	26
		2.1.1.1 Modelling Dynamic Systems with Differential Equations	27
		2.1.1.2 Making Differential Equations and Data Comparable	28
		2.1.1.3 Requirements for the Use of Differential Equations	29
	2.1.2	Transient and Steady States	30
	2.1.3	Defining Model Equations	30
	2.1.4	Systems to Which Theoretical Modelling Can Be Applied	31
	2.1.5	Compartmental Analysis and Inhomogeneity	31
2.2		Linearity and Non-Linearity	32
2.3		Empirical Modelling – a Description of System Response	34
	2.3.1	Empirical Equations and Curve-Fitting	34
		2.3.1.1 Spline Functions	35
		2.3.1.2 Self-Modelling Non-Linear Regression	36

	2.3.2	Transfer Functions	37
	2.3.3	Convolution Integrals	38
	2.3.4	Combining Subsystems	39
	2.3.5	Frequency Domain Analysis	40
2.4	Point Stability in Models		42
	2.4.1	Tests for Stability of Linear Models	43
	2.4.2	Stability of Non-Linear Models	44
2.5	Concepts of Feedback		45
	2.5.1	Biological Homeostasis and the Concept of Feedback	45
	2.5.2	Feedback Control	46
		2.5.2.1 Point Stability in Models of Negative Feedback	49
		2.5.2.2 Effectiveness of Feedback Loops	50
		2.5.2.3 Negative Feedback Loops and Their Mechanisms in Endocrinology	52
2.6	Biological Development and Mathematics Beyond Instability		54
	2.6.1	An Example of Parameter-Dependent Changes in System Stability	56
	2.6.2	Limit Cycles	58
	2.6.3	Stability Behaviour and Spatial Inhomogeneity	60
	2.6.4	Examples of Non-Linear Equations Showing Instabilities	61
	2.6.5	Generalized Descriptions of Instabilities in Biology	64
2.7	Finite Level Modelling		66
2.8	The Need for Statistics		69
	2.8.1	Transformation and Weighting	70
	2.8.2	Parameter Uncertainty	71
		2.8.2.1 Monte Carlo Simulation	71
	2.8.3	Testing Hypotheses	72
	2.8.4	Normal Distributions in Biology	73
	2.8.5	Statistics and Experimental Design	73
3	**Comparing Models with Experimental Results**		**74**
3.1	Analogue Simulation		74
3.2	Approximate Simulation by Digital Computer		75
3.3	Suitable Digital Computers		76
3.4	Estimation of Parameters		77
	3.4.1	Linearity and Non-Linearity in Parameter Estimation	78
	3.4.2	Defining the "Best" Fit of a Model to Data	78
	3.4.3	Methods of Parameter Search in Non-Linear Models	80
		3.4.3.1 Direct Search Methods	80
		3.4.3.2 Gradient Search Methods	81
3.5	Practical Details of Fitting Non-Linear Models to Data		82
	3.5.1	Weighting by Variance in the Data	82
	3.5.2	Measurement Error Estimated from the Fitting Process	83
	3.5.3	Constraining the Search	83
	3.5.4	Terminating the Search and Examining the Residuals	84
	3.5.5	Outliers	84
	3.5.6	Interpretation of Parameter Estimates	85

	3.5.7	Goodness of Fit of the Model	85
	3.5.8	Difficulties in Parameter Optimization	86
		3.5.8.1 Parameter Interaction and Sums of Exponentials	86
3.6	Models Containing Differential Equations		88
3.7	Using the Computer to Fit Models to Data		89
	3.7.1	Exponential Decay: Clearance of PMSG	89
		3.7.1.1 Application of Monte Carlo Simulation	91
	3.7.2	Growth of Elephants	96
	3.7.3	How Thick is the Wall of an Ovarian Follicle?	99
4	**Design of Analytical Experiments**		**103**
4.1	Principles of Design		103
	4.1.1	Randomization	103
	4.1.2	Replication	104
	4.1.3	Reduction of Random Variation	104
	4.1.4	Factorial Experiments	105
4.2	Sequential Design		105
	4.2.1	Design Criterion for Parameter Estimation	106
	4.2.2	Design Criterion for Model Discrimination	106
	4.2.3	Combined Model Discrimination and Parameter Estimation	107
	4.2.4	Termination Criteria	107
	4.2.5	Implementation	108
	4.2.6	A Computer Algorithm for Combined Design Criteria	109
	4.2.7	Does Sequential Experimentation Work?	110
	4.2.8	Testing the Design Criteria by Monte Carlo Simulation	110
5	**Dynamic Systems: Clearance and Compartmental Analysis**		**115**
5.1	Clearance		115
	5.1.1	Clearance of PMSG from the Blood	116
5.2	Compartmental Analysis		120
	5.2.1	Writing Equations to Describe Dynamic Systems	122
	5.2.2	Hormonal Influence on Zinc Transport in Rabbit Tissues	123
		5.2.2.1 Analytical Integration: Two Compartments	125
		5.2.2.2 Analytical Integration: Three Compartments	127
		5.2.2.3 Other Applications	131
	5.2.3	Numerical Integration of Dynamic Model Equations	131
		5.2.3.1 A Two-Compartment System	131
		5.2.3.2 A Three-Compartment System	132
		5.2.3.3 Comparison of Series and Parallel Models	133
	5.2.4	A Generalized Mammilary System	135
		5.2.4.1 Transport of Albumin	137
		5.2.4.2 Transport of PMSG	139
	5.2.5	Extension of the Generalized Mammillary System	141
6	**Ligand–Protein Interaction and Competitive Displacement Assays**		**143**
6.1	Interactions Between Ligands and Macromolecules		143

		6.1.1	The Binding of Ligands to Non-Interacting, Independent Sites 144

- 6.1.1 The Binding of Ligands to Non-Interacting, Independent Sites 144
  - 6.1.1.1 The Binding Properties of Human Pregnancy Plasma 146
  - 6.1.1.2 Binding Expressed as a Molar Ratio 151
- 6.1.2 Sequential Binding and Co-operativity 152
  - 6.1.2.1 Use of the General Binding Model 153

6.2 Competitive Protein-Binding Assays 155
- 6.2.1 Theoretical Models 156
  - 6.2.1.1 Effects of Labelled Ligand and Cross-Reactants . . 156
  - 6.2.1.2 Analysis of a Radio-Immunoassay for Testosterone . 157
- 6.2.2 Empirical Models 160
  - 6.2.2.1 Logit-Log and Non-Linear Regression Models . . . 162
  - 6.2.2.2 Simulation of the Testosterone Radio-Immunoassay . 164
  - 6.2.2.3 Spline Functions 167
- 6.2.3 Weighting 167
- 6.2.4 Sensitivity and Precision 168
- 6.2.5 Optimization of Assays 169

7 Mathematical Modelling of Biological Rhythms 171

7.1 Biological Rhythms: Experimental Evidence 171
7.2 The Contribution of Mathematics 173
- 7.2.1 Description of Rhythms 173
- 7.2.2 Mathematical Models of Response to Stimuli 174

7.3 Response of Rhythms to Stimuli – Rhythm Coupling 175
- 7.3.1 Phases Sensitive to Stimulation 176
- 7.3.2 Disturbances in Models Involving Limit Cycles 181
  - 7.3.2.1 Pulse Stimuli Causing Phase Changes 181
  - 7.3.2.2 Limit Cycle Interpretation of Phase Changes 182
  - 7.3.2.3 Application of a Limit Cycle Model 184
- 7.3.3 Entrainment of Oscillators by Rhythmic Forcing Functions . 185
- 7.3.4 Interactive Coupling of Limit Cycles 186

7.4 Rhythms, Endocrinology and Biological Control 189
7.5 Empirical Characterization of Rhythms from Data 191
- 7.5.1 The Sine Wave Model 192
  - 7.5.1.1 Temperature Variation During the Menstrual Cycle . 192
- 7.5.2 Auto-Correlation: Analysis in the Time Domain 194
- 7.5.3 Frequency Analysis of Rhythms 195
  - 7.5.3.1 Auto-Correlation and Frequency Analysis of Temperature Data 196
- 7.5.4 Bivariate Processes; Cross-Correlation and Cross-Spectra . . 198

8 Large Systems: Modelling Ovulatory Cycles 201

8.1 Modelling the Ovulatory Cycle 201
8.2 A Description of the Ovulatory Cycle 203
8.3 Use of Differential Equations with Cyclic Solutions 204
8.4 Use of a Threshold Discontinuity to Produce Cyclicity 208

8.5	A Physiologically Based Model of the Rat Oestrous Cycle	209
8.6	An Empirical Model of the Rat Oestrous Cycle Controlled by Time	211
8.7	An Attempt to Include More Variables	212
8.8	Eliminating the Differential Equations: A Finite Level Model	213
8.9	A "Complete" Description	217
	8.9.1 Testing the Model	220
	8.9.1.1 The Effect of Short-Term Random Oscillations	220
	8.9.1.2 Response to Infusions of Oestradiol and GnRH	221
	8.9.2 Further Modifications	222
8.10	Conclusions	223
9	**Stochastic Models**	226
9.1	Non-Parametric Statistical Models	227
	9.1.1 Comparing Two Independent Samples	228
	9.1.2 Comparing Two Samples Related by Pairs	229
	9.1.3 Comparing More than Two Samples with Related Individuals	230
	9.1.4 Identifying the Difference: Critical Range Tests	231
	9.1.5 Comparing More than Two Independent Samples	232
	9.1.6 Conclusions	232
9.2	Multivariate Analysis	232
	9.2.1 Principal Component and Factor Analysis	233
	9.2.1.1 Factor Analysis: Steroid Production by Ovarian Follicles	234
	9.2.2 Cluster Analysis	237
	9.2.3 Discriminant Analysis	238
	9.2.3.1 Application to Steroid Production by Ovarian Follicles	238
10	**Appendix A: A Summary of Relevant Statistics**	242
10.1	Variance, Standard Deviation and Weight	242
10.2	The Propagation of Variance	243
10.3	Covariance and Correlation	244
10.4	z-Scores, or Standardized Measures	244
10.5	Testing Hypotheses	245
10.6	Runs-Test	245
10.7	Chi-Square Test	245
10.8	Tests of Normality of Distribution	246
10.9	Comparing Two Parameters: The t-Test	246
10.10	Comparing Any Number of Parameters: Analysis of Variance	247
10.11	The Variance Ratio or F-Test	248
10.12	Confidence Intervals	249
10.13	Control Charts	249
11	**Appendix B: Computer Programs**	250
11.1	MODFIT: A General Model-Fitting Program	250
11.2	SIMUL: A Program for Monte Carlo Simulation	260

11.3	FUNCTN Subprogram RESERVR: Exponential Decay	266
11.4	FUNCTN Subprogram EXPCUBE: Growth of Organisms	266
11.5	FUNCTN Subprogram POLYNOM: General Polynomial	267
11.6	FUNCTN Subprogram FOLL: Growth of Ovarian Follicles	268
11.7	DESIGN: A Program for Efficient Experimental Design	268
11.8	FUNCTN Subprogram CA1: Compartmental Analysis	278
11.9	FUNCTN Subprogram CA2: Compartmental Analysis	279
11.10	FUNCTN Subprogram CA2A: Compartmental Analysis	281
11.11	FUNCTN Subprogram CA3: Compartmental Analysis	282
11.12	FUNCTN Subprogram MASSACT: Ligand Binding	284
11.13	FUNCTN Subprogram GENBIND: Ligand Binding	287
11.14	FUNCTN Subprogram RIA: Competitive Protein-Binding	288
11.15	FUNCTN Subprogram RIAH: Competitive Protein-Binding	289
11.16	FUNCTN Subprogram SIN: Rhythmical Data	290
11.17	FUNCTN Subprogram LIMIT: Limit Cycles	290
11.18	Other Programs for Fitting Non-Linear Models to Data	291
	11.18.1 SPSS NONLINEAR	292
	11.18.2 MLAB: An Online Modelling Laboratory	292
	11.18.3 SAAM: Simulation, Analysis and Modelling	292
	11.18.4 Other Programs	292
12	**Appendix C: Analytical Integration by Laplace Transform**	294
References		296
Subject Index		307

1 Modelling in Biology

A *model* describes, recites the characteristics of, or defines, the workings of a system.

Modelling is a fundamental human activity. We each carry in our mind a conceptual model of our "world", a conscious or subconscious structure of many levels, rational or irrational, formed from expectations, experiences and learning. All perceptions are compared with this malleable model and found to be irrelevant, confirmatory or contradictory. From the comparison can develop action, emotion, new models.

The activity of scientific investigation is an attempt to use controlled observations or experiments to rationally build or modify conceptual models derived from our imagination, experience and learning. Our perceptions may thereby become richer and more meaningful, and our expectations more reliable.

Much of this book is concerned with ways of comparing scientific observations with models. This is not a new pursuit; it is at the basis of all scientific investigation. The teaching of the necessary skills is essential to scientists in training, but too often the details have been expected to be acquired unguided while learning the all-important conclusions from the modelling efforts of others.

Every experimental design, performance and analysis involves modelling. One may unconsciously use models which follow the well-tried, acceptable paths of history. Or one can purposefully seek to reassess assumptions and to select anew from all conceivable possibilities, interactions, elements and conditions for study, those ever more appropriate to our increasing experience of the system of interest.

Even so-called facts are based on models. To quote von Bertalanffy (1973):

> According to widespread opinion, there is a fundamental distinction between 'observed facts' on the one hand – which are the unquestionable rock bottom of science and should be collected in the greatest possible number and printed in scientific journals – and 'mere theory' on the other hand, which is the product of speculation and more or less suspect... such antithesis does not exist... when you take supposedly simple data in our field – say, determination of Q_{O_2}, basal metabolic rates or temperature coefficients – it would take hours to unravel the enormous amount of theoretical presuppositions which are necessary to form these concepts, to arrange suitable experimental designs, to create machines to do the job – and this all is implied in your supposedly raw data of observation. If you have obtained a series of such values, the most 'empirical' thing you can do is to present them in a table of mean values and standard deviations. This presupposes the model of a binomial distribution – and with this, the whole theory of probability, a profound and to a large extent unsolved problem of mathematics, philosophy and even metaphysics.... Thus even supposedly unadulterated facts of observation already are interfused with all sorts of conceptual pictures, model concepts, theories... The choice is not whether to remain in the field of data or to theorize; the choice is only between models that are more or less abstract, generalized, near or more remote from direct observation, more or less suitable to represent observed phenomena.[1]

---

[1] Words taken from Ludwig von Bertalanffy; General System Theory (Allen Lane The Penguin Press, 1971; Penguin University Books, 1973) pp 163–164. Copyright by Ludwig von Bertalanffy, 1968. Reprinted by kind permission of Penguin Books Ltd., London, and George Braziller Inc., New York.

The simplest measurement is the outcome of an interaction between a measuring instrument and a model of a system, rather than a direct property of the real system itself. The way in which measurements are made depends on how the information is to be applied; a measuring tape is used differently in assessing the distance between two points depending on whether it determines the length of the path taken by an insect crawling over rough ground, or the same route travelled by a flying crow. Determinations of the "level" of a hormone depend on the model of its mode of action. The property of the hormone that we think is effective in producing a response dictates whether we measure its total molecular concentration in blood, the amount not bound to plasma protein or the rate of fluctuation in level.

Biological models reach the printed page in many forms. A model can be a simple mathematical equation such as $y = x^2$. It can be pages of closely packed, personalized symbols in fine print linked by multiple, angular arrows. Neither the use of complexity, nor the constraint of a model to an easily soluble mathematical equation guarantees its effectiveness.

There are other kinds of modelling which do not use mathematical equations. Sometimes models containing precise verbal statements may embody a biological concept in a more useful form than do mathematical equations (Williams, 1977). The response of one organism may be used to model that of another, as when drugs are administered to animals to test likely effects in humans. Mechanical or physical models may be studied where experiments on the system of interest would present insurmountable practical difficulties. The problems specific to these types of models will not be discussed here; our concern is with models involving mathematical descriptions. All models have in common an attempt to capture the significant aspects of a system in a form which is useful for investigating the properties of the system.

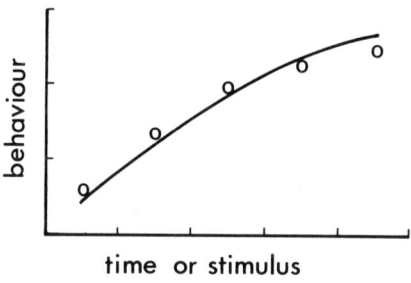

Fig. 1.1. Comparing experimental data with behaviour calculated from a model of the system. The *points* (○) represent the experimental measurements, and the *smooth curve* the model

1.1 The Nature of Scientific Models

A real system is a source of behaviour. We convert our observations of a system's behaviour into experimental data (either the variation of something with time, or in response to a stimulus). A model is a set of instructions designed by us to generate data resembling those of the real system. These instructions may merely describe the data, or they may embody our concept of what causes the behaviour. Comparison of the two sources of data, measured and generated (see Fig. 1.1), shows how compatible are the concepts of the model with experimental observations, and

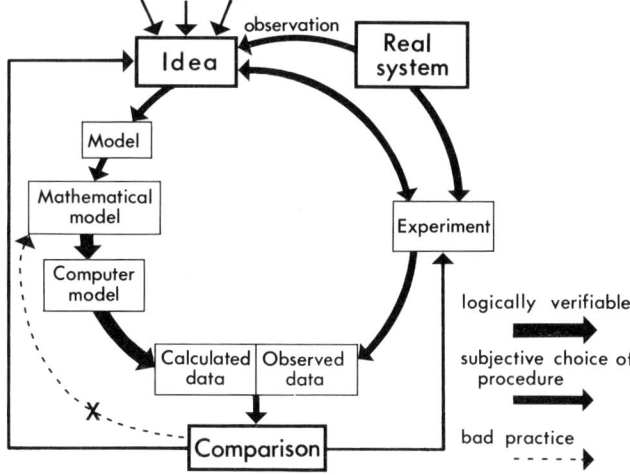

Fig. 1.2. The processes of mathematical modelling

whether our ideas are worth further development. Figure 1.2 shows a generalized scheme of the procedure of modelling mathematically. Other aspects of the modelling process illustrated in this diagram will be considered later.

1.1.1 Different Kinds of Models

Levins (1970) describes a model as an attempt to replace

> the universal or trivial statement "things are different, interconnected and changing", with a structure that specifies which things differ in what ways, interact how, change in what directions.

There are several different levels at which this model structure can be specified; the one selected depends both on the aims of the modeller and on the amount of information available about the system.

An *empirical model* is the most superficial. It describes accurately the values of a particular set of experimental data; under the same conditions, response to any suitable stimulus can be predicted from the model. However, the model *is not unique* and the particular mathematical form chosen may not reflect mechanims within the system. An empirical model bears little direct relation to the biological structure or to general physical laws. There may not even be a direct causal relationship between the stimulus and the response – merely a correlation.

A *theoretical model* (sometimes called analytical or mechanistic) *embodies our concept* of what causes the behaviour observed. The model description is based on biological and physical laws believed to be acting between components of the system. The consequences of the proposed mechanism can be calculated and agreement with experimental data strengthens the hypothesis. Prediction should be possible under a broader range of conditions than in empirical modelling. Two tendencies in theoretical modelling may be further distinguished: those that attempt to capture the essential, minimal aspects of the mechanisms required for reproducing the results, and those that try to be as complete as possible by simulating behaviour in terms of all known effectors and interactions. In building a model it is important to distinguish between empirical and theoretical aspects so that the ability of the model to explain, as opposed to describe, is not overestimated.

A third approach, known as *metaphoric* modelling, uses a *generalized description* of the system behaviour, without concern for details of the particular components. The belief underlying this kind of model is that any particular system behaviour can be classified according to the types of interactions involved. The consequences of these classes of interaction can be investigated mathematically, or are already known. The qualitative insights arising from these models may be surprising. By simply describing the dynamic type of the system the possibilities for its behaviour can be deduced, even without understanding the specific nature of the components involved. A description is made of the functional properties of a system rather than its structure. A metaphoric model becomes a theoretical one when the mathematical components are all identified with some observable entities in the system. However, the generality of such mathematical descriptions may make comparison of the model with any particular real set of data and real structural elements difficult. This is because those aspects of the system behaviour from which are derived the equations describing the dynamics, need not correspond in a direct and simple way to structural elements (although they will undoubtedly be a more complex function of them) (Rosen, 1977). Just as the reality of gravitational forces "applies to both the cosmos and to apples", physical disparity need not preclude powerful unifying concepts stemming from common organizational or control principles.

Some models combine aspects from several of these approaches. Examples of them all will be found throughout this book.

1.1.2 Reductionism in Biology

Another way of considering a system, biological or otherwise, is as a set of components that interact. A model attempts to describe relevant components and their interactions in such a way that it mimics the features of interest in the system. The finding and describing of components and their individual interactions is referred to in philosophy as reductionism.

Interactions between components often produce an organized total that is more than the sum of its parts. For example four isolated elements ○ ○ ○ ○ and their interactions ⧼ ⧼ ⧼ ⧼ when organized as a whole ▯ clearly take on new or emergent properties and possibilities (von Bertalanffy, 1973). The emergent behaviour relates to the consequences of interactions which were not understood in making the model description, but which ultimately affect the result. Such emergent properties can frequently be derived from mathematical models and are one of the main rewards of modelling. Many believe, however, that there are limits to such revelations and that in complex biological systems general principles of organization are unlikely to be revealed from the study of the minutiae of particular systems. An idea of general function, of course, necessarily precedes the construction of a detailed model. This does not deny that general principles, manifested in particular circumstances, cannot be described in terms of chemistry and physics. Crick (1966, p. 55) discussing replicating nucleic acids writes:

There is nothing, therefore, in the basic copying process, as far as we can see, which is different from our experience of physics and chemistry except, of course, that it is exceptionally well designed and rather more complicated.

Pattee (1970) and others contend that it is precisely "this exceptional design", those principles of adaptive self-organization or programming bringing about functions that distinguish living from non-living matter, which are the focus of the biologist's attention, and which cannot be revealed solely by reductionist study of biological systems in terms of physics and chemistry.

Are the laws of physics, chemistry and mathematics derived for inanimate matter sufficient to describe the properties peculiar to biological systems, such as self-organized responses to the environment, self-maintenance and development through the building of highly ordered structures, reproduction and evolution? Certainly, recent advances in these fields have produced generalized metaphoric models exhibiting strikingly "biological" behaviour (Sect. 2.6).

In conclusion, it seems that while reductionist analysis is necessary to confirm a hypothesis concerning the overall functioning of a system, an exclusively analytical emphasis will probably result in the loss of essential characteristics of the whole. This conflict between the need to test hypotheses using models in which specified biological components and interactions are compared with data obtained from real systems (theoretical modelling), and the difficulty of identifying the components of metaphoric models describing generalized organizational principles with real physiological structures, recurs in our discussions.

1.1.3 The Scope of Modelling

A model is a structure to play with – and in so doing to discover new behavioural possibilities of the system. A model is not definitive. It simply works out the consequences of proposed solutions to the perceived problem, in order to determine how these results compare with experimental observations. A model should be no more than a guide to constructive and efficient experimentation. It should lead to better models. It should grow, transform or become obsolete when tested, and yet have served its purpose well. It should never be finished or ready for publication in the "quod erat demonstrandum" form. Models are necessarily simplifications, concerned with one or a few very limited aspects of the system studied.

Whether models explain phenomena or merely describe them is a subjective matter. More relevant is whether they predict new, testable phenomena, show up deficiencies in current knowledge, suggest new experiments or create new perspectives that unify hitherto disparate facts.

An explanation renders phenomena more meaningful or intelligible. Obviously, whether something is made more meaningful depends on one's experience, learning and the paradigms of one's discipline of expertise. Bradley (1968) emphasizes the importance of tolerance between fields of learning. A model can still be very useful even if it is constructed without complete awareness of all the contextual material from another field. However, collaboration across disciplines may be more effective or even essential where models at one level (e. g. behavioural) are explained using the components of another discipline at a different level (e. g. biochemical).

An illuminating study of the historical usefulness of mathematical modelling in the development of ideas is presented by Provine (1977), applied to the subject of evolution. He concludes that although models that have been described may not correspond precisely to reality, nor all the claims made for them be justified, they have given observations a new significance by placing them in a framework of quantitative analysis. That is, mathematical modelling, even when applied to a field which is not readily quantifiable, has been shown to make experimental observations more meaningful or explicable. Modelling has offered effective guidelines based on experiment for the development of ideas. Provine gives the following illustration of the kind of contribution that mathematical modelling has made. Natural selection acting on the small variations known or reasonably supposed to exist in natural populations, was shown by this technique to be sufficient to account for evolution at the population level; Darwin's qualitative hypotheses were adequate and an additional factor proposed by disbelievers was not required.

Mathematical modelling in some form appears capable of making useful or essential contributions in most endocrinological investigations. For example, in a long list of problems related to contraception in the female reproductive tract, which according to Greep et al. (1976, pp. 138–147) require investigation, few topics are apparent in which mathematics would not be helpful.

1.2 Clarity from Complexity

A system needs first to be identified and distinguished from its surroundings in order to permit description, measurements and observations. In endocrinology such things as function, a chemical which can be analysed or physiological structures, may delineate a system for investigation. The system is described in more detail than its environment, the effects of which are held constant where possible, or lumped (defined in Sect. 1.2.4). Interactions within the system need to be stronger than those with the environment; weak interactions can be used to define the limits of a system. Exclusion of a component interacting strongly with the system precludes a viable model.

The selected system is made up of a set of components which interact. Components can be identified for systems as diverse as the chemical reaction between a substrate and its enzyme, or the interaction between the moon and ovulation in certain monkeys.

Any real biological system may contain a very large number of internal elements and interactions. In addition, many environmental factors influence biological systems: time, light, temperature, the availability of nutrients and the rate at which they are supplied, previous history and so on. And any individual biological entity may behave differently from another, which is apparently very similar.

The complexity necessary to describe such a system may seem unmanageable. Even computer technology may not be able to deal with all these factors within finite space, time and financial resources! Those most relevant to the behaviour of interest must be selected for experimentation and for devising a mathematical model. Selection of components ought to be an individual, creative activity; a model is a personal statement.

1.2.1 Experimental Frames

Complexity can be described as a function of the number of possible ways of interacting with a system. Modelling is an abstraction of experience, and limits these interactions by defining an *experimental frame* within which the model is expected to be effective. An experimental frame describes a chosen, limited set of conditions in which experiments or observations are carried out. Those factors known to influence the system but which are assumed to be constant, or are held constant, must be clearly stated. (Of course there may be other affectors which are unknown.)

A model of a system may be valid in one experimental frame (or set of conditions) but not in another. Real systems may have many possible experimental frames. As models satisfactorily reproduce experimental results from a progressively wider range of experimental frames, they become stronger or more "robust". The model becomes more general and therefore has richer, more meaningful things to say about the nature of the system.

One of the major aims of modelling is to make valid *general* statements about systems which apply to individuals or samples of individuals other than those actually measured. Bridgeman's operational philosophical principle, however, goes so far as to state that physical entities are to be described only within the operational contexts in which they are measured. No generalizations allowed! Should then predictions from successful modelling be applied only within the experimental frame in which they were tested? Certainly it is necessary to recognize that extrapolation is involved in using models outside their tested frames, and to proceed with suitable caution.

A more difficult problem is to ensure that all the effective agents are known and can be controlled under the chosen experimental conditions. A model will surely not describe the behaviour of a real system effectively where an unknown agent is influencing its function. Establishing physiological systems in the laboratory to elucidate "normal" behaviour contains traps of this kind. For example, concluding that biological clocks in crabs are internal because they persist when obviously linked external factors such as tides and light are removed, does not allow for the possibility of other external effects such as geomagnetism. One can never be sure that every possible condition relevant to physiological function has been accounted for. This is where imagination, experience and sensitive observation of the system outside controlled conditions are essential, and why biologists can never be replaced by mathematicians!

1.2.2. Variables and Parameters

Once the system has been identified, the experimental frame defined by selecting the range of behaviour of interest, and the components thought relevant to this behaviour are named, the relationships governing the interactions of these components must be described by mathematical equations. Concepts useful for clarifying mathematical relationships are discussed here. Choice of the mathematics appropriate to the perceived nature of the system is the topic of Chap. 2.

Variables are simply those measurable attributes of a system which vary. Those which are active in initiating or maintaining changes in behaviour of the system are called *independent variables*, while those which show that the behaviour is changed are called *dependent variables*. These variables have been distinguished in different disciplines by a variety of names:

Cause and effect,
Stimulus and response,
Input and output,
Independent and dependent variables,
x and y.

They can be discriminated by the property that whereas changes in independent variables alter dependent variables, changes in dependent variables will not usually influence the independent ones. For example, time is an independent variable. Its passing may result in a continuous reduction in the concentration of a hormone in the blood. But increasing the dependent variable – the hormone concentration – by other means will not reverse time. The dependence of y on x may be written in a generalized mathematical form, $y = f(x)$, meaning that y can be described by some particular, but here unspecified, function of x.

However, sometimes variables are interdependent, for example, in a reversible chemical reaction such as

$$\text{enzyme} + \text{substrate} \rightleftharpoons \text{enzyme-substrate complex}$$

or where the variables are part of a closed causal chain (feedback loop), such as in the model

$$\text{LHRH} \rightarrow \text{LH} \longrightarrow \text{oestradiol}$$
$$\text{(pituitary)} \quad \text{(follicle)}$$

The concentrations of estradiol and LH are postulated to mutually influence one another but, unlike the reversible reaction, at quite different places and by different mechanisms.

Parameters are factors which influence the behaviour of a system but which are held *constant* either naturally or by experimental design. Because they are constant, parameters characterize the behaviour of a model by constraining the form of its response. In the equation of a straight line $y = A_1 + A_2 x$, x the independent variable can take a range of possible values which produce a corresponding range of values of y, but the parameters A_1 and A_2 are held constant to give the line its particular form. Parameters may also be thought of as inputs which are invariant. It is wise to ensure that entities selected for description by this term actually are effectively constant within the chosen experimental conditions. The values of parameters are estimated when the behaviour of a model is compared with experimental data (Chap. 3). In theoretical models, parameters have real physical interpretations and therefore their estimates must be physically feasible if the model is to be acceptable. In empirical models parameters have no such physical meaning because the form of the equations is not related to the causal mechanism.

Other terms necessary for mathematical descriptions of the behaviour of systems are absolute constants such as π and e, and also statistical measures (Appendix A and Chap. 9).

A technique providing a useful internal check that particular equations contain sufficient variables and parameters is dimensional analysis, outlined by Riggs (1963).

1.2.3 Diagrams

A diagram showing interactions of components in a visual form is a powerful aid to comprehension and simplification. A particularly useful notation for showing causal relationships is the symbol and arrow diagram described by Riggs (1970). Block diagrams, (discussed in Sect. 2.3.4), analogue notation (Roberts, 1977, Chap. 10) and flow diagrams (Davies, 1971, pp. 32–36), are other helpful means of presenting and comprehending connective links between variables in models.

1.2.4 Lumping

Although a great deal of detail may be known about relationships governing the behaviour of a system, inclusion of every detail of a complex mathematical equation may be unnecessary or unhelpful, or even preclude the possibility of any investigation because of limited resources of time or computation.

Lumping is a process of simplifying models by combining elements into a single variable, or by simplifying interactions. For instance, instead of dealing with a large number of single molecules and their interactions, we can lump them into some sort of average, such as a probability function like concentration or pressure. Similarly, concentrations of several kinds of substances and their interactions can be lumped and treated as a "pool". An illustration from the study of the metabolism of cells might be that all molecules relating to the breakdown of nutrient carbohydrate be lumped together into a single pool, with inputs and outputs suitable for the pool as a whole. If the focus of the model is some other property of the system, this simplification may be appropriate, and much time and effort is saved by not describing mathematically each individual enzyme in the chain and its interaction with substrate and affectors. If this initial simplification does not reproduce experimental data, a more complex treatment should be tried.

The relationship between input and output in a "pooled" system may often be an empirical equation that summarizes many unknown intermediate steps in a simplified, fixed mathematical form. Of course, the lumping method necessarily assumes that intermediate steps are uninfluenced by any other changes in the system. The validity of this assumption may be hard to check when the natures of the intermediate steps themselves are unidentified. In such cases lumping may weaken the model.

One or more variables or parameters that are thought to be less important within the experimental frame of interest can be omitted altogether. By testing the effects that changing the values of parameters have in model behaviour, some parameters or variables may be revealed as irrelevant within the chosen experimental frame. These may then be lumped or discarded. Methods of choosing the model which best fits the data from several models with different structures and parameters are discussed in Chap. 4. Another simplification, sometimes appropriate, is to restrict the range of the independent variables or experimental frame so that interaction terms, or even the effects of some components, are made negligible.

Selection of the time frame of interest usually results in helpful lumping. Variables influenced only by time intervals much longer than that selected can be lumped as constant; variables responding relatively very quickly can be assumed to be already at equilibrium, or regarded as being instantaneous switches between one type of behaviour and another. If one is examining enzyme reactions in the millisecond

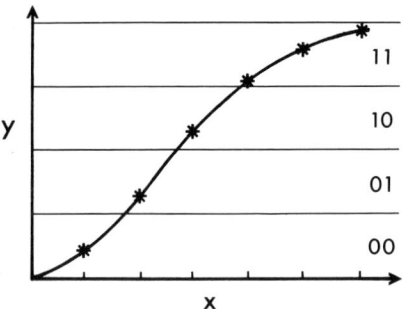

Fig. 1.3. Data *points* (*) described by selected finite levels rather than by values on a continuous scale

range, the replication rate of a cell over hours is probably not relevant, and vice versa.

The complexity of a mathematical function can sometimes be simplified without loss of accuracy. Linear approximations (Sect. 2.2) simplify by removing interactions within the model.

Finite level modelling (Sect. 2.7) can be used to simplify calculations by restricting the range of numbers used to describe variables. For example, in Fig. 1.3, if the response of y to varying x provides results as shown, instead of fitting a curve to the points, four states might be distinguished, one low, two intermediate and one near or at the maximum. Using binary notation, all data can be designated by one of these four states – 00, 01, 10 or 11. This may not really be as gross a simplification as it appears, because experimental error could make the finer distinction of y values effectively meaningless.

1.2.5 Hierarchical Levels

The concept of *hierarchical levels* overlaps with that of lumping and is useful for simplifying biological models. Any system, animate or inanimate, can be described in terms of separate subsystems which, in interaction, determine the behaviour of the total system. Each of the subsystems might likewise be described in terms of smaller components, and so on, at successively more detailed levels. For example, an endocrinological system is composed of organs and other morphological structures that interact (via hormones). These in turn may be made up of different cell types. Each cell is composed of substructures, each of which contains different molecules and macromolecules. Each molecule is composed of atoms which inter-relate, and so on, into more detailed realms of physics. Any of these subsystems at any level may be studied by itself, and the results will be useful in understanding the next less detailed or higher level.

It is customary to simplify models by describing their behaviour at a particular level in terms of components at the next, more detailed (lower) level. Movement from one hierarchical level to another has similarities to the lumping process in that a many-to-few "mapping" or transformation occurs. Many attributes at the one level flow together into a small number of sufficient attributes at the next higher level.

In apparent contrast to this simplification, however, subsystems clearly can be combined in many ways to produce an increased variety of structures and behaviours. This is why it is more difficult to predict the form of unknown behaviour at higher levels from details at lower levels, than it is to devise an explanation for observed higher level events in terms of lower level components. It has been suggested that in biology these many possible structural forms have not been realized because of *constraints* imposed during the course of evolution. Combination of simpler forms that were successful as self-maintaining organisms in earlier environmental conditions, may have allowed emergence of new functions and forms not available to the parts. But many combinations will not have provided for adaptation to additional environmental pressures and will have been removed by selection processes. Those retained will have provided the starting point for further changes, and the arrow of time has moved on irreversibly.

The structural hierarchy requires the introduction of *control hierarchies*, in which collective upper level structures provide constraints controlling the details of behaviour of lower level structures, so that organized coherent performance of function occurs in place and time. For example, an endocrine system is at one level of a control hierarchy in which hormones provide information or messages for selective control of specific parts of the total system at appropriate times. The nature of control hierarchies, for which language and its syntax have been used as a simile (Waddington, vol. 4, 1972), is a major focus of interest in biology.

1.2.6 Stochastic and Deterministic Behaviours

Stochastic and deterministic behaviours are useful concepts related to the idea of hierarchy. *Stochastic* behaviour is, in the short term, unpredictable – the nature of the outcome is governed by chance, and a probability only can be placed on the occurrence of any particular event. The toss of a coin gives an unpredictable and therefore stochastic result. The use of mathematical theory is not, however, precluded by such uncertain results (see, for example Chap. 9). Statistical theory, statistical mechanics and Markov probability chains are used to study probabilistic situations. The study of stochastic processes shows that over a long time, or with large numbers of events, some have determinate outcomes. (For instance, a perfectly weighted coin will fall heads up in 50 percent of an infinitely large number of tosses.) In the long term, some stochastic processes have a small number of discrete outcomes, while the outcomes of others are widely distributed, or chaotic.

Deterministic behaviour is predictable and reproducible, and each measurement obeys some natural law or mathematical equation. For example, on varying the volume of an ideal gas V at constant temperature T, the pressure P behaves deterministically: $P = nRT/V$. Of course, no real measurement is entirely deterministic because all are subject to stochastic uncertainty. Uncertainty is usually neglected initially when modelling almost deterministic data; statistical theory is then used to calculate the effects of the uncertainty (Sect. 10.1).

The ideas of stochastic and deterministic behaviour are related to those of hierarchies because many stochastic events can produce a single deterministic outcome. While detailed measurements of a small number of events at close range yield chaotic or stochastic results, the same events, when viewed from a greater distance or over a longer time interval so that very large numbers of events are included, may give rise to a deterministic or predictable average. For example, the effect of the range of momentum of many individual gas molecules is experienced as a simple pressure measurement. Whether systems and transitions are particulate and unpredictable (stochastic), or continuous and predictable (deterministic), depends on the relative distances, time intervals or numbers of events that are measured. Random elements or events at one level become the organized processes of the next, less detailed hierarchical level (Sect. 1.2.5).

1.2.7 Problems of Individuality

Mathematical conclusions in models are completely general. They apply to anything conforming to the stated conditions. However, in biology, the experimental data which render the mathematical model tenable come from a particular individual biological entity, or a selection from a class of individual entities. How does the model apply to other entities of the same class? In some scientific modelling the class of entities is homogeneous and completely definable (such as all solutions of a pure chemical at a specified concentration, temperature and pressure). A random sample (a particular solution) provides the experimental data. In this case, the model will apply to any other members of the class (any solutions of the specified type) within the limits of confidence determined by the usual parametric statistical methods designed for such cases (Appendix A). Some biological modelling approximates this situation.

In other cases, uncertainty in biological experiments includes not only experimental error but also individual variation. If this variation is relatively small and takes one of the forms which can be summarized statistically (such as being normally distributed), then there is little difficulty. However, variation frequently arises because individuals are unknowingly combined which belong to two or more separate classes not having some properties in common; these may produce different quantitative or qualitative outcomes. This kind of variation comes from the simplifications which are often necessary in designing the model. One or more additional unknown factors influence the behaviour of some of the individuals. In this case non-parametric statistics are more appropriate (Sect. 9.1). Because biological systems are so complex, the complete definition of the class to which a model applies may be extremely difficult.

The investigator must be sensitive to the reasons for variation so that experiments can be as controlled as possible. For instance, the effects of previous history on current performance can be considerable. Variation over long or short-term cycles may inadvertently be included in the differences between individuals, making error unnecessarily or even ludicrously large. For example, the hormone content of blood may vary with the stage of the life cycle, reproductive cycle, circadian or lesser cycles. If a model is devised to describe data from blood withdrawn always at one time of day, a falsely narrow range of hormone may be found. If blood is pooled from several individuals then information about behaviour with time may be lost; rhythms, and factors influencing them, may become undetectable. The answer to this problem is to carry out a wide range of sensitive, exploratory experiments testing the class of individuals to which the model is hoped to apply.

The use of large numbers of individuals, and the inclusion of controls which have not received the stimulus being investigated, are attempts to detect and allow for individual variations in response. Finite level modelling can assist by removing fine distinctions between results (Sect. 1.2.4 and 2.7); a response may simply be classified as being present or absent, high or low. Similarly, the technique of self-modelling (Sect. 2.3.1.2) can extract general mathematical relationships from data while accomodating individual variation.

Definition of the limits of the class of individuals to which a model is expected to apply, is particularly important in biology. So many factors can influence the state of biological entities, and they can be so heterogeneous, that one may be investigating a class with only one member, an individual. While precise mathematical description can often be derived for an individual, we usually seek more generally applicable models. We look for common characteristics between individuals, not idiosyncrasies. Modelling at the metaphoric level (Sect. 1.1.1) is concerned with finding classes of systems exhibiting homologous forms of behaviour and organization, rather than investigating the behaviours peculiar to individuals with parameters and variables identified for small classes only. However, if these metaphoric models are to be more than qualitative speculations they must be compared with real systems.

1.3 Experimental Data

Experimental data is required for testing a model. Needless to say, the support given to a model by experimental results can be no better than the quality of the data used. Beyond the scope of this book are the choice of experimental method and apparatus, the initial conditions of the system and any experimental changes used in the process of collecting results. However, mathematical theory can contribute usefully in determining the amount of data required, and also in choosing the most effective values of the independent variables for differentiating between possible models (Chap. 4).

There are different kinds of experimental data and these require different mathematical approaches. For example, many endocrinological investigations are concerned with detecting the presence or absence of an effect in response to experimental manipulation. Precise, quantitative measurements are either unobtainable or inappropriate. Finite level modelling (Sect. 2.7) and non-parametric statistical methods (Sect. 9.1) can be useful here. As understanding of endocrinological processes increases more subtle models are needed. The demand has grown for more precise measurements made under more carefully controlled conditions. This book is mainly concerned with methods of analysis suitable for this more detailed data.

1.4 Predictions from Models — Simulation

Simulation means calculating the response of a model by substituting values for its parameters, and a range of values of the independent variables. It is thus possible to investigate the characteristics of the model under a variety of conditions. The behaviour of the real system can, of course, be studied only by experimentation.

Simulation has several important applications. Testing the responses of a model provides an understanding of its potential, which may not be apparent from the equations. If predictions from the model are confirmed by experiment, the confidence in the model is greatly enhanced. The significance of sections of the model to its overall behaviour can be investigated and simplifications achieved. The stability of the model to perturbations can also be tested, and fundamental constraints on the values of the parameters and variables necessary to maintain the desired behaviour made apparent.

Simulation can be used to investigate the effects of experimental uncertainty on the characteristics of a model. In this way it is possible to conserve resources by determining, before experimentation is begun, whether the precision of measurements is great enough to yield useful information. It is also possible to predict the number of experiments required to reach a given level of precision in the results, or to differentiate between models. Where experiments are impossible, time-consuming, costly or unethical, simulation using a probable model can suggest efficient ways of tackling the problem, and possible outcomes.

Simulation is used frequently in this book and its capacity to provide new interpretations of phenomena and suggest novel and productive experiments will become apparent.

1.5 A Model of Complexity Producing Organized Simplicity

Regardless of how one might lump and simplify models of living organisms, real systems are composed of millions of chemical entities. These components have even more millions of ways of interacting with each other, and yet again more possibilities for sequencies of interactions. For example, the micro-organism *E. coli* has been estimated to contain two thousand genes, and human beings two million. If gene behaviour is modelled in binary terms (i. e. the gene is either active or inactive), then for a mere 1,000 genes, there are $2^{1,000}$ or approximately 10^{300} possible combinations (or states) of active and inactive genes. What would happen if any of these states could occur at any one time, and in any sequence over a period of time?

The number of possible modes of behaviour of the genes alone in any one cell could very well be greater than the 10^{23} μs estimated to have passed during the entire existence of the universe. Therefore for processes taking longer than a microsecond (genes need 5–90 s to become active or inactive) a primordial cell might not yet have returned to a state previously occupied. That is, the cell might not yet have completed a cycle. But a characteristic of living cells is their stability (adherence to a limited number of modes of behaviour), and reproducibility of behaviour states. The behaviour of simple cells of the same genetic type becomes even predictable under some conditions (their replication time, for instance).

How is it that with all these myriads of possibilities only a few sequences of behaviour are persistently, predictably and repeatedly expressed? Kauffman (1970) among others, has devised metaphoric models to investigate such complexity. The interesting results of one such model of gene interaction, which is applicable also to other types of molecules in biological systems, show that simplified, stable processes can be expected to occur in multicomponent complex systems as the logical consequences of certain constraining conditions outlined below. Furthermore, the time course of cycles of behaviour in Kauffman's models of genes, parallels and predicts the time required for cell replication. A brief description of Kauffman's

A Model of Complexity Producing Organized Simplicity

modelling follows to show how even such a simple, abstract model can have non-intuitive, aesthetically pleasing results – that complexity can lead to organized simplicity.

The components in the model need not be specified except that they show binary behaviour, i.e. they are either active or inactive, as denoted by the values 1 or 0, respectively. The value of every component is made to be dependent upon the values of two other components in the previous time interval. (Dependence of most components on more than three, or less than two other elements, does not give systems with the required biological properties.) All values of components are computed at successive time intervals, $t = 1, 2, 3, \ldots$.

The two inputs to each element are chosen at random, and the effect of the two inputs on the output of every component is also chosen randomly to be any one of all the possible Boolean functions (described below) of the inputs. Once these interactions are decided upon, the net of linked components remains fixed in choice of inputs to each element, and in their effect on the output.

There are three particular examples of Boolean functions shown in Fig. 1.4. In the general case, two components a and b each with a value of 1 or 0 together can be in one of four possible states at any one time t. Each of these states determines a value for variable c which may be either 0 or 1, at time $t + 1$. The Boolean function chosen for c defines the four output values of c in response to all of the four possible input states from a and b. It can easily be seen that there is a total of sixteen different ways of choosing response sets for c (i.e. Boolean functions) with two input components. In general there are 2^{2^n} Boolean functions for n components.

A simple illustration of such a net (Kauffman, 1970) is given below. The model contains three binary components A, B and C, interconnected as shown in Fig. 1.4. The Boolean function chosen for each component is shown beside it.

There are $2^3 = 8$ possible states of the total system (ways of choosing three values of 0 or 1) for A, B and C, which are shown at time t on the left of Table 1.1. The values of each component in the next time interval (on the right of Table 1.1) can be computed from each of these possible states using the Boolean functions given in Fig. 1.4. Figure 1.5 traces the sequence of state changes at successive time intervals and is derived from Table 1.1.

Any of the eight possible states is shown to move rapidly into a cycle of three states, which is then continuously repeated.

Randomly connected nets of different sizes have been tested by Kauffman and others. Those where most components are connected to two others tend to have

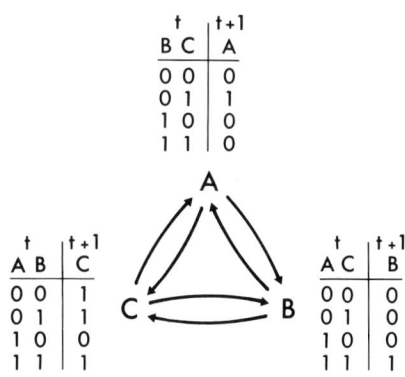

Fig. 1.4. A net of three elements with their chosen Boolean functions. These describe the outputs resulting from each set of two input elements

Table 1.1. State changes at the next time interval for all possible values taken by the net of three elements shown in Fig. 1.4

t			t+1		
A	B	C	A	B	C
0	0	0	0	0	1
0	0	1	1	0	1
0	1	0	0	0	1
0	1	1	0	0	1
1	0	0	0	0	0
1	0	1	1	1	0
1	1	0	0	0	1
1	1	1	0	1	1

properties similar to biological systems. Nets of 1,000 elements possess about 10^{300} possible states, but a typical net of this size, in which each element depends on two others, cycles between only twelve of these states. For each net size tested, the distribution of cycle lengths is markedly skewed toward short cycle lengths. Equilibrium states (those which successively become themselves) are common (as you will discover if you choose other Boolean functions in the previous example). By projection from these results, nets of one million elements possess cycles of about 1,000 states in length, illustrating an extreme localization of behaviour among $2^{1,000,000}$ possible states. Nets of 1,000 elements have only about sixteen distinct cycles (as opposed to states) available. Those of one million have 500 different cycles. If "noise" is introduced by allowing a few random components to change their values, the states rapidly return to the cycle from which they came, showing very stable behaviour with properties like biological homeostasis. As Kauffman concludes, these results suggest that, in biology, high molecular specificity is necessary, not only for precision of product formation, but also to give a low number of specific connections between components so that chemical oscillatory behaviours (biochemical cycles) in these systems are brief and stable. A characteristic of any biochemical net of high specificity, where macromolecules are directly affected by a small number of other components, should be its highly localized, apparently directed, behaviour – the task of evolution in selecting organized simplicity out of complexity may have been less difficult than we thought. This is but one example from a number of models on this theme.

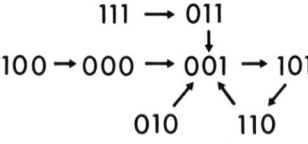

Fig. 1.5. Sequence of state changes at successive time intervals for the net shown in Fig. 1.4. Each *arrow* indicates one time interval

1.6 Subjectivity in Modelling

A model is a simplification of our perception of reality. That "the world" does exist, and that it is not capriciously organized, experimental scientists would surely agree (at least much of the time). Parts of existence can be described to a moderate level of satisfaction in a condensed algorithmic fashion, within certain conditions. However, perception itself involves unconscious modelling and is therefore distorted and filtered by knowledge, beliefs and previous experience: "in science it is often true that believing is seeing" (Yates et al., 1972). We are likely to notice what we look for, in the sense of seeing what is not there and, unless we have built the idea into our model first, we may not see what is. One of the delights of mathematical modelling is that predictions can be non-intuitive, and indeed we might well refuse to believe some experiments if we were to observe the results before predicting them. A scientist cannot disentangle his study of nature from his own interaction with nature. Whether a factor is observed and registers as significant is determined by one's own previous learning. Laszlo (1972) suggests that the brain is the major organ of adaptation through sensory input causing physiological effects. Our senses are highly tuned to perceive what is necessary to aid survival. Therefore we are hardly likely to make objective or isomorphous observation of events.

The act of abstracting (i.e. modelling) our perception adds further approximations and distortions. The need to test and place strains on a model, and to compare it sensitively and objectively with experimental data is, therefore, paramount.

It can be productive to have several models of the same phenomenon with different perspectives, each describing observed results. Conscious efforts to restate the problem in another form can sensitize one to new possibilities of interrelationships. Can a different level of modelling be used (Sect. 1.1.1), or the model be made more general or specific, simpler or have other experimental frames? Can the results of modelling similar systems be usefully applied, or can the results of modelling this system be extended to another problem? Levins (1970) suggests that "truth is the intersection of independent lies". It is certainly likely that a closer approximation to the truth may lie at the intersection of models with different perspectives, but it must be borne in mind that we are adept at finding many ways of restating the same old idea.

The usefulness of a model is strongly related to the imaginativeness of its concepts, to the depth of the perceptions involved, and to new viewpoints described. Confirming established preconceptions tends to be sterile.

At the same time modelling is a necessary adjunct to a creative idea because it can place the idea on a firm experimental basis. It requires that the idea be stated in a precise, unambiguous form. Areas deficient in understanding become apparent, as does the need for new experiments to clarify issues. Models can support or demolish ideas by suggesting testable hypotheses.

The results of testing a model, as opposed to conceiving an idea, determines the historical fate of the model. Newton, defending himself against Robert Hooke's accusation that his *Mathematical Principles of Natural Philosophy* merely explored the mathematical consequences of Hooke's own idea, said:

Mathematicians, who find out, settle, and do all the business, must content themselves with being nothing but dry calculators and drudges; and another, who does nothing but pretend and grasp at all things, must carry away all the invention. (Provine, 1977)

Hooke, "pretending and grasping at all things" could neither deduce nor accurately predict, as did Newton, the behaviour of the planets, the moon or the seas, in an experimentally verifiable way. A little dry drudgery made all the difference between real advances in knowledge and eventual obscurity for the idea (or perhaps notoriety, as for catastrophe theory; Sussmann and Zahler, 1977: but see Sect. 2.6.5).

1.7 Mathematics in Modelling

Early in the human approach to quantitation, numbers were apparently used only as adjectives, or even as indistinguishable parts of words for the objects themselves. Thus the word for "two-men" perhaps bore no resemblance to that for "two-trees". Abstraction of the number property that groups have in common (possibly using the fingers as a generalized model), and the naming of numbers as entities in themselves, allowed the concepts necessary for mathematics to develop (Aleksandrov et al., 1969).

Mathematics is a further abstraction, seeking to save direct enumeration for every possible situation by preserving the form of the answer for future use. By substituting relations for values, we symbolize and definitely fix all numerical operations which follow the same rule. We write a relation between the quantities under investigation in the form of an equation. The object of solving the equation is to find what values of the dependent variable will satisfy this relation.

In mathematics, the relationships of abstract concepts, one to another, have been explored in great depth. If a model conforms to a known mathematical equation, then a range of consequences, relationships and possibilities has already been worked out in an abstract, generalized form by logical deduction. Mathematics is useful to biologists not just in quantitation but also in the mathematical properties of logic, rigour, precision, deductive powers, the indisputable character of its conclusions and in the exceptionally broad range of its application. Mathematics opens up unsuspected possibilities for explanations of biological observations, and for exploration of non-intuitive kinds of behaviour.

Nevertheless, mathematics is concerned with possibilities rather than actualities; its results must be interpreted and compared with the biological reality to assess whether they are meaningful in each particular case. The mathematical operations used in equations need to be shown to apply sufficiently accurately to the real system to be useful, or be explicity stated as assumptions. For instance, one plus one does not equal two if the numbers refer to the mixing of equal volumes of water and alcohol.

The act of defining precisely the biological meaning of symbols in a mathematical equation, determining those components which vary dependently and independently or are held constant, what values, dimensions and range of values they have, and the exact way in which they are to be inter-related in a model, is a very useful exercise for revealing the extent or deficiencies of our knowledge of a system. Such an activity may often suggest meaningful experiments to perform before further use of mathematics.

Having derived equations to describe the system, the logic of mathematics can reveal inconsistencies and redundancies in the mathematical description, and hence in the understanding of the interactions. While it is easy to modify the form of the equations to improve the comparison of their predictions with experimental measurements, any changes should be guided by sound biological reasons (Fig. 1.2).

A model can be logically falsified only in the sense that it may be shown to be mathematically illogical (mathematics has nothing to say about the biological logic). The hypothesis that a model is mathematically an effective description of the biological experimental data *can* be tested for falsity, or at least a probability placed on this hypothesis being true by correct use of the theory of statistics (Chaps. 3 and 4; Appendix A). It is in the testing of such hypotheses that ideas are given an experimental basis. Attempts to test more than a few hypotheses about the system, or to calculate the values of too many unmeasurable components by matching model performance to experimental data, will not yield useful results.

Only parts of the process of modelling can be subjected to the scrutiny of irrefutable mathematical logic. Much of modelling is determined by subjective choice based on such criteria as "appropriateness" or "greater relevance" (see Fig. 1.2, and Sects. 1.2.1 and 1.2.4). Criteria for selection of models used in other disciplines, such as optimal performance under some specified conditions, or the principle of parsimony (selecting the simplest form) may not be valid in biology; by the theory of evolution, present forms of biological mechanisms have developed irreversibly by being selected for "fitness" to some undetermined environmental constraints, many of which may no longer exist. Constant reference to the biological system is necessary in using mathematics to give these choices a firm basis on biological reality, and to avoid uninterpretable mathematical tautologies.

Mathematics generalizes. It draws conclusions where the symbols can apply to any type of entity that obeys the defined conditions. However, while the concept of gravity applies to both the cosmos and apples, these two systems have many essential characteristics that are not shared. It is a mistake to assume that mathematical conformity implies identity or even similarity of the systems in any other respect (von Bertalanffy, 1973). Nevertheless, focussing of attention on common aspects may be rewarding. The discovery that the behaviours of certain biological systems are described by the same mathematical form may demonstrate a previously unsuspected but fruitful relationship of behaviour and organization in these systems, even though the structural components themselves are very different. Such unifying concepts have proved most effective in physics.

Biology is now posing a major challenge and stimulus to the theory of mathematics to investigate and find conditions for, and consequences of, the kinds of interactions and behaviours found in living organisms. In technological development we have been able to design machines using the mathematical skills available; problems have not been tackled until suitable mathematical approaches have been developed. However, in attempting to explain biological behaviour we cannot constrain the design of model systems to fit mathematical theories already devised. Unlike technological research, the aim of biological investigations is not to achieve some final output. We try to understand the how and why of biological function, and this may not be amenable to procedures we already know how to manipulate. Some mathematical methods are remarkably powerful but many biological situations are not yet able to be effectively modelled mathematically.

Some limitations in existing methods of dealing with our perceived nature of biological systems are discussed in Chap. 2.

Reading mathematical texts is not easy for probably the majority of people trained in biology. On scanning a few pages of (initially) incomprehensible hieroglyphics it is clear that mathematicians think by using symbols in place of words, and that accumulated experience of these symbols makes the equations very much more meaningful than they appear to a biologist. When describing mathematical models to a wide audience, a careful verbal explanation of the mathematical operation, or reason for it, assists those not versed in mathematics to make the effort to comprehend the significance of an unfamiliar operation. An added difficulty is the proliferation of terminology currently encountered. Symbols that are familiar in one discipline are frequently used quite differently in another, and even normal everyday words are redefined at the beginning of a text to have unfamiliar significance. Constant recourse to definitions, repeated readings and a simple text of mathematical formulae, definitions, operations and usages appear to be the only solution, but one requiring considerable enterprise. Such effort is unlikely to be made unless the non-mathematical reader has been convinced by prior explanation that it is certain to be fruitful to his or her own discipline.

Collaboration with mathematicians also has difficulties in communication. The mathematician may not comprehend the complexity and sensitivity to conditions and stimuli of biological systems, while biologists rarely seem to realize the advantages of planning experiments using mathematical criteria to maximize effectiveness, and in analysing the results. To be sufficiently familiar with a system and sensitive to its changing behaviour, so that relevant components and conditions can be selected and valid simplifications made, a modeller must also be an experimentalist, or ought to collaborate with one.

As a result of divergent experience, each researcher may be aware of only a fraction of the implications contained in data received from other fields. Nevertheless, the biologist remains responsible for the biological appropriateness of the mathematics, and needs to be able to listen to, read, interpret and criticize mathematical results.

1.8 Computers and Models

Use of computer techniques greatly facilitates thorough investigation of the properties of models, and their match with experimental data. The advantage of the computer lies in making possible investigations which would not otherwise be attempted. Complex model structures can be studied easily. In addition, restrictions are removed from the forms of interactions which can be conveniently postulated. Many interactions common in biological systems do not produce responses which can be described by a general mathematical equation suitable for hand calculations; each value of the response must be recalculated for each set of input values and parameters. Such repetitive numerical manipulations are performed effortlessly by computer.

Few systems of interest are sufficiently simple to permit intuitive predictions of responses to be made. Computers are particularly well-suited to exploring the possible range of non-intuitive behaviour. The model and conditions can be easily modified and the effects of these changes on calculated responses rapidly compared. The speed with which the behaviour of a model can be experienced is of the utmost value in its investigation. Nevertheless, the computer can only provide particular solutions; it is incapable of formulating or even recognizing a generalization. Generalizations stem from the mind of the investigator.

The computer not only has the power to provide numerical data with great speed and accurancy, but also to present it in a form intelligible to the user. While we are inept at comprehending the significance of lists of figures, our ability to assimilate pictorial information is very great. Figure 1.6 shows two pictures of the steroid molecule cortisol drawn by computer from a list of atomic co-ordinates, or positions of the atoms in space. By rotating one of the images slightly the computer has been programmed to convey the illusion of three dimensions. This program allows the image of the molecule to be redrawn for viewing from any angle, to be magnified or reduced.

The computer offers speed and accuracy, but skill and experience are needed to attain these goals. Programming computers, and proving that programs are free of errors, demands expert knowledge, and can be time-consuming. The greatest care must be taken to ensure that the input data is absolutely faultless – the machine cannot correct mistakes. This need for meticulous attention to detail runs contrary to the practice of simplifying and approximating necessary in biological research. The resources of the machine are not unlimited; investigations of models must be confined within the time available on the computer and its storage space. Financial considerations are important as the overhead costs of computers are very high.

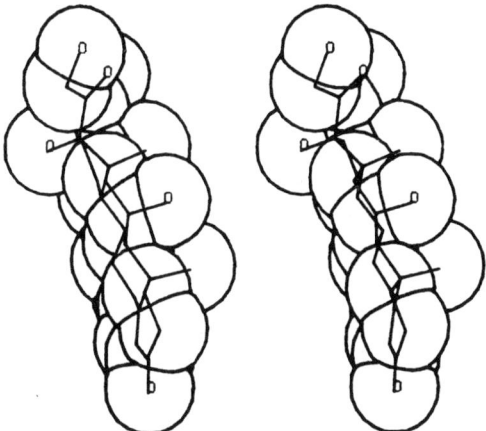

Fig. 1.6. Stereo-diagram of the three-dimensional structure of the cortisol molecule, viewed from above. Only the carbon and oxygen (O) atoms are shown. The diagram was drawn by a Data General Nova 2 mini-computer equipped with a visual display unit, using a modfied version of the program described by Warme (1977). The outlines of the space-filling ball model are superimposed on the molecular skeleton, which shows the bonds between the atoms. The diagram may be seen in three dimensions by relaxing the eyes and focussing on a distant object above and behind the page. When the page, held vertically, is raised into the line of vision a third central image will be seen in three dimensions. Persistence may be required intially to achieve this effect; alternatively, a viewer can be used. The molecular co-ordinates were determined by X-ray crystallography (Roberst et al., 1973)

Most important of all, however, is the need to keep the aims of modelling in view. It is essential to be ready always to modify or even abandon a model in light of its performance. Elegant computer programs are not the goal; the machine is a tool to be used to test the validity of concepts, not an end in itself. The very real dangers of investing computers with definitive authority or even mystical powers are discussed by Weizenbaum (1976). Computer programs are themselves models and the products of programmers; they are therefore prone to the same simplifications, fallacies and insensitivities as other human ideas. A thorough appreciation of this is essential if one is not to be at a disadvantage in assessing the validity of conclusions in publications describing experiments analysed by computer.

1.9 Description of Models

The energy and personal gratification achieved by constructing and testing a model must not remain localized at its creator. To ensure that results are correctly understood, applied and acclaimed, careful and complete communication is essential (see, for example, Zeigler, 1976). In one of the best of all possible worlds, the description of a modelling exercise might include the following.
1. The purpose of the model. This should fit the model into the reader's "world" model; the latter should be permanently influenced as a result.
2. Verbal description of the model. This includes:

   a) The naming and description of static entities in theoretical modelling. Components – named, described and given a relationship to parts of the real system. Variables of each component (inputs, outputs and inaccessible variables), and parameters – the range of each and its role in describing components and mathematical symbols used.

   The choice of which elements shall be variables held constant and the ranges of values of interest, defines the experimental frame. The experimental frame chosen determines how relevant the modelling exercise will be to the functioning of the real system.

   b) The description of "dynamic" interactions between components, or their communication with each other and how these are interpreted mathematically, or both. Comments on the lumping of variables, parameters and data. Simplifications used in writing mathematical equations.

   c) A clear statement of assumptions involved and estimates of their validity or relative validity. Experimental data supporting the assumptions. A clear description of empirical parts of the model. Omissions from the model.

   d) Diagram showing relationships within the model.

   The aim of this verbal description is to place the particular conditions, components and interactions in a broader field of possibilities. A description of types of models tried and discarded while devising the one presented, along with the reasons for their failure, can also be of interest.
3. A mathematical description (usually equations) in which omissions, redundancies, inconsistencies and ambiguities have been remedied.
4. A description of how the equations are interpreted by the computer program or other simulation technique. A full description of the program and machinery allows the reader to judge for him or herself the effectiveness of the procedure, just as the description of apparatus, materials and methods are necessary in presenting

experimental work. Programs must be verified so that errors in the program are not confused with mistakes in the model.
5. Description of experimental data with which the model is compared, and the methods used to obtain it.
6. Simulation results, comparison with experimental data, and analysis, with comments on the significance of the variables and parameters to the total response of the model, and the likely effect of experimental and random errors.
7. Conclusions on the range of application and validity of the model. Predictions and experimental verification.
8. Comparison of the model with past models, and suggestions for future modifications and experiments.

1.10 Modelling in Perspective

To stimulate insight and to dispel mirages, experimentation and model building must be concurrent. A sensitive experimental understanding is necessary to judge what classes of system should be selected for study, what simplifications are meaningful, and to know the detail from which to select, add to, or modify models. Handling of the system provides insight into selecting relevant experimental frames. If we wish to "understand" the hows and whys of a biological system, all physiologically relevant frames or situations in which the system functions need to be defined and studied using theoretical models. This is a different exercise from describing empirical relationships mathematically in limited, well-known experimental frames, or ones for which the mathematics can be solved simply.

The testing of a system experimentally outside normal physiological conditions in order to elucidate normal functioning mechanisms, occurs frequently but is probably erroneous. Concentrations and components should be within the limits of those found in functioning organisms because overdose, presence of an unusual or absence of a usual component, may create a quite different mechanism of operation. For instance, extensive calculations and experimentation were performed on haemoglobin to determine the detailed reaction rate kinetics with oxygen before the marked influence of 2,3-diphospho–glycerate, a conspicuous component of red blood cells, was discovered (Benesch and Benesch, 1967). A mathematical description of the rate of growth of insect larvae in laboratory experiments as a function of food supply, temperature and so on, would contribute little to an understanding of mechanism if, in natural conditions, larvae were to use cues from their food supply to hasten or retard their maturation so as to ensure that the adult emerges when the food plant is in flower (Williams, 1977). Biological systems are very complex and often can be modelled only under highly circumscribed conditions. Excessive confidence in the range of application of the model is both unwarranted and irresponsible.

The invention of experimental techniques, and the discovery and characterization of components (the reductionist approach), are essential prerequisites for, and concurrent activities with, successful modelling. The following parable of the biochemist who set out to discover the workings of a motor car (elaborated by Dalziel, 1973) illustrates how dependent is successful modelling upon reductionist discovery of parts, suitable techniques for finding them and inspired concepts of possible modes of interaction.

The biochemist homogenized a car in an aqueous medium and observed a rapid evolution of gas, which he measured in a Warburg manometer. Hopefully, he thought that this gas production drove the car but eventually realized that it was caused by the action of the battery acid on the metal of the car body. An enzymologist fractionated the car and isolated the intact battery. In suitable kinetic experiments he showed that it would cause a small wheel to revolve, concluded that the car was electrically driven, and predicted that a careful search beneath the accelerator pedal would reveal a variable resistance.

This parable also illustrates how quite logical attempts at modelling could be wildly untenable if predictions are not tested by experiment. Models ought to become obsolete.

The two models proposed above are perfectly valid beginnings to solving the problem. The use of the word "concluded" is the major error. The parable also illustrates the slowness with which understanding can be expected to be wrenched from systems that are complex relative to the tools and ideas available for their study. "Conclusions", however innovative or attractive, should be viewed with scepticism when their consequences have not been tested.

Modelling can be a very rewarding occupation. It is extremely pleasant to devise an ingenious explanation that ties assorted pieces of information into an aesthetic whole. For this reason, it is very easy to ignore other possibilities or to be biased in selecting information to support the model. Models can indeed act as blinkers. For those with a jaundiced view of the fruits of modelling, it appears that, for biological systems, the mathematics is so compliantly complicated that yet more cunning manipulations can always be found to prove any purpose, support any prejudice or prop up any misguided investment of time, energy or emotion. Models need to be strained and put under pressure where they are most sensitive if they are to develop and serve their true purpose.

A related fallacious use of models is to consider the reality as being "nothing but" the model or properties it embodies. The model must not assume a metaphysical reality.

> What is man, when you come to think upon him, but a minutely set, ingenious machine for turning, with infinite artfulness, the red wine of Shiraz into urine?

This quote from Isak Dineson's story *The Dreamers* in *Seven Gothic Tales*, given to us by D. S. Riggs, illustrates the fallacy of approaching a real system solely from the viewpoint of a simplified model.

Models are limited by our imaginative conception of the purpose of their overall activity or components. We are unable to describe meaningfully situations where the function of the whole, or of some component, has not been comprehended.

One of the major causes of problems in the application of technology to natural and biological phenomena has been the lack of sensitivity to, and dearth of inspired concepts on, the nature of the functioning of biological systems. This has lead to gross oversimplification and underestimation of many biological and human components in systems. Excessive faith has been placed in models emphasizing the technologically more accessible aspects of interference in natural and social events. For example, technological interference in the birth processes is judged almost exclusively on the infant mortality outcome to the detriment of morbidity and the normal development of the maternal role; analyses of side-effects of contraceptive methods have been carried out in terms only of gross pathological results.

Scientists have a strong responsibility to look beyond the pleasing, the accepted, the expected and the easily accessible in biological modelling.

1.11 Advantages in Modelling

From the foregoing sections, some possible advantages of modelling are summarized as follows.
1. Models test hypotheses. They provide means of studying underlying and inaccessible structures of systems.
2. Mathematical descriptions of relationships of system components may lead to new, non-intuitive predictions of behaviour under novel conditions, and suggest significant experiments to perform.
3. Models may explain observations or make them meaningful and intelligible.
4. Models may give guidelines to efficient experimentation where answers are immediately significant. They optimize resources.
5. Those aspects of a model most important to the system's function can be discovered through trial calculations. Fundamental constraints to the functioning of the system may also be identified.
6. The precision required in stating ideas about a system in mathematical form can clarify concepts.
7. A book-keeping function can be performed by modelling. A condensed, perhaps pictorial description of systems about which there is much diverse experimental data, can usefully and succinctly show which components are currently known to interact and to influence each other, even if the information is far from complete.
8. Empirical models may suggest interactions between components to look for.
9. A model can be used as a surrogate where actual experiments are impossible, time-consuming, costly or unethical. Models may suggest consequences of such experiments and hence ways of tackling problems.
10. Modelling techniques give guidance in studying very complex systems.
11. A good model identifies clear-cut problems for future research.

Stimulating reading on the topics mentioned in this chapter will be found in the works of von Bertalanffy (1973) and Zeigler (1976), and those edited by Matthews (1977), Mesarovic (1968), Solomon and Walter (1977), and Waddington (1968–1972). The book of Ashby (1956) is recommended as an introduction in non-mathematical terms to many of the concepts in this, and the following, chapter.

2 Mathematical Descriptions of Biological Models

The major aim in mathematical modelling is to obtain *equations describing the behaviour of a system* under all relevant conditions. This information may be quantitative or qualitative. It may be derived from a theoretical basis, in which the mechanism is analysed in terms of known or proposed interactions between components, from an empirical basis in which certain stimuli are shown to produce particular responses without reference to actual mechanisms, or from a metaphoric viewpoint in which equations have the same dynamical properties as the system, but with no detailed physical basis for their particular form.

In this chapter we sketch briefly some of the mathematical approaches which have been used in seeking this objective in biological modelling. The topics covered are far from comprehensive and the treatment is not rigorous. Instead, the intention is to show a range of possibilities, to stimulate interest in methods that the biologically trained reader may not have considered, and to indicate some of the potentials and limitations of current techniques when applied to biological systems. For details of how to use the techniques the reader may consult other chapters of this book or refer to specialized texts, reviews and papers.

The mathematical forms used for modelling should show the same properties as the system being investigated. They should be isomorphous or, in mathematical terms, have a "one-to-one mapping". Biological systems are usually non-linear (the components interact strongly), and open to the flow of matter and energy. They maintain themselves near a non-equilibrium steady state (Sect. 2.6), oscillate or change abruptly (at thresholds); they are inhomogeneous, discrete, stochastic and individual. In contrast, mathematics deals readily with functions that are linear, closed, reach equilibrium, are integrable, homogenous, continuous, deterministic and that describe infinite sets. It is important to be aware of the approximations and assumptions involved in using such mathematical functions to describe biological systems. Most mathematical methods have been developed to answer problems in physics, chemistry and technology. Awareness of the need for mathematics that can elucidate the properties peculiar to biological systems is comparatively recent.

2.1 Theoretical Modelling – Analysis of Mechanism

This section discusses differential and algebraic equations mostly from the viewpoint of theoretical modelling. These equations are also useful in other kinds of modelling.

2.1.1 Differentials

In modelling a system theoretically, it is frequently simpler to use descriptions involving not the absolute value of the dependent variable y, but instead the amount

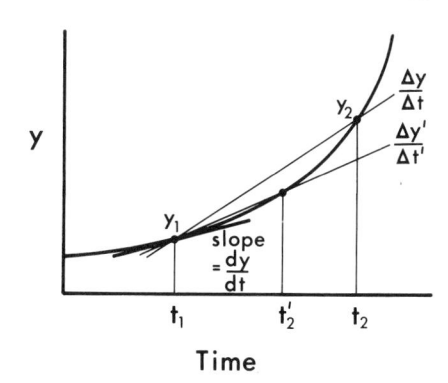

Fig. 2.1. Concept of a differential illustrated

of *change* in y over a measure such as time. Time appears as the independent variable in the following description although another measure such as distance or concentration should be used if appropriate. [While elapsed time may be important biologically at the level of chemical reactions, it is frequently not the decisive variable in the macroscopic behaviour of biological systems (see, for example, Sect. 8.6); sole dependence on elapsed time has probably been selected against during evolution (Williams, 1977).]

Change of y with time may be written

$$(y_2 - y_1)/(t_2 - t_1) = \Delta y / \Delta t. \tag{2.1}$$

Figure 2.1 shows that $\Delta y/\Delta t$ will vary depending on the time interval $t_2 - t_1$. Therefore the rate of change in y should be measured over an interval of time so small that all possibility of error due to variation of $\Delta y/\Delta t$ during that time is eliminated. The differential form of the equation is used

$$dy/dt = (y_2 - y_1)/(t_2 - t_1) \tag{2.2}$$

as $t_2 - t_1$ becomes "infinitely" small. The smallness of the time interval in differentials caused Newton's critic Bishop Berkeley to remark that they are "the ghosts of departed quantities." While dy and dt may have almost departed, the ratio they leave behind, dy/dt, is the slope of the tangent to the curve at y_1. If dy/dt can be measured reasonably precisely, then differentials have very concrete uses in describing the behaviour of systems. In some biological systems, however, insufficient events occur within Δt to give a clearly determined average value of y and these should not be modelled using differential equations (Sect. 2.1.1.3).

2.1.1.1 Modelling Dynamic Systems with Differential Equations

One reason why differential equations are used in building models is that there are a number of physical laws describing interactions between components which can be expressed by such equations in a particularly direct and generalized mathematical form.

[A differential equation has the property that it generalizes the forms of the corresponding algebraic equations; it removes the necessity to include a particular value of y measured at a given time t. The essential behaviour of the equation $dy/dt = -Ay$, for example, is independent of time and absolute values of y; it summarizes all algebraic equations of the form $y = y_0 e^{-At}$, whatever the value of the constant y_0 at t_0.]

Rates of diffusion, chemical reaction, heat flow, evaporation and change of momentum are examples of laws characterizing the behaviour of systems changing with time (dynamic systems). The law of mass action is one particularly useful in biological systems. This states that the rate of a simple chemical reaction is proportional to the molecular concentrations of the reacting substances, at least in dilute solution. When Y is formed from a single reacting species X, dy/dt is proportional to x, x and y representing concentrations of X and Y. That is, $dy/dt = Ax$, where A is a proportionality constant, known as the rate constant of the reaction. Alternatively, the rate of removal of Y by, for example, diffusion through a membrane, may be proportional to the concentration present. That is, $dy/dt = -Ay$, where the negative sign indicates that y decreases with time.

Differential equations can be written readily to describe the rate of formation or disappearance of substances from complex biological reaction schemes, using the laws of mass action and diffusion. All the ways of forming or removing each substance are summed to find the rate of change of its concentration. The way in which this is done is illustrated in Chap. 5, applied to dynamic models of the clearance, distribution, and metabolism of hormones and other substances in the body.

2.1.1.2 Making Differential Equations and Data Comparable

The major difficulty introduced by the use of differential equations in describing interactions in a model is that the dependent variable dy/dt is no longer expressed in a form which can be compared directly with experimental results, represented by values of y. Therefore, either (1) the results must be converted into differential form by estimating the slope of the tangent at each data point, or (2) the differential equations of the model are converted into absolute values of y, i.e. integrated. (Just as the formation of the generalized differential equation eliminates the need for the particular value of y included in the algebraic equation, so the reverse process, integration, requires the inclusion of a known value of y, and the time at which it occurs.) Gold (1977) describes the basic concepts of differentiation and integration in non-mathematical terms.

The first method involving the calculation of the tangent at each data point is prone to large uncertainties because of error in the experimental data. The precision of this process can be improved by fitting an empirical polynomial equation to several experimental points about the one of interest and then, by differentiating this equation, calculating a smoothed value of dy/dt at that point (see, for example, Swartz and Bremermann, 1975). These values become the experimental data for direct comparison with the differentials in the model.

The many methods devised for the second approach, integration, have been repeatedly described in mathematical texts. There are a few differential equations for which the corresponding integrated, generalized algebraic equation is known theoretically. Several techniques are available to assist in the integration of particular kinds of differential equations (e.g. Laplace transformation, Sect. 2.2). Otherwise, integration must be done numerically, which is equivalent to summing the area under a graph of the differential equation, a lengthy calculation because of the need for accuracy. There are a number of "hand" techniques for integrating numerically (some are described by Riggs, 1970). Fortunately, computers are ideal for tedious arithmetic and the availability of these rapid, accurate machines and well-designed integration algorithms has made possible the investigation of very much more complex models than before.

Difficulties have frequently occurred in integrating equations describing physiological systems by numerical methods because the differential equations are *stiff.* This means that the equations include regions where the rate of change is relatively abrupt. Recently, mathematical methods have been developed to ease this problem (Sect. 3.6).

2.1.1.3 Requirements for the Use of Differential Equations

The differential equations described above are known as "ordinary"; their variables are continuous, deterministic and homogeneous. Systems described by them must have the same properties. Discontinuous, stochastic and inhomogeneous systems can be investigated using other mathematical methods or concepts, some of which are indicated below.

When a system is *continuous*, changes in the dependent variables can be drawn as smooth, continuous curves; within very short time intervals before any value y_1 is reached, y has values very close to, and approaching, y_1. A system is time-continuous if changes in variables can occur at any time. In a *discontinuous* or *discrete* system, dependent variables can change between only a finite number of values or at particular times. Real systems behave discretely with respect to the dependent variable if small numbers of events are considered, but many can be approximated as continuous when each individual event produces a very small effect on the total system. For example, although the occurrence of pregnancy is numerically a discrete event in a group of women, it may be treated as being continuous in a very large population where the fractional change in numbers due to one pregnancy is very small. In contrast, while a woman can become pregnant time-continuously (that is, at any time) within a few fertile hours each month, viewed from the duration of a year, these widely separated intervals might be approximated as time-discrete. The requirement that the behaviour of the system be continuous as a whole, does not invalidate discrete treatment of continuous systems, such as in sampling at discrete time intervals during experiments and interpolating, or integrating equations numerically by summing the area under the differential curve at discrete (but small) time intervals. Difference equations (e.g. Sect. 2.6.1), finite level algebra (Sect. 2.7), and automata theory can be used to describe discrete systems.

In a deterministic system, at every value of t, the dependent variable has a precise value uniquely determined by the previous state; possible variation in the dependent variable at any particular value of t is very low. In stochastic systems, a probability only can be placed on any particular outcome. Determinism is often achieved by averaging large numbers of stochastic events (Sect. 1.2.6); if an insufficient number of events occur within each time interval of measurement then the variables of a system are indeterminate. The dynamics of stochastic systems can be studied using methods such as the Ito calculus. Statistical mechanics and Markov chains are concerned with probabilities of system behaviour.

Variables must also be homogeneous, in that individual particles must be identical, behave independently of each other and be spatially "well-stirred". High concentrations, for example, render the laws of mass action and diffusion inapplicable owing to interactions. Measured overall concentrations may not be relevant in highly structured cell components where the local concentration of a substrate near an enzyme might depend on local diffusion conditions, or supply from the reactions of a neighbouring enzyme. Variables must be homogeneous also with respect to time; i. e. their behaviour must obey the same constraints regardless of the time interval chosen to observe them. Differential equations of the kind known as "partial" can be used to study the dynamics of some kinds of inhomogeneous systems (examples are in Sects. 2.6.3 and 2.6.4).

2.1.2 Transient and Steady States

Systems can display transient or steady state behaviour. A change in the input to a system will produce a change in the output with time which is called a *transient* response. If the input remains constant the transients may approach constant values as time increases, although other forms of behaviour are possible (Sect. 2.6). When constant values are thus attained by all the variables, these values describe a *steady state* of the system. The rates of change of variables, i.e. the values of dy/dt, are necessarily zero at any steady state; the values of variables at steady states may therefore be calculated by equating differentials to zero. The mathematical description of the disturbance which displaces a system from its steady state is known as a *forcing function*. When studying the dynamics of a system, we are interested in describing the mechanisms which produce the transient behaviour. Steady state behaviour alone is often easier to investigate but less informative.

The steady state is clearly hypothetical in a biological system. It may possibly be approximated in laboratory experiments but in natural surroundings it is most unlikely that all inputs are constant or zero long enough for the system to become unchanging.

The description or "explanation" of transient and steady state behaviours of systems is the object of all the kinds of models described in Sect. 1.1.1.

2.1.3 Defining Model Equations

In addition to differential equations describing the dynamics of a system in terms of interactions between the variables, there are usually other relationships which can be expressed as algebraic equations. By the nature of the system, many variables and parameters (Sect. 1.2.2) are constrained in the values they may take, thus reducing the number of calculations and the effort required in comparing the model and data. For example, conservation laws may apply when a measure such as total mass of a reacting substance remains constant with time. Variables describing concentrations cannot become negative; there may be limits on the magnitudes of parameters or variables; or the values of some parameters may either be known or can be estimated in separate experiments. In addition, integration of any differentiated variable requires knowledge of a measured value of that variable at a known time, thus constraining the generalized differential equation to particular values. These initial values may be treated as unknown parameters if they cannot be measured.

Some of these equations will be redundant, their values being derived one from another. In the model of any system there are a minimum number of variables which must be defined in order to completely describe the state of the system at a particular time. These variables are called *state variables*. The other variables can be derived from known values of the state variables. Two states of the system having the same values for the state variables are indistinguishable. The state variables are related by a minimum number of equations called *state equations*.

In many cases, the state variables will be directly observed in experiments; otherwise the observed quantities will be related to the state variables by additional equations which may contain yet more parameters, known or unknown.

These state equations must be "solved". That is, differential equations must be integrated and the state variables expressed in terms which allow direct comparison with the experimental data. This comparison involves estimating values for the parameters which minimize the difference between model and data (Chap. 3). If a computer is used, numerical integration and solution of algebraic equations are carried out at the same time as parameter estimation. If suitable parameters cannot be found, the model is shown to be inadequate. In theoretical modelling these parameters have physical meaning and the values found must therefore be feasible in reality.

2.1.4 Systems to Which Theoretical Modelling Can Be Applied

Differential and algebraic equations are used in theoretical models where the nature of relevant components, variables and their interactions are postulated. In studying biological systems, there is often insufficient information to adopt a theoretical approach that is more than superficial. As experience and understanding of a system increases a theoretical analysis becomes more rewarding, and can be expected to play an increasingly important part in endocrinological studies.

Extensive theoretical studies have been made of the dynamic behaviour of enzymes and metabolic pathways, particularly glycolysis (introduced by Heinrich et al., 1977). Among other requirements for the simple application of differential equations, the enzymes in these models are assumed to be mixed homogeneously, and effects of diffusion or spatial dependence of metabolite concentrations are neglected. Computer methods have been used to investigate a very detailed theoretical model of complex enzyme systems by Garfinkel and his collaborators (Garfinkel et al., 1977). Other theoretical studies of metabolic systems have been carried out with analogue computers by Heinmets (1966), and interpreted in terms of carcinogenesis.

2.1.5 Compartmental Analysis and Inhomogeneity

Compartmental analysis, which is considered in detail in Chap. 5, can provide a simplified approach to the problem of inhomogeneity in describing the dynamics of components in biological systems. A minimal number of compartments is assigned to chemically identical components. The dynamic behaviour of each is distinct, and is characterized by different differential equations and parameters. The compartments are linked by transport processes, often diffusion. Identification of the compartments with physiological components is usually very difficult, so this kind of modelling cannot be classified unequivocally as theoretical. Where the simplification of the compartmental approach is too gross, partial differential equations must be used allowing continuous variation not only with time but also with space (Sect. 2.6.3).

2.2 Linearity and Non-Linearity

The mathematical concept of linearity is very important in modelling biological systems because the linearity of a system determines both the kinds of behaviours available to it, and the mathematical approaches which can be used in investigating these. Only certain kinds of interaction are linear, producing responses which can be readily characterized and predicted. Non-linear interactions have the potential to give rise to complex, non-intuitive behaviours which are of great interest in biology because of their rich variety of form.

Consider a simple system with one independent variable x which is constant with time. The dependent variable y will also be constant. If x is changed to a new constant value, y will change with time (transiently) and may also reach a constant value at a new steady state. In a *linear* system the total change in y is *proportional* to the change in x. That is, a graph of a set of x values, each held constant, versus the resulting steady state values reached by y is a *straight line*. The steady state responses of this system (and its transients) are proportional to the stimulus.

While physiological systems can show regions of linear response they usually have physical limits of size. Increasing stimuli will, in general, eventually saturate the system so that the response cannot increase proportionally and it therefore acts *non-linearly*. (An example is the response of the adrenal to stimulation by ACTH, shown by Urquhart, 1970.) It is in the saturating region that the system may display either significant changes of function or become non-functional. In the latter case, the normal physiological behaviour may be confined to the unsaturated region where responses can change sensitively with varying stimuli.

In many biological situations strong interactions between components in a system tend to yield non-proportional steady state responses which can be modelled as exponentials of the independent variable (as in equations describing growth), squared or other power terms (as in the phenomenon of allosterism or co-operativity) or variables multiplied together (as in chemical reactions); simple examples are given by Gold (1977, pp. 114–144). All biological systems should be assumed to be non-linear unless experimentally proved otherwise, and then taken as linear only within the range tested.

Linear techniques of analysis, as in Sects. 2.3.2 and 2.3.5, have been well developed in other fields of science, such as engineering. They provide a convenient approach also to those non-linear systems which can be approximated as linear, by using sufficiently small changes in input to ensure that departure from linearity is not great. Such methods will not, however, reveal anything about the often important properties of these systems which arise solely from their non-linearity.

Linear systems can be modelled using linear equations. Linear equations contain linear operators. An *operator* is a mathematical concept meaning simply an instruction to perform some defined mathematical operation on the associated variable. For example (Riggs, 1970), operator L acting on x might be defined as

$$L(x) = 5x^2 + 2. \tag{2.3}$$

If $x = 2v$, then

$$L(2v) = 5(2v)^2 + 2$$
$$= 20v^2 + 2. \tag{2.4}$$

An important operator defined previously is the differential d/dt. Another frequently encountered operator to be discussed below is the *Laplace transform*. This operator converts a time dependent equation (in mathematical terms an equation in the time domain) into an equation dependant on s, i.e. an equation in the s or complex frequency domain. The Laplace transform of x (a function of time) is defined as

$$\mathscr{L}[x(t)] = \int_0^\infty e^{-st} x(t) \, dt$$
$$= \breve{x}(s). \tag{2.5}$$

A linear operator has the following important property. If $L(x) = a$ and $L(y) = b$, then $L(x+y) = a+b$. That is, the result of summing separate operations on two or more functions is identical to operating on the same functions added together. This very useful property is called the *principle of superposition*; it can be used to test whether any equation is linear. By this definition $y = e^{-At}$ does not show a linear relationship between y and t because $L(t_1) = e^{-At_1}$, $L(t_2) = e^{-At_2}$, but $L(t_1 + t_2) = e^{-A(t_1 + t_2)} = e^{-At_1} \cdot e^{-At_2} \neq e^{-At_1} + e^{-At_2}$. Note, however, that the differential of this equation is $dy/dt = d(e^{-At})/dt = -Ay$ (Sect. 2.1.1.1) which does show a linear relationship between *rate of change* of y and y, that is, between rate and the whole function (e^{-At}). The differential is a linear operator, as is the Laplace transform.

Linear relationships greatly simplify the mathematical treatment of models. If several stimuli are superimposed on a linear system then the response is the sum of the changes produced by each stimulus applied separately. The system may also be analysed in terms of simple subsystems which can be recombined simply to find total functioning. Regardless of the order in which linear components act, the outcome will be the same.

Because of the property of superposition, when an independent variable is made to vary sinusoidally then, within a suitable range of frequencies of stimulus, a linear system will produce a sinusoidal response having the same frequency as the stimulus, but usually with a different amplitude (Sect. 2.3.5). Application of a sinusoidal stimulus is frequently used to test for regions of linear response in real systems (Basar, 1976).

Although a stable linear system may have many components, the dynamic changes of its variables, i.e. its transients, can be expressed simply in terms of decaying exponentials, and on occasions, damped sinusoids (Jones, 1973, p. 293).

Non-linear systems do not have these convenient, simple characteristics. The response of a non-linear system at the steady state is not proportional to the stimulus. In non-linear equations the effects of several inputs cannot be summed, and the outcome will differ if the order of applying stimuli is changed. Furthermore, the response of a non-linear system to a sinusoidal input, or indeed any other input, may take many forms which vary with the initial state of the system; it is even possible to obtain continuously oscillating outputs from a constant input (Sect. 2.6.2).

Before the general availability of computers, other techniques had been developed to ease the problem of integration but, apart from numerical methods, these could be applied only to linear systems and a few selected non-linear ones. The Laplace transform is one of these techniques suitable for solving linear equations; it has the advantage of converting differential equations which are functions of time, into linear algebraic equations as functions of s, which can then be solved directly for the dependent variable without integration. The variable s is complex, having the form $s = \sigma + j\omega$ where σ (the neper frequency) is the frequency at which an exponential change is occurring and is identical to an exponential rate constant (parameter A_2 in Eq. (2.7) below), j is the imaginary number equal to the square root of -1, and ω is the radian frequency at which a sinusoidal change is occurring. Conversion of a time dependent linear function into a function of s is accomplished by application of the Laplace transform [Eq. (2.5)], or more conveniently by referring to standard results in published tables. Initial conditions of differential functions are included in their transformation. After solution of the resulting equations, the dependent variables as functions of s are converted back into the time domain for comparison with experimental data by means of tables of inverse transforms. An application of this technique is illustrated in Appendix C. Certain conditions required for the use of Laplace transforms are met by most functions of time that are important in analysis of linear systems (Riggs, 1970).

2.3 Empirical Modelling – a Description of System Response

In biological systems, there is frequently insufficient information about possible components and interactions to be able to postulate equations, either algebraic or differential, to describe underlying mechanisms. The system must be investigated instead from the "outside". The mechanism is treated as an unknown "black box" (Fig. 2.2) and its response to imposed stimuli is studied. This is frequently the only possible approach to studying endocrine systems and many examples are given throughout this book. If an equation is written to represent the action of the "black box" system in converting input into observed output, it must necessarily be empirical, and therefore non-unique. Equations suitable for describing experimental data empirically are discussed below, followed by mathematical techniques for investigating systems where detailed mechanisms cannot be postulated.

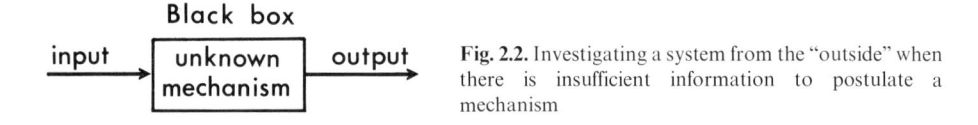

Fig. 2.2. Investigating a system from the "outside" when there is insufficient information to postulate a mechanism

2.3.1 Empirical Equations and Curve-Fitting

In a graph, the behaviour of observed data is conveniently summarized either by joining the measured points with straight lines, or by drawing a smooth curve. This allows values between points to be estimated and is known as *interpolation*. The simplest kind of curve that can be drawn through points for purposes of interpolation is a *polynomial* of order n

$$y = A_1 + A_2 x + A_3 x^2 + \ldots + A_{n+1} x^n. \tag{2.6}$$

The values of the parameters $A_1, A_2, \ldots, A_{n+1}$ are chosen to make the curve fit as closely as possible to the points. Suitable computer techniques for finding parameters in these and other equations using the criterion of least squares best fit are described in Chap. 3.

The choice of a polynomial model is entirely arbitrary. Mathematical experience has shown that curves of an amazing variety of shapes can be represented approximately by polynominals with positive, negative or fractional powers when appropriate values are given to the parameters. The straight line is a particular case where only the first two terms in Eq. (2.6) are retained. The simplest equation comparable with the error of the experimental data should be chosen; two to four parameters are usually sufficient to describe a simple curve.

However, polynomials do not provide good models for many of the relationships between variables found in biology. The following exponential equation is often appropriate

$$y = A_1 e^{-A_2 t}, \tag{2.7}$$

frequently written $y = A_1 \exp(-A_2 t)$, where A_1 and A_2 are parameters and t is the independent variable time. A great many practical cases can be dealt with by means of some variant of Eqs. (2.6) or (2.7). Graphs illustrating the forms these expressions may take are shown by Worthing and Geffner (1943, p. 57). Empirical curve-fitting is introduced by Riggs (1963, pp. 49–58), and useful assistance in choosing suitable empirical functions are given by Riggs (1970, pp. 515–531). Sigmoidal, humped and many other curves can be described by either polynomial or exponential functions. Sine functions give useful descriptions of rhythmical processes (e.g. Batschelet, 1974).

No mechanistic inference can be drawn from the form of an empirical equation because it is not unique. Complex interactions in a system can give an apparently simple empirical relationship. The use of empirical equations limits prediction to precisely those experimental conditions used in obtaining the data; extrapolation is out of the question. An empirical equation fitted to data from an experiment investigating a single independent variable may not be helpful in describing physiological behaviour in which many variables change simultaneously (Sect. 4.1.4). Uses of empirical functions are described below and in Chaps. 3 and 5–8.

2.3.1.1 Spline Functions

The shape of the response of a system often differs markedly from one region of values of the independent variable to another. When this occurs, simple functions such as those mentioned above may provide inadequate descriptions of experimental data. The behaviour of simple functions in a small region determines the shape of the curve everywhere – their form may be too restrictive. *Spline* functions do not have this limitation; they generate piecewise short lengths of (usually) cubic polynomials that give the best fit to *localized* sections of the data. These equations are then joined together smoothly so as to yield a single empirical function, accurately describing the disjoint data.

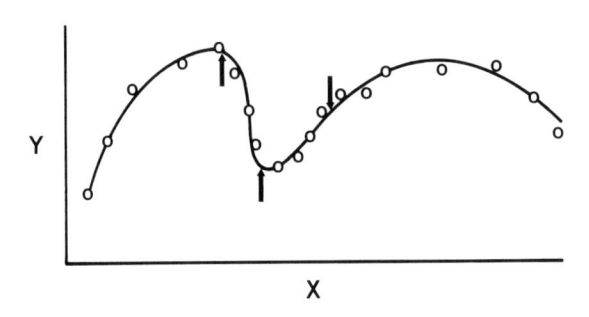

Fig. 2.3. A spline function fitted to data. The positions of the knots are shown by *arrows*

For example, consider the data in Fig. 2.3. It would be difficult to fit a single polynomial because of the curious, abrupt changes in shape. Instead, the data points are divided into sections at suitable values called *knots* and a cubic polynomial is then easily fitted to each intervening section. Smooth joining of the sections is ensured mathematically by making the slope of the cubic at the end of one section identical to that of the ajoining part. The smooth curve shown illustrates a hypothetical spline function, consisting of four separate cubic sections, each with four parameters. It is smooth, and fits the data well (as it should, with 16 parameters). This quality of fit could not be as easily achieved by other means.

Splines are simple polynomials and are thus easy to manipulate. Their statistical properties are convenient and rigorously defined, and their slopes readily calculated. Splines are therefore extremely flexible and convenient for the empirical description of disjoint data. Practical details of their use, such as how to choose the most appropriate number of knots and their locations, are given by Wold (1974), and Spath (1974) who provides useful computer programs.

2.3.1.2 Self-Modelling Non-Linear Regression

This technique, devised by Lawton et al. (1972), is capable of summarizing the common characteristics, or "shape", of the results from a group of individuals, which is often lost by simple averaging. In this respect the method is a generalized form of linear principal component analysis (Sect. 9.2.1).

Self-modelling embodies two quite distinct ideas. The first is that of a *shape invariant model* which adjusts the individual responses to common axes. That is

$$y = A_1 + A_2 \, g\left[(x - A_3)/A_4\right] \tag{2.8}$$

where A_1 and A_3 are shift or location parameters defining the position, and A_2 and A_4 scale parameters affecting the choice of scale for each sample of data on the y and x axes, respectively.

The second idea concerns the nature of a function $g(x)$, which defines the *shape* common to all the samples of data. It may be a postulated theoretical model or, if unknown, approximated by an empirical function, perhaps a spline. The originators of the technique advocate the use of linear splines (i.e. linear interpolation) where there are many data points; otherwise cubic splines might be more suitable.

Two things are achieved by this means. The "best" shaped model is found by fitting splines and, simultaneously, at the most four parameters in the shape invariant model are found which adjust each curve so that all can be superimposed on a common shape.

This method, as yet little used, offers the considerable advantage of readily extracting the essential features of a family of curves. Several clear illustrations are given by Lawton et al. (1972); for a physiological application, in which the ventricular pressure in individual baboons was compared, see Levine et al. (1977).

2.3.2 Transfer Functions

The mechanisms and components of many endocrine systems are largely unknown and the "black box" approach (Fig. 2.2) must be used to study their behaviour. If the response of a system can be described by *linear* equations, investigation of a number of interesting properties is possible. For example, an equation may be determined which is characteristic of the system, and which enables the response to any suitable input to be predicted. This function is known as the *transfer function*, relating change in input to change in output.

Transfer functions of linear systems are frequently determined in the s domain, which has the advantage of avoiding integration. This means that the input and output functions measured as usual in the time domain are transformed by Laplace operators and combined to yield the s domain transfer function

$$G(s) = \frac{\text{Laplace transform of output}}{\text{Laplace transform of input}} = \frac{\breve{y}(s)}{\breve{x}(s)}. \tag{2.9}$$

To determine a transfer function, empirical equations are fitted to the usual time-dependent set of experimentally measured input and output data, the resulting equations transformed term by term using Laplace tables, and combined as above. The response of the system to any other (Laplace transformable) input can then be found from the equation

$$\breve{y}(s) = G(s)\,\breve{x}(s) \tag{2.10}$$

followed by inverse transformation of $\breve{y}(s)$ into the time domain for comparison with experimental data.

This apparently complicated procedure greatly simplifies calculation of the effect of passage of a single input through a series of subsystems. The overall transfer function in the s domain of concatenated subsystems is merely the product of the individual forms of $G(s)$ determined for each subsystem. Responses of subsystems linked in more complicated ways can also be calculated.

When using Laplace transforms it is always required that starting conditions be zero so that effects from previous unknown inputs are not included in measurements. In biological experiments this usually means that the system must be in a steady state (Sect. 2.1.2) at the start of the first input, and differences between the initial steady state and the resulting effects are used to determine $G(s)$.

The system must also be shown to be linear over the range investigated; if it is non-linear a different transfer function will be determined for each state (set of values of variables) of the system.

In a linear system the effects of several inputs can be simply summed.

The usual kinds of experimental input function used are step (⎯⎺), pulse (⎯⎺⎯), ramp (⎯╱), sinusoidal or impulse of infinitely short duration (↑). The *impulse* or *delta function* has the special property that the response to a unit impulse input is $g(t)$, the inverse of the Laplace transform of the transfer function $G(s)$ [Eq. (2.9)]. In practice, a delta function is approximated by any injection or infusion input of short duration relative to the time of onset of the response, and to the smallest time constant of the system.

For example, in Sect. 3.7.1 and 5.1.1 the results are given of fitting an empirical equation to data describing the clearance of a reproductive hormone from blood plasma after injection. The curve took the form $y = 6.1 \exp(-0.6t) + 19 \exp(-0.022t)$, where the units of y were i. u. PMSG/ml and time t was measured in hours. The injection can be treated as an impulse function. The Laplace transform of the empirical equation fitted to the experimental data becomes the transfer function $G(s) = [6.1/(s+0.6) + 19/(s+0.022)]/38,000$ [Eq. (2.9)]. Using this and Eq. (2.10), it is possible to determine the concentration of the hormone in plasma during and after *any* infusion or combinations of infusion schedules for which Laplace transforms can be found. Using computer methods of numerical integration it is possible to solve the same problem in which any form of input is used, as described below.

In the above example the same empirical equation was found to fit experimental data after injection of two different amounts of hormone (Sect. 5.1.1). This indicated that the clearance system probably acted linearly, and was not saturated at the concentrations used.

The methods of linear systems analysis have yielded useful physiological information even from markedly non-linear systems, such as the response of perfused canine adrenal to ACTH (Urquhart and Li, 1968; 1969). Here the time and intensity characteristics of the transient and steady state responses to a variety of input functions were determined. It can also be instructive to find those ranges of input values to which a system responds without saturation, and the effects of drugs and experimental manipulation on these limits. Although a unique mechanism cannot be identified using empirical equations, it may be possible to suggest models compatible with the data, and to design experiments to distinguish between them. For example, Urquhart and Li (1968) suggested several models for adrenal response to ACTH, some based on biochemical synthesis of cortisol; these models were tested with their data.

Another example of the use of these techniques in endocrinology was a study measuring the responses of adrenalectomized rats to infusions of corticosterone using several kinds of input functions (Papaikonomou, 1974, Chap. 10).

2.3.3 Convolution Integrals

In determining an output using the transfer function [Eq. (2.10)], it may be difficult to convert the product $G(s)\bar{x}(s)$ into a form found in tables of inverse Laplace transforms. In that case the convolution integral can be used, which has the form

$$y(t) = \int_0^t g(\tau) x(t-\tau) d\tau \tag{2.11}$$

where τ is a variable of time described below. Notice that this integral is entirely in the time domain and the advantage of the s domain in avoiding integration is lost. Such an integral is, however, readily calculated numerically from experimental data by the careful application of suitable algorithms for the computer.

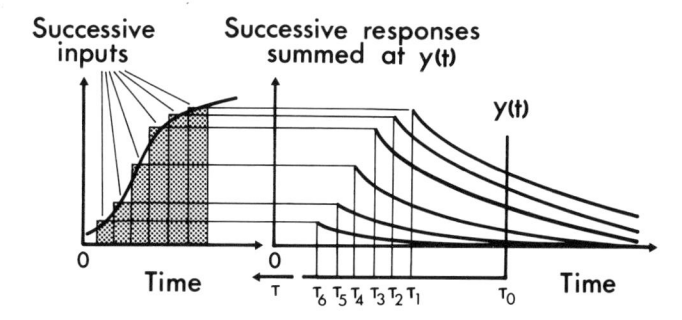

Fig. 2.4. A convolution integral illustrated as the sum of responses to successive impulse inputs. Adapted from Sollberger, 1965, with Kind permission

The convolution integral can equally well be derived from consideration of the input as a sum of succesive impulses or delta functions. The total response at time t is then the sum of all values that the individual responses to each impulse input have reached at time t. The actual value of an individual response at time t to a particular impulse depends on how much earlier (measured by τ) the impulse input occurred (see Fig. 2.4). Recent stimuli contribute relatively most to the response, while earlier ones add less as the time of their application recedes.

Convolution integrals, and the reverse form deconvolution integrals, have a number of very practical uses in those endocrinological systems which can be approximated as linear. An input, output or transfer function can readily be calculated by computer if the remaining two functions are known.

For example in Sect. 8.9, a convolution integral has been used in a model describing the current effect of a reproductive hormone $[y(t)]$ on target tissue. Not only the instantaneous level of hormone $[x(t)]$ is considered but also previous contributions from the levels of hormone in the recent past $[x(t-\tau)]$. These effects of earlier levels decline with time as described by $g(\tau)$.

The reverse process of deconvolution can be used to find the production levels of a physiological substance which cannot be measured directly, but only after its concentration has been modified by other body processes. Rebar et al. (1973) have determined details of the pulsatile secretion of a reproductive hormone from the pituitary, which represents the unknown input $x(t)$, by measuring the resulting hormone concentrations in blood plasma, the output $y(t)$. The transfer function $g(t)$ represents removal of the hormone from the circulation by metabolism, excretion and so on, and was measured separately.

An example of the use of deconvolution to determine a transfer function involving fluorescence decay times in biological materials is given by Johnson and McIntosh (1976).

2.3.4 Combining Subsystems

Transfer functions can be useful in studying the behaviour of models of systems formed by combining subsystems or components. *Block diagrams*, frequently encountered in texts on control theory, use transfer functions to describe relationships between subsystems. Each is represented by a box linked by input and output arrows to other boxes, to "summing" points, or to inputs or outputs external to the system (Riggs, 1970). The links between components must be unidirectional, not reversible; any reversible interactions must be lumped into one block. An example is given in Fig. 2.6.

If the system is linear or can be approximated as linear, a transfer function, $G(s)$, may be written in each box. These functions may be found experimentally or postulated on theoretical grounds. For any input to each subsystem the transfer function determines an output, which then acts as input to the next block. Being linear, the transfer functions are combined as appropriate to determine the overall response of the system to *any* given Laplace transformable input, without the need to calculate the effect of each individual component as the input moves through the system. The output description is also generalized, and does not require a new equation for each set of inputs.

These diagrams are used frequently to illustrate methods and principles of mathematical treatment applied to generalized systems or to physical analogues such as the ubiquitous flow of water from tanks, found in texts on control theory. When representing biological systems, problems of non-linearity may occur. In such cases blocks tend to be occupied by undefined transfer functions, non-linear functions or graphs showing an approximate shape of the non-linear response to input. Non-linear components cannot be simply combined into overall transfer functions for the system.

This representation may be useful when determining the behaviour of subsystems which can be removed, e.g. by ablation or by selective blocking with drugs; comparison of the transfer function of an intact linear system with that of the modified one, reveals the behaviour of the affected part alone. With non-linear behaviour this removal technique may make it possible to identify the subsystems causing the non-linearity. A biological example of this approach is mentioned in Sect. 2.3.5.

2.3.5 Frequency Domain Analysis

Frequency domain analysis is concerned with characterizing the responses of an experimental or model system to the *periodic* or rhythmic aspects of input functions. Input–output analysis in this domain is similar to that in the s domain to which it is related (Riggs, 1970).

The main aim is to determine how passage through a system modifies the amplitude and phase of a periodic input when the frequency of this input forcing function is varied. (For the meaning of terms used to describe periodic functions, see Fig. 7.1.) Linear systems have the property that periodic inputs of *constant amplitude and frequency* produce periodic outputs with the *same frequency* after the transients die down. Passage through a system usually causes the *phase angle* of the input to be shifted by delay, and the *amplitude* of the signal to be altered by an amount which varies with the input frequency ω. The relative amplitudes $G(j\omega)$ (also known as gain) and phase angles $\varphi(\omega)$ of input and output are characteristics of the transfer functions and time constants of the components making up the particular system; they therefore provide a generalized description of its behaviour. Graphs of log $G(j\omega)$ and $\varphi(\omega)$ vs. log (ω) are known as *Bode diagrams* and their interpretation can yield much useful information about the system. The characteristics of different subsystems may be distinguishable in these diagrams. Additional concepts relevant to frequency analysis are discussed in Sect. 7.5.3.

Frequency analysis is applicable to linear systems or those which can be approximated as linear when input signals are small. It cannot deal with spontaneously oscillatory systems.

The application of periodic rather than step inputs may be advantageous in biological systems, most of which "adapt" slowly to a constant input, making it difficult to measure the new steady state. The response to an oscillating input is measured only when the system has reached a sinusoidal steady state. If the baseline of the response can be made to approximate the unstimulated level, the effects of adaptation are avoided; alternatively, measurements made at a new steady state will include adaptation properties. The major difficulty with biological systems is that they may alter their properties within the time required to test responses to a range of frequencies.

Rather than using periodic inputs and measuring output data at the steady state, it is possible to obtain the frequency characteristics of a linear system from analysing the transient responses to step or impulse inputs.

An example of a biological use of this technique follows. Basar (1976) proposed that any mechanism postulated to explain the functioning of a system must have similar time and frequency characteristics to those observed for the system as a whole. He applied frequency analysis to non-linear systems in order to gain insight into possible mechanisms inside biological "black boxes". By comparing the frequency characteristics of the auto-regulation of blood flow through rat kidney with other systems, both intact and when inactivated by drugs, he was able to suggest a working hypothesis for this mechanism. Although it appears from their physiological structures that the auto-regulation of blood flow in the coronary system may have a quite different mechanism from that in the kidney, the distinctive non-linear frequency characteristics shown by responses from both perfused organs stimulated with step or impulse changes in blood pressure, were very similar when analysed by Bode diagrams. Furthermore, these characteristics correspond closely to those of the contraction response of smooth muscle to stretch. Addition of the drug papaverine to paralyse vascular smooth muscle in both kidney and coronary systems eliminated the non-linearities in the responses in both in a similar way, and identified the passive non-regulating frequency characteristics of the organs. This evidence suggested as a working hypothesis, but did not prove, that the auto-regulatory mechanism in both systems is largely due to vascular smooth muscle contraction in response to blood pressure.

In another interesting study Urquhart (1970) has used frequency analysis to examine the responses of cortisol secretion from isolated perfused adrenals when stimulated with sinusoidally varied concentrations of ACTH in blood. The ability of the gland to respond sinusoidally to the oscillating input decreased markedly at rates of more than one peak every 10 min.

A major problem in measuring both frequency characteristics and transfer functions in the s domain in some biological studies may be that the parameters change too rapidly for initial conditions to be established, for steady states to be obtained or for frequency responses to repeat themselves. Where cyclical changes occur in parameters (driven, for example, by biological rhythms) these may be included in the model in addition to changes in the variables under investigation.

The use of frequency analysis in studying feedback systems and their stability characteristics is discussed below.

2.4 Point Stability in Models

An important test of any model in biology is that it should display the same characteristics of stability as the real system. Biological systems are, in general, very stable when disturbed and their models should be shown to behave similarly.

The concept of stability has several meanings. Here a system is said to show point stability if, when displaced from a steady state by an instantaneous disturbance, it returns towards the same state as time increases. Systems may return to a steady state either monotonically or by damped oscillations. *Structural* stability requires a more stringent test; it applies if a system maintains the same overall qualitative dynamic behaviour in the presence of any small disturbance or variation in system structure. Biological systems are generally structurally stable.

An analogy often used is to picture a stable steady state as being at the bottom of a bowl-like depression. When a ball, representing current values of the variables, is displaced from the centre, it will roll back down or around the bowl to reach the steady state. In terms of the equations of a model of the system, the path traced by the ball is called the *trajectory* and represents the values taken by the perturbed variables as time increases. Each initial state of the ball determines a trajectory depending on the shape of the bowl, which is itself defined by the parameter values and forms of the equations.

If when perturbed the system does not return to the same state, but the disturbance is amplified either monotonically or by oscillations, then the system, and its steady state, are *unstable*. The analogy is a ball disturbed from balance on the top of a hill (Fig. 2.5 a).

The term *equilibrium* in classical thermodynamics applies to systems isolated from the environment when variables become constant with time; dy/dt therefore equals zero. Open systems (as exemplified by a living cell) exchange matter and energy with their environment and are thereby continuously disturbed from equilibrium. If the exchange of matter is constant, however, a steady state (Sect. 2.1.2) may be reached in which inflow balances the drive to equilibrium and variables take constant values. Differentials of variables will in this case also equal zero. Classical thermodynamic equilibria in ideal systems with no interactions between components produce *neutral stability* which is like that of a ball placed on a

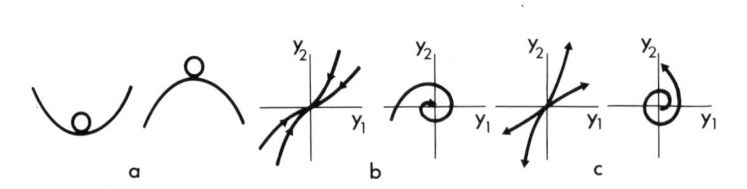

Fig. 2.5a-c. Stability and instability in dynamic systems. **a** Topological metaphor. **b** Trajectories of stable systems in phase space showing monotonic and oscillatory returns to the steady state. **c** Monotonic and oscillatory trajectories of unstable systems disturbed from the steady state

flat surface; it will remain wherever placed, having no preferred position. Although this kind of stability is rarely encountered in reality, classical physics is based upon it and has had much success in explaining in these terms such phenomena as planetary motion and the behaviour of gases which can be approximated as ideal (Goodwin, 1970). In biological systems, however, the space describing all posible values of the variables (phase space) is not thus evenly populated with neutral steady states. There are attractor areas and preferred orbits because of the openness of the systems, and the interactions between components. As discussed later, the topology of stability in biological systems is full of "mountains, valleys and ridges".

The steady states of model open systems exhibit interesting "biological" behaviours. For example, in linear systems, and those with only one accessible steady state, these states are independent of the initial conditions; i.e. they have properties of equifinality (von Bertalanffy, 1973). This means that regardless of its starting position such a system will eventually reach the same steady state. Consider a very simple open system in which y is imported at a constant rate R and removed at a rate proportional to its concentration with rate constant k. Then $dy/dt = R - ky$. At the steady state the differential is zero and then $y_\infty = R/k$. This value is completely independent of the initial value of y. It is dependent on the reaction rates which in a cell are determined by the characteristics and concentrations of enzymes, and by transport properties. In contrast, the values of variables at thermodynamic equilibrium in a closed system are independent of the presence of catalysts; the natures of catalysts and their effects on rate constants are here irrelevant.

Non-linear systems, unlike linear ones, may have several steady states, and the one approached depends greatly on initial conditions. In some conditions non-linear systems may have very interesting forms of stability other than a single point, which has only one set of output values corresponding to each set of input values (Sect. 2.6).

2.4.1 Tests for Stability of Linear Models

Linear systems are stable if with finite inputs a finite output is maintained as time increases to infinity. Therefore, when differential equations of a dynamic model are integrated, the equation describing the output, y, cannot contain terms such as At or $e^{\lambda t}$ where $\lambda > 0$, because these functions increase indefinitely with time.

Consider a linear model of a system at a steady state where all the variables are made equal to zero by subtracting their actual values. Disturbances to the model and the resulting responses are measured as differences from this steady state, $y' = y - y_\infty$. A test demonstrating the stability of the model is therefore to show that the trajectory of y' is described by equations containing terms $e^{\lambda t}$ where the values of λ, the eigenvalues, are always negative; such a function moves towards the steady state where $y' = 0$ as time increases, thus reducing the effect of the disturbance. Eigenvalues are the roots of the "characteristic equation" of the model; this equation is derived from the differential equations describing the unforced response of the model, where the differentials are made into variables, λ, for which values are sought. Thus parameters of the model equations of a system determine the eigenvalues. The "unforced" or "natural" response of the system is that occurring on application of an impulse input where the forcing function is applied instantaneously before the response begins. The characteristic equation is therefore related to the transfer function from which it may be determined (Riggs, 1970, pp. 164–166). In an unforced system, s in the denominator of the transfer function becomes equivalent to the eigenvalues. Changes in the stability of the model can be investigated by determining the effect on the eigenvalues of varying the parameters.

Eigenvalues can be real or complex numbers. If all eigenvalues (roots) of the characteristic equation describing a linear system, or a system approximated as linear, have negative real parts, the model behaviour is stable. If a root has a positive real part the behaviour is unstable, the initial disturbance increasing with time. If the roots are complex, the trajectory of the response to an impulse disturbance is oscillatory. The damping time constant is dependent on the real part of the root, and the oscillating frequency on the imaginary part (Fig. 2.5). Other linear tests of stability based on frequency analysis are described in the discussion on feedback loops (Sect. 2.5.2.1).

Without actually calculating eigenvalues it is possible to determine whether they have negative real parts using the Routh-Hurwitz method (Riggs, 1970, pp. 172–176).

2.4.2 Stability of Non-Linear Models

In linear models the test described above give results applicable to any size of perturbation; such models are said to be globally stable. In non-linear models there may be more than one steady state, not necessarily having the form of a single point, and tests must therefore be local, i.e. applicable only to the area around the steady state of interest. The linear tests described above can be used also for analysing the stability of single point steady states in some non-linear models (Rosen, 1970) which have been approximated as linear. (This could be done, for example, by expressing the equation as a Taylor series in which all but the linear terms are ignored.) The stability results so obtained will, however, apply only to perturbations which leave the variables sufficiently close to the steady state so that the linear approximations are valid. Larger perturbations may cause quite different stability properties to be exhibited. Using the analogy of May (1973), if the locally stable valley bottom were inside the peak of a volcano, then although small disturbances would return to the valley floor, large perturbations may carry the system over the crater's lip to spill out in the terrain below. Similarly, on disturbance away from an unstable steady state point, the trajectory of values of the variables may move towards another region where stable behaviour becomes possible (Sect. 2.6).

Another technique for testing a larger, but defined region around a steady state single point of a non-linear model, involves the use of Lyapunov functions (Walter, 1972; Rosen, 1970). If disturbances within an area about the steady state point do not result in the variables going beyond some other vicinity around this point, then the model of the system is stable in this region. The chosen Lyapunov function defines the limits of the regions of disturbance and model stability which are tested.

The extent of interaction of components (defined by the parameters of the equations) determines the stability properties of a model. It is therefore necessary to map the responses of non-linear models numerically over a range of parameter values to get an idea of the possible behaviour of the variables. Each response must be calculated individually using a particular set of values for the parameters; in contrast to linear models, the global behaviour cannot, in most cases, be described.

Tests of a non-linear model for structural stability can be informative. An example is given in Sect. 8.9.1.1 where stochastic variation of an input variable was simulated by adding a small random term to equations describing the concentrations of some variables in the menstrual cycle. The resulting changes in the overall response were comparable with natural variations.

2.5 Concepts of Feedback

2.5.1 Biological Homeostasis and the Concept of Feedback

Biological systems cannot maintain their consistent behaviour by adhering strictly to internal rules in disregard of their environment, because they are open systems dependent on an inflow of materials and energy. Neither can they compliantly respond to imposed conditions, as suggested by the response models of Fig. 2.2, because the stimuli continually change without reference to their survival. Heat, light and nutrients are not supplied at a constant convenient rate; they may be deficient, or in excess, or supplied randomly, in gradients, or in cycles. Biological systems require mechanisms for sensing and responding appropriately to a large number of environmental cues simultaneously, in such a way that their self-organization is controlled, either in those steady states necessary for survival, or by developing in a genetically directed way.

These activities are familiar to endocrinologists because endocrine systems and their hormones are instrumental in detecting environmental conditions, in maintenance of the stability known as "homeostasis", and in development.

Even the reproductive function is a mechanism for a form of homeostasis, but at a different hierarchical level from stability in the internal environment of an organism (Laszlo, 1972). Here the entire organism is reconstituted from some of its specialized cells and the remainder of the parent organ eventually decays ("dies"). Individual mortality is the price species pay for their environmental adaptation. Ageing and death are balanced by birth and growth and the species maintains the organization characterizing its genotype.

What has mathematics to contribute to these concepts of biological stability and development? In Sect. 2.5.2 we shall concentrate mainly on homeostasis, while in Sect. 2.6 mathematical concepts of development are elaborated. Von Bertalanffy (1973) argues that open systems can have inherent properties of stability caused by the energy relationships in the interactions involved, these being reflected in the stability behaviour of the equations describing such systems. A particular process need not be inherently stable, however, if there is a sensing mechanism which detects the current state of the system and environment, or both, and modifies future performance to make output conform to some predetermined standard. A moving bicycle represents a very unstable system unable to progress for long without the brain of the rider making it responsive to internal and external events, thereby giving it stability under a reasonably wide range of conditions. Such a control mechanism, known as feedback, may not itself supply the energy necessary to bring about self-regulation, but instead serves to alter the system's use of available energy resources. Both kinds of mechanisms leading to stability appear relevant to biological function.

2.5.2 Feedback Control

The concept of feedback has been developed mainly in the field of electrical engineering to solve problems such as the maintenance of a particular controlled response in the face of changeable inputs. The systems usually considered were composed of simple linear electrical components. From the above discussion, the concept of feedback might be expected to be useful also in biology for describing possible mechanisms for maintaining stability of components. However, application of the mathematical developments is generally less easy in endocrinology than in physical systems because of the ill-defined components, interactions and even function of biological systems, and the complexity of interactions and non-linearities involved. Descriptions of feedback control in biology are given by Riggs (1970; 1977) and Jones (1973); Rassmussen (1974) provides an endocrinological discussion.

In feedback the simple unidirectional relationship of input to output, cause and effect, described in Sect. 2.3 is modified; the output feeds back to influence the way in which the system responds to input — a rate constant (parameter) used in the equation describing the effect of stimulus is no longer constant but becomes a function of the output. Reversible reactions are, however, excluded from the definition of feedback.

Negative feedback occurs where an increase in output reduces the response to input

$$A \xrightarrow{+} B \xrightarrow{+} C$$
$$\underline{}$$

An increase in A causes an increase in B, which in turn augments C. Increase in C then reduces A. Intuitively, it appears that a system described by such a model would tend to reduce output to levels lower than if the feedback loop were not operating, or were open. Several endocrine systems have been modelled in these terms (references above). Positive feedback occurs when an increase in output produces an increased response to input

$$A \xrightarrow{+} B \xrightarrow{+} C$$
$$+$$

A system modelled thus would be expected to produce higher levels of output than if the loop were open, and it might become unstable, the response increasing until some physical limit is saturated, some resource totally consumed, or a new form of system behaviour becomes thermodynamically more favourable (Sect. 2.6).

Feedforward in a chain of reactions is also possible. For example, positive feedforward implies that an increase in A

$$\overset{+}{\overbrace{A \xrightarrow{+} B \xrightarrow{+} C}}$$

accelerates the conversion to C, thus producing a rapid amplification of the initial stimulus, such as the cascade effect in blood clotting, or the release of insulin in response to increase in glucose concentration. In biological systems feedforward reactions are uncontrolled and are thus probably part of a negative feedback loop.

Empirical or theoretical transfer functions in the s domain and frequency analysis are often used in studying linear feedback systems, or those approximated as linear. The feedback may also be ignored and "black box" methods used to describe simple overall input–output behaviour (Sect. 2.3). However, the mathematics may become simpler and more relevant to the actual mechanism when the system is described as subsystems linked together into a feedback loop. Theoretical modelling of feedback using differential equations is also possible if sufficient information on components and interactions of the system is available or can be postulated, and other requirements for the use of these equations are satisfied. In most biological systems, insufficient information is available as yet to take a direct theoretical approach to investigating feedback control by hormones. Metaphoric modelling using non-linear differential equations is discussed in Sect. 2.6.4 for situations where feedback produces the interesting response of stable oscillations. In Sect. 1.4 is described a very general metaphoric model of another mechanism for producing stable homeostatic responses in complex systems.

In feedback control theory based on physical systems, conventional negative feedback is represented as shown in Fig. 2.6. There is a fixed reference value in the system and a mechanism for comparing this reference value with the output, by way of the feedback loop. The difference between the reference and output values (the actuating error) is used to alter the way in which the input stimulus is processed to produce output response.

In Riggs' (1970) "moist and mobile" world of living things fixed reference values seem rarely to occur. The controller may be hard to identify or meaningless, and it may not act immediately after the subtraction process. A more appropriate representation, therefore, for a simplified biological feedback system might be that shown in Fig. 2.7 in which there is merely a causal loop. Note that changes in any component in such a loop will cause changes to varying degrees in all other components.

The characteristic features of a negative feedback loop are as follows. (1) Each process has inputs and outputs coupled cyclically so that the output of one process

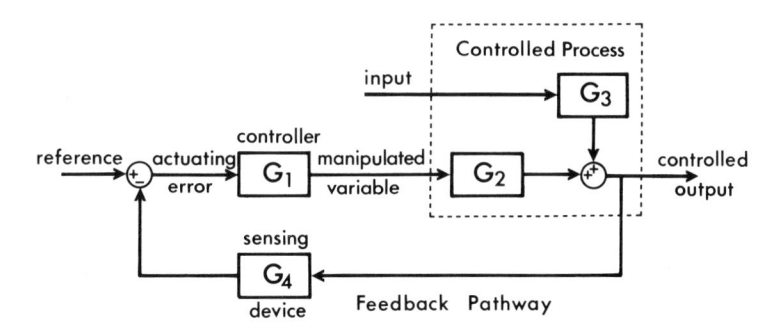

Fig. 2.6. A conventional negative feedback system; G_1, G_2, G_3 and G_4 are transfer functions. Adapted with kind permission from Riggs, 1970, Control theory and physiological feedback mechanisms. Copyright by The Williams & Wilkins Co., Baltimore, Md.

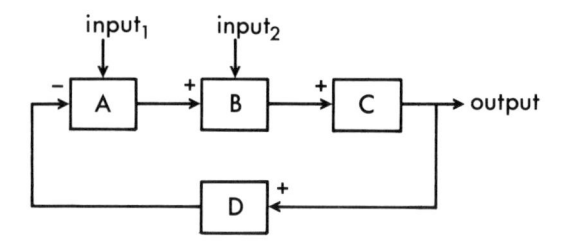

Fig. 2.7. Simplified representation of a biological negative feedback system; A, B, C, and D are transfer functions

becomes the input to another, (2) there are an odd number of processes in the loop where increase in input produces a decrease in output (sign reversal) and (3) at least one process in the loop is irreversible.

These features may be used to identify feedback loops. Simple examination of input–output data does not confirm feedback because the same characteristics can be displayed by a suitably designed system without feedback. Negative feedback is suspected where the output remains nearly constant over a wide range of conditions. The identification of the sign reversal process is usually an important step in investigating a suspected feedback system.

A sign reversal process is illustrated by Riggs (1970) in a model of the regulation of the osmolarity of extracellular fluid by antidiuretic hormone. While increase in osmolar concentration of extracellular fluid acts through the pituitary to increase secretion of the hormone, the resulting increased reabsorption in the distal segments of the nephron will, be sign reversal, decrease the osmolar concentration of the fluid. This serves to decrease the activity of the pituitary in producing hormone.

Known forms of sign reversal processes in endocrine control loops act through inhibition of the hormone secretory process by the target cell response (insulin system), inhibition of an enzyme converting a hormone precursor to hormone, as for angiotensin, or by feedback of either response or hormone production on the hypothalamus, as in the systems producing vasopressin and cortisol (Rassmussen, 1974).

What sort of behaviour is introduced by the presence of negative feedback loops in a model of a system?

The major effect is to decrease the sensitivity of the system to changes affecting the independent variables. Any real system will, however, have limits on its capacity to stabilize itself; there will be minimum or maximum values where feedback ceases to operate. For example, when maximal response to a hormone is reached, further increases in hormone production will be ineffective in producing stability; the loop in the model acts as if open. The effectiveness of feedback is measured as gain or the related quantity, magnification. These characteristics of the feedback loop are determined by the relative rates of the individual reactions involved (which are related to the parameters of their descriptive equations), the non-linearity of the reactions, and the number of steps in the loop. The higher the gain of a system, the more closely will the dependent variables return to their unperturbed values when a constant disturbance is applied. High gain produces faster response to disturbance, but makes oscillatory or unstable behaviour more likely.

There are, therefore, three important questions which can be asked mathematically of biological systems where the presence of feedback has been identified.

(1) Under what conditions is the system stable? (2) How effective is the feedback loop when disturbed in returning the system to its previous state? (3) What sort of mechanisms might be involved, and what are their properties? These points are discussed in the following sections.

2.5.2.1 Point Stability in Models of Negative Feedback

Experimentally it is interesting to determine the limits of feedback control in response to stimuli in biological systems. What levels of stimulation has the organism been adapted to deal with?

Linear tests for stability (Sect. 2.4.1) can be used on models of feedback loops either by analysis of the signs of eigenvalues obtained from theoretical equations, or from calculating s from the transfer function of the unforced system. With non-linear systems the stability characteristics determined using linear approximations apply as before only when small disturbances about the particular steady state are investigated; each steady state will have a different transfer function, changes in which can influence the stability characteristics.

The higher the gain of a negative feedback system, the faster it returns to the steady state. With sufficient gain, linear models with more than two components can be made to exhibit damped oscillatory responses. With three or more components, damping lessens as gain increases until a critical value is reached where instability ensues. Instead of each loop variable diminishing to a constant value, oscillations grow as far as the physical constraints on the system will allow, a new stable behaviour such as a limit cycle occurs (Sect. 2.6.2), or the system is destroyed. Greater damping of an oscillatory response occurs if the time constants in a feedback loop differ greatly; this has an effect similar to reducing the number of reactions in the loop, thus enhancing the stability behaviour of the model.

The stability of linear feedback models is often determined from analysis in the frequency domain rather than as a function of time. In frequency terms, instabilities can arise when the subtraction of the return signal through a negative feedback loop produces a signal that is in phase with the input signal, thus increasing its amplitude. Under the right conditions these resonant frequencies may result in ever increasing amplitudes and instability. Resonant frequencies, and the conditions under which they may lead to instability, are revealed by Bode diagrams (Sect. 2.3.5) or Nyquist plots (Riggs, 1970). (These approaches are equivalent to determining eigenvalues in the time domain.) Experimentally, the presence of resonance in these diagrams is indicative of a feedback loop. Destabilizing resonant frequencies will be selected by the system from any real input signal which necessarily contains noise at many frequencies; instability is a property of the design of the model and cannot be avoided by attempting to impose inputs at other frequencies. Frequency analysis of stability may be applied to suitable heavily damped, non-linear systems in which linear approximations are appropriate.

Instability in feedback loops is increased by the presence of transport lags caused by such processes as diffusion or transport of materials in blood. Such delays are common in biological systems (unlike electrical ones). They introduce an increase in phase lag of the return signal which may be similar to the time constants of other processes involved. Delays of this kind must, therefore, be considered in assessing the instability of any model of a system.

The stability properties of a particular feedback loop will be influenced by any other loops interacting with it. The effects on stability of the inclusion of further feasible loops in a model of a biological feedback system needs to be considered.

It is of interest to determine parameter values producing unstable behaviour in the model of a negative feedback loop. Such instability can lead to stable oscillations in the values of the variables with many of the properties of biological rhythms (Sect. 2.6.4 and Chap. 7).

2.5.2.2 Effectiveness of Feedback Loops

Qualitative evidence of an inhibitory reaction in a causal loop of biological reactions must not be assumed to mean that this feedback causes stability. Several feedback loops may contribute to the observed stability, or spurious interactions or responses may have arisen from non-physiological doses or conditions used for testing. It is advisable to establish quantitatively, under normal physiological conditions, the range of effectiveness of any proposed stabilizing mechanism for comparison with actual performance. For example, according to Stear (1975), F. E. Yates measured the effectiveness of the feedback between the adrenal cortex and the hypothalamus, in which cortisol inhibits the secretion of corticotrophin releasing factor. Even though appropriate connectivity between these hormones and organs had been demonstrated, the open loop gain measured (0.3) over the time scale thought to be relevant was inadequate to account for the observed physiological responses.

Open loop gain (OLG), frequently called gain, is a measure of the effectiveness of feedback and describes the relative magnitudes of a signal before and after traversing the whole feedback loop once. A negative feedback loop is shown in Fig. 2.8, in block diagram form. G_1 and G_2 are transfer functions describing the transformations of the values of X_1 into X_2, and X_2 into X_4. If the loop is opened, a constant signal inserted, and the output measured at the other side of the opening point after the system has reached the steady state, the transfer function equals the open loop gain. That is, $\text{OLG} = G_1 G_2$.

Magnification (Mag) is a related quantity, equalling $1/(1 + \text{OLG})$ for negative feedback. It measures the relative ability of a feedback loop to decrease the response to a constant disturbing input (step input) when the loop is operating, in comparison with when the loop has been opened by, for example, destroying the interaction between two of the components.

A generalized causal loop is shown in Fig. 2.9. In this loop

$$\text{Mag} = \left. \frac{\delta L_i / \delta X_i |_{\text{closed}}}{\delta L_i / \delta X_i |_{\text{open}}} \right|_{\infty}. \tag{2.12}$$

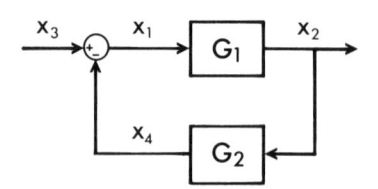

Fig. 2.8. Gain of feedback systems; G_1 and G_2 are transfer functions

Concepts of Feedback

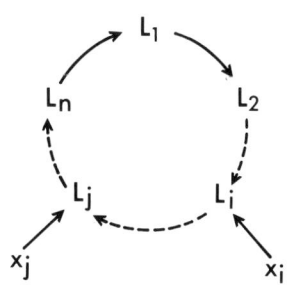

Fig. 2.9. Generalized feedback loop. Symbols X represent inputs and L loop components

Both measures may be applied at the steady state to linear systems, and also to highly damped non-linear systems approximated as linear by the use of small input signals. In the latter case the gain and magnification will be different for each steady state investigated. Rhythmical and unstable systems cannot be thus measured.

There are several ways to determine open loop gain or magnification on suitable systems. Frequency analysis produces Bode plots which can be used to display the way in which gain varies with the frequency of input. In biological systems gains and magnifications may be obtained by measuring changes in response to a constant input signal with the loop closed (intact), and after opening by surgery or drugs. These responses must be measured at the same steady state, but it is frequently difficult or impossible to return the system to the same state after destroying interactions in the feedback loop.

Riggs (1977) describes a potentially very useful method of obtaining gains at steady states with the feedback loop left intact. This technique can be used even if most of the components in the loop and their interactions are experimentally inaccessible, or even unidentified. It is required, however, that all inputs to the loop are controlled so that a steady state can be maintained. In addition, two components of the loop must be measurable, and each must have a different input by which it alone can be directly manipulated. Changes in input x_i (Fig. 2.9) to one loop component, L_i, will be shown in the resulting steady state values of the other component, L_j. These changes will depend on the transfer function of the intervening part of the loop. For a series of step inputs to L_i, therefore, a mathematical expression can be obtained to describe the observed steady state responses of L_j

$$L_j(\infty) = f_1[L_i(\infty)]. \tag{2.13}$$

Conversely, the transfer function describing the remainder of the loop will influence the way in which the steady state values of L_i are altered by changes in step inputs to L_j

$$L_i(\infty) = f_2[L_j(\infty)]. \tag{2.14}$$

Simultaneous solution of these equations yields the "overall steady state" called the *operating point* of the system at which input and response values coincide for each L. The open loop gain at this operating point is then the absolute value of the product of the differentials of the two functions at the operating point

$$\text{OLG} = \frac{df_1[L_i(\infty)]}{dL_i(\infty)} \cdot \frac{df_2[L_j(\infty)]}{dL_j(\infty)}. \tag{2.15}$$

In linear systems this value is a constant for all operating points. A study of the variation of OLG or Mag with conditions for non-linear biological systems is itself of great interest.

One or both functions describing the mutual influence of L_i and L_j may be obtained by fitting empirical equations to suitable experimental measurements on steady state changes. Or, one or both equations may be known theoretically, or proposed analytically from a knowledge of the mechanisms involved. With theoretical equations *and* the possibility of experimental determination of OLG, a theoretical model can be tested.

Riggs (1977) describes a possible use of this method to investigate the gain in the feedback loop controlling plasma Ca^{2+} with parathyroid hormone. First, Ca^{2+} or a calcium chelating agent is infused at various constant rates to force the steady state of Ca^{2+} to change. At each steady state the concentration of Ca^{2+} and parathyroid hormone is measured to yield the curve of the relationship $PTH = f(Ca^{2+})$. An infusion of the hormone would yield the corresponding curve for Ca^{2+} changes at the steady state. This information is sufficient to determine the OLG of the feedback system.

Riggs (1970) describes approaches to multiple interacting feedback loops under the same conditions of step inputs, steady states, and operating points applicable to those systems which can be approximated as linear.

2.5.2.3 Negative Feedback Loops and Their Mechanisms in Endocrinology

The nature of feedback loops in endocrinology in particular, and biology in general, presents some difficulties in devising models and experiments based on feedback control theory.

For example, many biological systems react to a disturbance by returning rapidly and efficiently to constant values of the dependent variables, which implies high gain. Yet, contrary to prediction of the theory applied to simple engineering regulators with high gain, biological systems are extremely stable. This is probably because living organisms contain multiple interlocking feedback loops all influencing the regulation of any one variable. Several homeostatic systems serving apparently different purposes, and responding to different stimuli, all influence each other by having common active materials or providing precursors to them. For example, there are often two antagonistic hormones which provide the feedback mechanism regulating a variable. These are, however, rarely direct antagonists; the action of one can often produce additional disturbances which stimulate other systems. Stear (1975) has proposed models of the types of feedback and feedforward mechanisms theoretically required to produce uncoupling of systems interacting in this way, such as thyroid and adrenal control.

Feedback loops like that shown in Fig. 2.7 may be a gross simplification. Jones (1973) describes some of the processes which could be involved in regulating body heat; he draws a diagram similar to Fig. 2.10 to show that in any process there may be several kinds of effectors of the regulated process and many receptors of several different kinds to detect the results. All of these activities, plus many other input signals, more or less obviously related, may be received by a controlling organ such as the hypothalamus where genetic information, previous experience and current stimuli are integrated and acted upon.

Concepts of Feedback

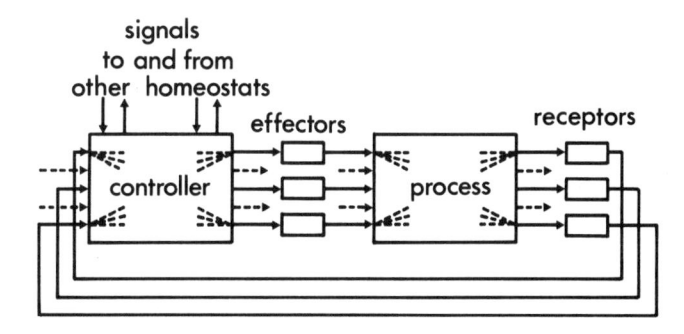

Fig. 2.10. Homeostatic feedback in biological systems. Adapted from Jones, 1973, with kind permission

Stimulus–response activities in endocrine systems are often very complex. Not only may several hormones be involved in controlling one function but each may activate many types of tissue in different ways, as does oestradiol. Furthermore, there are many instances of hormones having several kinds of action on the one type of target cell, each with different time constants and mechanisms. These produce from a single tissue multiphased overall responses spanning a considerable time period. There may be an immediate action in which the time constants of some chemical processes in cells are altered, inactive precursor cells may be activated by hormone more slowly, and responding cells may be stimulated to undergo mitosis producing activity over a yet longer time span. All need considering and making quantitative in a description or model of the hormone activity.

Measurements of steady states may not be practical in endocrinological investigations. Many systems do not return immediately to a steady state after a stimulus is withdrawn, but may be altered in activity over days or even permanently – a unidirectional change under hormonal control as in growth and differentiation. Some systems may be constantly disturbed by either random inputs or those from circadian or other rhythms. Internal or environmental sources may change parameters, which may vary with age, species, individuality, current treatment, blood flow, lighting and feeding regimes, reproductive state, time of year, competition of other body systems for energy resources, changes in removal rates, and so on. Adaptation of the system to stimuli may occur depending on the amount of stimulation recently received.

Furthermore, while electrical circuits are designed for particular purposes, the functions served by biological systems or components are not always evident. Melatonin, prostaglandin and relaxin are in this category. Therefore it may be difficult to identify and include in a model all relevant components and interactions, stimuli and responses, or even to know what stimuli are appropriate to the activation of a feedback system.

In spite of these difficulties, concepts of control theory provide a structure for directing experimentation, and increase awareness of possibilities. Each system must be approached using current ideas and information in order to determine which simplifications are appropriate to its investigation. Knowledge of how overall dynamic stability and development is maintained is required if we wish to understand endocrinological systems. Where this aim cannot yet be attempted, identification of components, stimuli and the nature of their interactions, followed by quantitative descriptions of the non-linearities of transient and steady state responses in the subsystems making up feedback loops, provide absorbing study.

The kinds of subsystems involved in endocrine loops for which qualitative and quantitative studies are required include the following: the nature of hormone interactions with extracellular receptors, the ensuing intracellular messengers and their interactions with intracellular receptors to produce responses in target organs, the natures and effects of responses, and substances bringing about the inhibition of hormone secretion. Transformation of steroids by liver and kidney, or the activities of organs which convert prohormones to active forms, are important; peripheral metabolism of hormones can strongly influence the overall process.

Rassmussen (1974) describes different types of feedback control operating in endocrine systems and discusses the mechanism of hormone action on enzymes, genes and membranes, and their relationship with energy metabolism. As a first approximation, it might be expected that the response to hormones could be modelled using simple Michaelis–Menten type relationships [Eq. (2.25)]. However, a proportional response between the concentration of a hormone and its effect (below the saturation region) is not usually observed. Instead, it is common to find receptor responses which are explicable in terms of co-operativity. This cooperativity causes strong non-linearity (Sect. 2.6.4).

Examples of generalized models of endocrine systems based on control theory have been described by Rassmussen (1974). Riggs (1970) has investigated the construction of many models of biological systems showing feedback loops, including antidiuretic hormone, insulin, parathyroid hormone and thyroid stimulating hormone. Jones (1973) has also applied feedback control concepts to several biological systems. Other examples are a model of the biphasic non-linear response of insulin to glucose and amino acids, put forward by Bergman and Bucolo (1973), and models of interactions simulating transient responses observed in endocrine and metabolic systems when stimulated by step inputs, described by Licko (1975). Chapter 8 discusses models of ovulation in which feedback is used to control rhythmical changes in the values of variables.

2.6 Biological Development and Mathematics Beyond Instability

The outstanding characteristic of living things is their organization, both of structure (in space) and in function (through time). This organization can be maintained and can evolve as a stable process in spite of widely varying environments. Models of biological systems must exhibit similar properties and have similar responses to random or other influences. The study of stability and development of biological systems and their mathematical representations, both qualitatively and quantitatively, is a rapidly advancing field.

Stability and evolution of biological systems are not explicable in terms of the classical laws of thermodynamics and statistical mechanics. These laws state that an isolated system (not exchanging matter or energy with the environment) cannot increase its total organization with time, but must evolve towards a stable equilibrium state of maximum disorder or entropy. Destruction of order always occurs near the equilibrium state. If dS is the variation of entropy during a time interval dt then dS is always ≥ 0 in an isolated system.

Biological systems are not isolated. They maintain themselves by exchanging matter and energy with their surroundings; i.e. they are open. With a continuous inflow of matter a system must be displaced from its equilibrium condition. With constant inflow it may, however, reach a steady state where the disturbance from inflow balances the drive to equilibrium (von Bertalanffy, 1973).

Prigogine and others (see, for example, Glansdorff and Prigogine, 1971, or, for a simplified description, Prigogine et al., 1972) have developed the idea that with sufficient inflow of negative entropy an open system may become more structured. If dS_i represents the sum of internal entropy change arising from reactions, diffusion and so on, then $dS_i \geq 0$. But the inflow of entropy from the environment dS_e has undefined sign. Thus it is possible, under certain conditions of inflow, that the total entropy of the system $dS = dS_i + dS_e \leq 0$, and therefore structure may arise and be maintained. Such a condition can only occur far from equilibrium because of the required exchange with the environment. At the point where ordered structures may arise, the original behaviour of the system becomes unstable and the system evolves through instability to a new, more structured, stable state.

The physical example usually quoted to illustrate this type of change is the onset of thermal convection in a fluid heated from beneath. Below a critical temperature gradient, the energy is distributed in random thermal motion. Above the critical value such a situation is unstable, and macroscopic highly ordered convection patterns begin spontaneously to emerge and develop towards a new stable behaviour.

Note the change in hierarchical level of order in this transition from microscopic order on the molecular level, to macroscopic order of observable convection patterns. Note also that a threshold or critical value of input was necessary for change to occur. Both these kinds of behaviour are observed qualitatively in biological systems.

Because any real system is stochastic, i.e. it is subject to random fluctuations of variables and parameters, there is always a finite probability that the critical state for instability will be reached. Such random fluctuations are normally damped, but if they reach the critical points positive feedback may bring about new macroscopic ordering of the system. Does evolution therefore occur through random fluctuations (Prigogine et al., 1972)? Statistical mechanics is a technique for studying dynamic systems for which initial conditions cannot be completely specified, i.e. they are not deterministic. An extension of this approach has been hailed as that most suited for studying biological behaviour (Yates et al., 1972). At the present stage of development, the restrictive conditions required for application of its theories make useful investigation of biological problems difficult (Rosen, 1970, Chap. 9).

Interactions such as those found in biological systems have been shown (using deterministic mathematics) to produce, beyond their critical instability conditions, a wide variety of possible kinds of behaviour exhibiting structures organized in both space and time (Sect. 2.6.3). These forms of organization can arise even from initially random or homogenous mixtures. The behaviours of such systems are surprising; they would be difficult to derive intuitively without the aid of mathematics and their conceptual and mathematical implications are currently attracting much interest.

The problems in applying these ideas quantitatively to development and control of actual biological systems appear, however, to be immense, although some exciting first steps have been made in modelling theoretically simpler real systems of chemicals and biochemicals, as mentioned below. A more empirical approach has been taken in investigating biological systems with such behaviour for which the components cannot be postulated (Winfree, 1977, in his studies of circadian rhythms).

2.6.1 An Example of Parameter-Dependent Changes in System Stability

Before dealing briefly with some of the concepts that have been used by both biologists and mathematicians to describe the behaviour referred to in the previous section, a heuristic example is given to illustrate in practical terms the existence of instability points leading to new and unexpected results. It must be emphasized that these changes in behaviour result from strong interactions between the components of a system, and therefore the equations describing the models are non-linear. The stability characteristics of a model can be changed by varying the parameter values defining the extent of these non-linear interactions.

The example chosen for illustration is a difference equation described by May (1976), in which events occur in discrete steps. This form of the equation makes it particularly easy to follow the trajectory at successive time intervals towards stable, or away from unstable states, but analogous behaviour, less easy to illustrate graphically, could occur with more strongly non-linear interactions described by several inter-related differential equations.

The difference equation of interest describes the number of objects at the next time interval, $N(t+1)$, as a function of the number of objects now, $N(t)$. The objects may, for example, be insects breeding seasonally where generations do not overlap. This type of equation has had interpretations in many disciplines, including genetics and epidemiology. The basic non-linear equation is

$$N_{t+1} = N_t(A - BN_t), \tag{2.16}$$

or, to generalize, and release it from dependence on absolute values of N, we make $y = BN/A$ obtaining

$$y_{t+1} = Ay_t(1 - y_t) \tag{2.17}$$

where y has values between 0 and 1. Values of y_{t+1} plotted against y_t yield a humped curve (Fig. 2.11). The behaviour described is that of a population increasing in the next generation when small, but decreasing when large. The steepness of the hump is "tuned" by the parameter A which also determines the possible kinds of behaviour of the system. In Fig. 2.11, $A = 2.8$.

Taking an arbitrary value of y_t at $t = 1$, it is possible to follow the trajectory described by values of y in succeeding generations. For example, with an initial value of $y_{t=1} = 0.1$, the value of y in the next time interval $(t+1=2)$ can be found on the curve at y_2. Taking y_2 now on the y_t axis, $y_{t+1=3}$ has the value labelled y_3, and so on. It can be seen that succeeding generations show damped oscillations which approach a constant value of y, y_∞, such that all $y_t = y_{t+1}$. Alternatively, this point may be found by simply plotting the line $y_t = y_{t+1}$ which is at an angle of 45° to the axes, and finding the intersection with the curve described by Eq. (2.17). Thus this

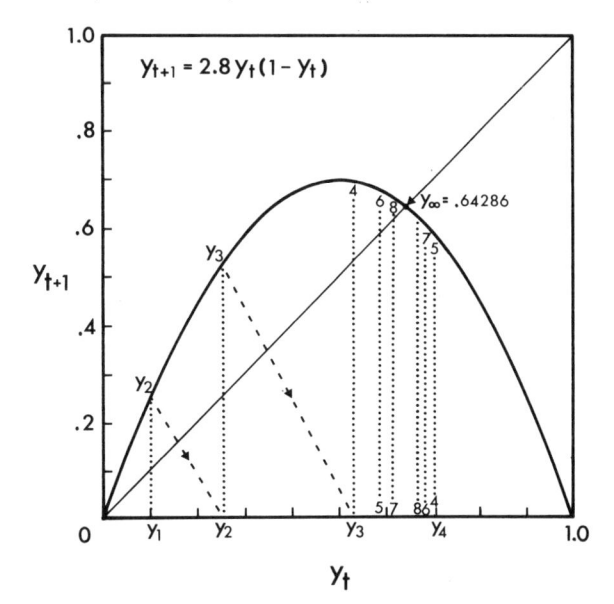

Fig. 2.11. Illustration of a stable steady state. The numbered y values trace the trajectory moving from $y_1 = 0.1$ *towards* y_∞ *with time*

value of y_∞ is a stable solution of the equation, as indeed is the trivial case where $y_t = y_{t+1} = 0$.

By increasing the value of parameter A, a different type of behaviour can be produced. In Fig. 2.12, $A = 3.4$ and $y_{t+1} = Ay_t(1 - y_t)$ as before. Proceeding with the trajectory of y as above, it can be seen that the numbers in succeeding generations do not move towards the solution that was previously stable, but move away from it and towards two values, one on each side, between which a stable oscillation occurs. The original stable state is now unstable and another stable behaviour has evolved. The value of the parameter A at which this new behaviour is first produced is called a *bifurcation point*.

As A is increased further these two points will become unstable and will bifurcate to produce a cycle of population values of y containing four points. Further increase in A will rapidly produce further bifurcations giving cycles of 8, 16, 32, 64 and so on, up to 2^n points. At higher values of A, cycles of every period can occur, as well as aperiodic trajectories where no matter how many generations are produced, a repeating pattern of numbers never occurs. In aperiodic cycles, and those containing many separate points, the behaviour of the system appears chaotic and a stochastic description is likely to be appropriate, in spite of the underlying deterministic equation. Further,

> it may be observed that in the chaotic regime arbitrarily close initial conditions can lead to trajectories which, after a sufficiently long time, diverge widely. This means that, even if we have a simple model in which all parameters are determined exactly, long term prediction is nevertheless impossible. In a meterological context, Lorenz has called this general phenomenon the 'butterfly effect': ... the fluttering of a butterfly's wings could alter the initial conditions, and thus (in the chaotic regime) alter the long term prediction. (May, 1976)

The behaviour of physiological systems, nevertheless, appears in general to be more firmly controlled than this.

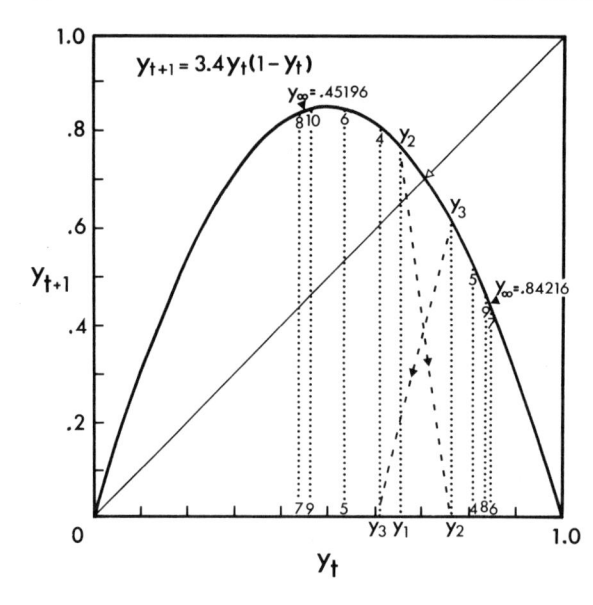

Fig. 2.12. Illustration of an unstable steady state with stable, oscillatory response. The equation represented is the same as that in Fig. 2.11. but with a different value for the parameter. The trajectory from y_1 moves with time away from the region of the unstable steady state towards two new, stable values

Difference equations with delays between events are less stable than their continuous differential analogues, in which the time interval between events ("generations" in the above example) becomes infinitely small. A simple non-linear differential equation will show trajectories converging on a stable point, or diverging from an unstable steady state. A minimum of two coupled differential equations are required before stable oscillations, known as limit cycles, can occur. Three or more coupled non-linear differential equations may show chaotic behaviour, depending on their parameters. Models of reaction–diffusion systems can be in this latter category. Because physiological processes are determined by chemical reactions coupled with diffusion processes, these possible outcomes may be biologically very relevant, and should be part of our thought processes in devising models. Some aspects of the behaviour of reaction–diffusion systems are discussed below.

Practical considerations arise from these possibilities. For example, the behaviour of a system which is stable or oscillatory in the natural state, might be rendered inexplicably chaotic in the laboratory by an inadvertent change in a bifurcation parameter. Also, it is possible for deterministic systems under controlled conditions to produce apparently random responses. Olsen and Degn (1977) report the observation of this kind of chaotic behaviour in the concentration of dissolved oxygen during reaction with certain concentrations of the enzyme horseradish peroxidase, in the presence of constantly infused NADH.

2.6.2 Limit Cycles

In the preceding example of a non-linear difference equation, there was initially a stable steady state to which all starting values of y converged with time. As A increased, this single steady state became unstable, and any initial value moved towards a stable oscillation between two discrete values of y. The analogous situation with non-linear first order differential equations requires at least two

Biological Development and Mathematics Beyond Instability 59

interacting components. The stable, continuous oscillations in variables which can arise when parameter values make a single steady state unstable, may be represented as a function of time like the example in Fig. 2.13. They are usually plotted as a limit cycle in phase space (Fig. 2.14) where the heavy line represents concurrent values of the phases of y and z. The values change constantly with time and traverse the loop once each cycle. This kind of stable behaviour is called a *limit cycle* because, when the system is displaced from these values of y and z to a point either inside or outside the cycle, the variables will move back towards the cycle as time increases. More than two interacting components can give similar stable oscillating responses. If the variables are set to values corresponding to the unstable steady state, known as the *singularity* of the cycle where $dy/dt = dz/dt = 0$, they remain fixed with time. A slight disturbance, however, sends the variables spiralling out towards the stable limit cycle (Fig. 2.14). Changing the parameter values may suppress the oscillatory behaviour; the dotted line in Fig. 2.14 shows how new parameter values in the equations produce a trajectory moving towards a stable steady state. It is also possible theoretically to find multiple stable and unstable limit cycles surrounding a single steady state point.

Limit cycles are of particular interest in biology because their rhythmic properties, and the stability of the rhythm to disturbances, are very similar to the multifarious oscillations displayed by living systems, of which more are being discovered as observers become aware of their existence. Some limit cycles may also have their frequency influenced (entrained) by external stimuli. Chapter 7 discusses some models of biological rhythms in terms of these interesting properties of limit cycles. Cronin (1977) provides a mathematical discussion of some relevant points.

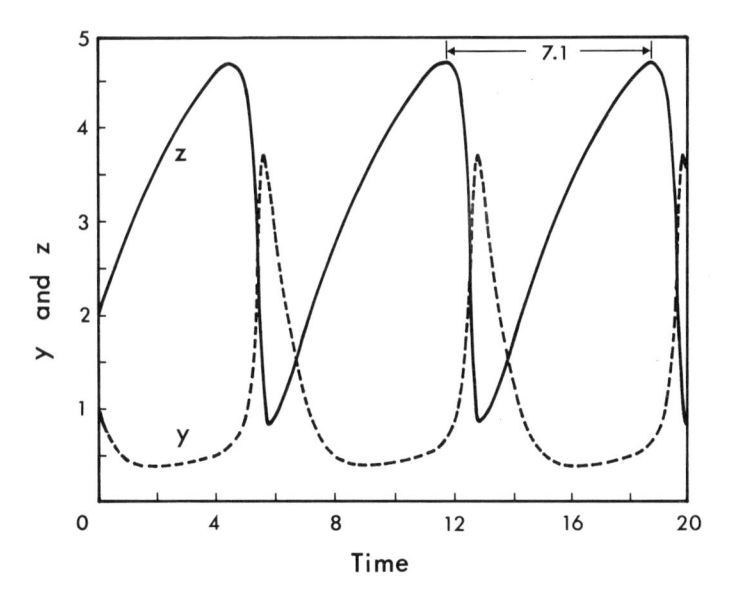

Fig. 2.13. Values of the variables of a limit cycle as a function of time, as defined by Eqs. (2.19) and (2.20) with diffusion terms omitted. Parameters A and B equalled 1 and 3, respectively. The period of the cycle is approximately 7.1 time units. Values of y and z were calculated by computer using program SIMUL run with option (1) (Sect. 11.2) together with FUNCTN subprogram LIMIT (Sect. 11.17)

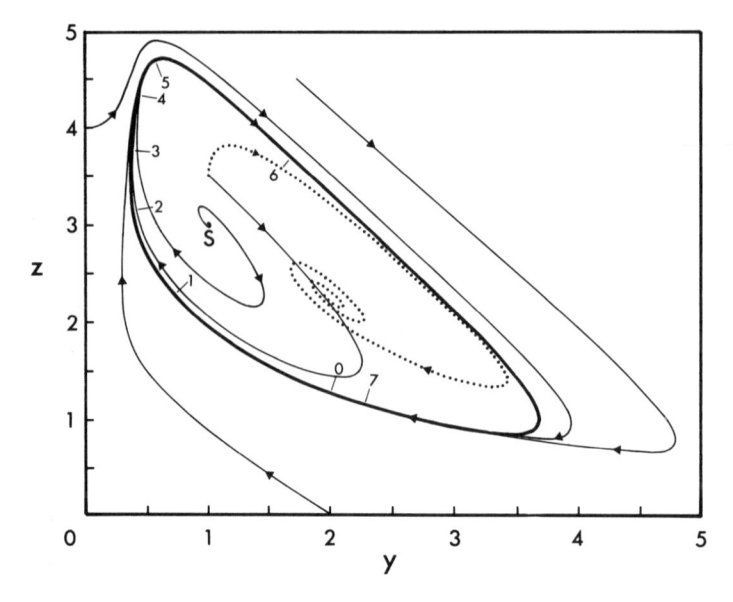

Fig. 2.14. The limit cycle of Fig. 2.13 displayed in phase space (*heavy line*). Equal time intervals are marked on the cycle (0 to 7). Also shown (*light lines*) are trajectories approaching the limit cycle from initial values both inside and outside the cycle. When begun at precisely $y=1$ and $z=3$ (S), the trajectory remained constant at this point. In the trajectory illustrated starting near S, the initial values were displaced slightly to $y=1.001$ and $z=3.003$. The *dotted line* represents the trajectory of the equations when $A=2$ and $B=4.5$. With these values of the parameters, the trajectory showed damped oscillations moving towards a stable steady state. The values of y and z were calculated by computer (see the legend to Fig. 2.13)

2.6.3 Stability Behaviour and Spatial Inhomogeneity

Most of the literature on limit cycles is concerned with biochemical reactions between enzymes and substrates or ecological problems such as predator–prey interactions. Approaches to both types of systems usually assume that the reactants are spatially homogeneous, and that the systems are "well-stirred".

Biological systems in general are not well-stirred. Membranes, separate cells and cellular structures, and different concentrations of both large and small molecules are found on each side of the membranes. Nutrients, hormones and waste matter diffuse through tissues producing concentration gradients. Thus concentrations of substances may vary not only with time but also with up to three dimensions of space. Compartmental analysis represents a linear simplification of this problem which is achieved by lumping (Sect. 2.1.5 and 5.2). A more detailed approach, allowing the continuous variation of variables over space, requires the use of partial differential equations describing rates of change in concentrations with respect to both time and space.

Equations for models of such systems include two kinds of terms: one describes diffusion and the other describes reaction rates in the usual way. If concentrations are not too high, diffusion can be approximated by Fick's law and

$$\delta x_i/\delta t = D_i \nabla^2 x_i + V_i(x_1, \ldots, x_N) \qquad (2.18)$$

where D_i is the diffusion coefficient for x_i, ∇^2_{xi} is the sum of the second order partial differentials of x_i with respect to space, and V_i is the function describing the biochemical reactions in terms of the independent variables. The rates of the chemical reactions are assumed to obey mass action laws, and will usually be some non-linear algebraic function of the other chemical species x_1 to x_N.

Mathematical theory gives little help in determining generalized behaviour from this kind of equation. Investigations have been made on particular examples using numerical calculations (see below). It has been shown that there are several qualitatively different dynamic behaviours possible. These depend on the particular form of the kinetic equation, the relative sizes of the diffusion and rate parameters, the starting conditions, the amount the system is displaced from equilibrium, and the conditions obtaining at the boundary of the space considered. The types of behaviour which may be shown are: (1) simple homogenous approach to point stability, (2) homogenous (space independent) oscillations of the values of components, i.e. limit cycles, (3) spatial variation of component values which are constant with time (standing waves) and (4) many different changes in component values that depend on space, and also vary with time (propagated waves).

Furthermore, these spatial and time variations in component values may arise from disturbance of an initial state that is homogeneous in space and constant in time. The descriptions of such theoretical phenomena have obvious potential implications for understanding the processes of development, differentiation and control observed in biological systems. These mathematical results are non-intuitive. They arise simply from describing a system as being non-linear and open. Yet they provide a new way of approaching hitherto unexplained empirical observations, and scope for new directions of research. Observations of these more complex spatial behaviours in real systems are few, and investigations of real systems within these terms are just beginning. The mathematical theory defining the kinds of systems which can produce these results, and the necessary and sufficient conditions which bring them about, is being developed, stimulated by the problems presented by biology.

The system most extensively studied by experiment is the Zhabotinski-Zaikin reaction (Kopell and Howard, 1973; Winfree, 1974 a). This shows spatial and temporal variations in chemicals displaying contrasting colours in response to disturbance from homogeneity.

2.6.4 Examples of Non-Linear Equations Showing Instabilities

The stability behaviour of an autocatalytic reaction has been intensively investigated by numerical calculations. This system gives the simplest form of differential equations yielding instabilities. It is represented as a series of chemical reactions as follows

$$A \to Y$$
$$B + Y \to Z + D$$
$$2Y + Z \to 3Y$$
$$Y \to E$$

where the third step shows autocatalysis and the system is open to A, B, D and E. At or near equilibrium the system displays a unique steady state. To place the reaction as far from equilibrium as possible E and D are removed as soon as they are formed so that they become vanishingly small. If the reactions are made irreversible, the rate constants are set to 1, the diffusion coefficients D_A and D_B are made infinite so that these substances are always homogeneously distributed, and only one spatial dimension r is considered, the equations for this system can be written (Sect. 5.2.1) as

$$\delta y/\delta t = D_y \delta^2 y/\delta r^2 + A - (B+1)y + y^2 z, \quad (2.19)$$
$$\delta z/\delta t = D_z \delta^2 z/\delta r^2 + By - y^2 z. \quad (2.20)$$

A third equation can be written if D_A is assumed to be finite

$$\delta A/\delta t = D_A \delta^2 A/\delta r^2 - A \quad (2.21)$$

in which, although independent of y and z, A is no longer a constant parameter. When the substances are perturbed from the steady state, this system may amplify fluctuations to give a variety of new final states, which depend on the initial disturbance and on the parameters A, B, D_y, D_z and D_A.

For example, when D_y and D_z are very large (implying rapid diffusion in a homogeneous medium), the diffusion terms can be ignored, and with infinite D_A and B at certain values the resulting steady state can be a spatially homogenous, stable limit cycle (Fig. 2.13). With A, D_A and D_y constant, and with certain values of D_z and B, standing waves are produced (Fig. 2.15). With other values of D_z and B, propagated waves appear, which are shown at three time intervals in Fig. 2.16. For a fuller description see Prigogine and Nicolis (1971).

This kind of scheme involving product activation of the enzyme phosphofructokinase without spatial variations, has been proposed to account for the well known oscillations observed in glycolosis (Heinrich et al., 1977). Higgins (1967) shows, in systems described by two controlling chemical reactions, those combinations of activation and inhibition, both between the reactions and auto-regulatory, which can produce limit cycle behaviour. A pair of differential equations of this kind describing activation has been used by Kauffman to model metaphorically the dynamic characteristics of mitosis of the slime mould (Sect. 7.3.4), which has interesting implications for biological control.

Another type of biochemical interaction, a model of which is known to produce non-linear equations with similar properties of instability, is substrate inhibition of enzymes combined with diffusion. B. Bunow and colleagues (personal com-

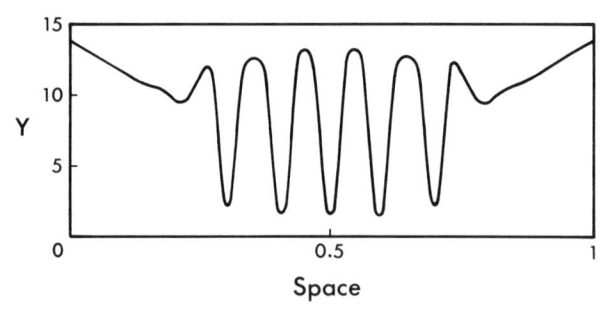

Fig. 2.15. Stable standing waves of the concentration in y (dependent on space but not time) produced at a steady state of Eqs. (2.19–2.21) when the boundary concentration of $A = 14.0$, $D_A = 197 \times 10^{-3}$, $D_y = 1.05 \times 10^{-3}$, $D_z = 5.25 \times 10^{-3}$, $B = 26.0$, and the boundary conditions of $y = 14.0$ and $z = 1.86$. Redrawn with kind permission from Prigogine and Nicolis, 1971, Biological order, structure and instabilities. Q. Rev. Biophys. 4: 107–148. Copyright by Cambridge University Press

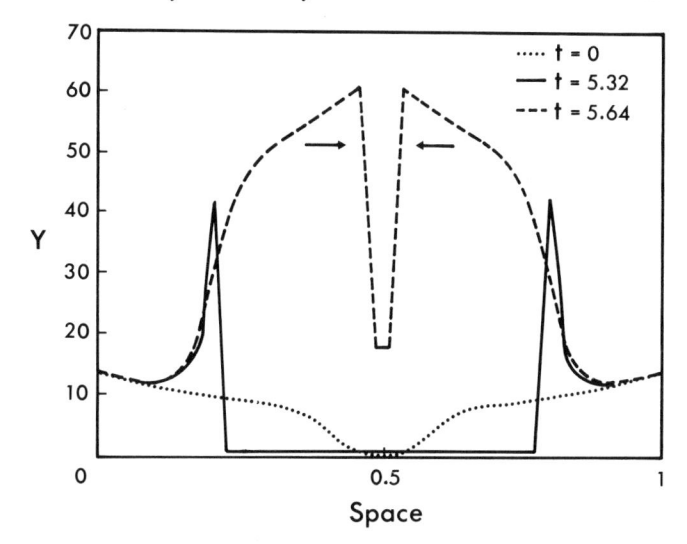

Biological Development and Mathematics Beyond Instability

Fig. 2.16. Propagated waves of concentrations of y (dependent on space and time) produced as a stable steady state of Eqs. (2.19–2.21) under the same conditions as in Fig. 2.15 but with $D_z = 0.66 \times 10^{-3}$ and $B = 77.0$. The concentrations of y are drawn at three time intervals during a cycle of the wave formation having a period of about 8.4 arbitrary time units. This cycle is repeated continuously. Redrawn with kind permission from Prigogine and Nicolis, 1971, Biological order, structure and instabilities. Q. Rev. Biophys. 4: 107–148. Copyright by Cambridge University Press

munication, 1978) are studying, both theoretically and experimentally, the way in which conditions and disturbances affect the spatial and temporal behaviour of such an enzyme when immobilized on a membrane. The enzyme peroxidase is of this type, and is known to yield oscillating concentrations of reaction products, as well as exhibit chaotic behaviour (Olsen and Degn, 1977).

Many other reaction schemes alone or combined with diffusion have been shown by numerical calculations to exhibit behaviour of the limit cycle type, or spatial inhomogeneities, or both. One kind of system which can yield stable oscillating steady states may be particularly relevant to some kinds of endocrine function. This is the non-linear negative feedback loop (Sect. 2.5), usually studied in terms of an enzyme chain in which a product inhibits either an earlier reaction step or the synthesis of the enzyme through gene repression. The steady state of negative feedback loops becomes unstable at a critical degree of inhibition, and is more likely the greater the number of steps in the loop (Walter, 1972). The form of the rate equations, set up in the usual way (Sect. 5.2.1) for such a loop containing three chemicals, might be

$$dx_1/dt = f(x_3) - B_1 x_1, \quad (2.22)$$
$$dx_2/dt = A_2 x_1 - B_2 x_2, \quad (2.23)$$
$$dx_3/dt = A_3 x_2 - B_3 x_3. \quad (2.24)$$

The term $f(x_3)$ describes the production of x_1 and its inhibition by x_3, and might have the form $f(x_3) = A_1/(1 + x_3^\varrho)$, where ϱ describes the co-operativity of x_3 in producing inhibition. When $x_3 = 0$ the production of x_1 is a maximum at A_1, but as

x_3 increases the reaction is inhibited. The higher the value of ϱ the more likely is a single-valued steady state to become unstable, and stable oscillations to arise. With a loop of three reactions, ϱ is required to be equal to 8 for instability of a single steady state, while with ten reactions ϱ need be only 1.6 if all the rate constants are equal (Heinrich et al., 1977; Walter, 1972).

Schemes such as those described above have been used in metaphoric modelling where similarities between the dynamic behaviours of equations and of real systems have been investigated, although the parameters and variables may not have been identified with physiological components. An example is discussed in Sect. 8.3.

2.6.5 Generalized Descriptions of Instabilities in Biology

The concepts described below have not, in general, been given quantitative interpretations meaningful in terms of physiological components. Models using them have been metaphoric (Sect. 1.1.1), or even verbal with no quantitative application.

Waddington's (1957) metaphor of an epigenetic landscape was designed to summarize his observations on the differentiation and development of living systems. His description bears obvious similarities to the thermodynamic metaphor developed by Prigogine, from a quite different conceptual basis (introduction to Sect. 2.6). Waddington proposed that slight variations in the cellular materials initially available to genes were the cause of large and clear cut differences between the forms taken by the developed tissues. Once started on a particular path of development this path is strongly favoured, and the system will return to it even if temporarily perturbed. He described the system behaviour by an analogy frequently used since: the possible states available to the system are represented as a landscape of valleys and ridges, and the current state of the system as a ball which rolls down the valleys to a stable state. The valleys branch, so that when started from slightly different places the system may take one of several different courses to reach different final states. Notice that in this metaphor (and others) the development is not reversible. Having chosen a particular path, the other possibilities open at this junction are no longer available, although other choices are yet to come. Time moves in one direction, and the present and possible future states of organization in the system are a product of its history. This analogy can describe only three dimensions; real systems may have many more. It is, nevertheless, a helpful metaphor which aids thought about biological stability and development. In comparison with the thermodynamic metaphor, Waddington's landscape is the surface defined by the thermodynamic trajectories of the system. The valleys are attractors and the branching points are bifurcations. This concept has much in common with topology, a branch of mathematics concerned with the properties of surfaces in many dimensions.

Thom has developed this metaphor mathematically. His catastrophe theory (Thom, 1975) is concerned with the effects of perturbing certain types of relatively simple non-linear mathematical models exhibiting structural stability (Sect. 2.4). These models have more than one stable attractor surface for the values of the variables. The attractor surfaces, equivalent to the surfaces described by Waddington, are found by equating the differentials to zero. When perturbed through a point of instability on one equilibrium surface, the trajectory comes under the influence of another equilibrium surface exhibiting different behaviour, to which it makes a rapid transition. Thom's theory of catastrophe provides a complete classification of the transitions that may occur at points of structural instability in certain limited systems containing no more than four control parameters, and described by ordinary differential equations. Periodic variations (limit cycles) and spatial variations of the variables (involving partial differential equations) have not been thus classified. Systems in which all rapid reactions are reversible (as may occur in biochemical reactions) cannot undergo catastrophes.

One of the simplest forms of catastrophe behaviour is exhibited by the cusp model which contains one behaviour variable x, and two control parameters A and B related by the quartic function $x^4/4 - Ax - Bx^2/2$. It is characterized by the following types of dynamic behaviour. (1) At certain values of the parameters two forms of behaviour become possible from the same state of the system. (2) Sudden transitions may occur between them (3) at points which differ with the direction of the change. (4) No compromise behaviour is possible from these states and (5) small perturbations in the initial state of the system can result in large differences in the final state after a given disturbance. Heinrich et al. (1977) illustrate this theory in terms of large differences in rates of dynamic processes in a system. In such cases the behaviour of the system is dominated by the slow processes because the fast ones are "in equilibrium". However, if the slow trajectories move the values of variables towards areas which are unstable for fast trajectories, then these rapidly change the system to a neighbouring slow trajectory which is relatively stable for all reactions.

Although identification of parameters and equations in any real system appears to be exceedingly difficult, the classifications of catastrophes have provided a qualitative means of describing discontinuous, more complex behaviours than can be dealt with using simpler concepts. Examples of qualitative interpretations of the heart beat and nerve impulse, and of animal and human behaviour, using this theory, are given by Zeeman (1972; 1976).

Bifurcation and catastrophe theories are similar. They analyse how variations in the values of parameters affect the types of behaviour of the total model system. A comparison between the two approaches has been made by Nicolis and Auchmuty (1974). Bifurcation theory is applicable to a broader range of system types. A simple heuristic example of how variation of parameters can produce a bifurcation was given earlier (Sect. 2.6.2).

Automata theory and finite level analysis (Sect. 2.7) are concerned with these changes from one state, or form of behaviour, to another (i.e. threshold transitions), and how they affect the overall behaviour of the system. For example, genes may be classified as being either active or inactive, and the relationship of the timing of transitions to system behaviour investigated. Use of differential equations to give a detailed description of the dynamics of each transition is not relevant in such studies.

The Raschevsky–Turing metaphor had earlier proposed that positive feedback was important in the differentiation of cells (Rosen, 1977). In the later metaphors described above, positive feedback occurs after instability is reached. The trajectory of a perturbed system diverges from the unstable steady state to reach a new stable state. Rashevsky's model is described as follows. If an open solution of reacting substances, such as an enzyme and substrate, is totally homogenous it will remain so for ever. If, however, a slight inhomogeneity of substrate arises and the higher concentration formed inhibits the reaction, then substrate will accumulate at this point. Eventually a much higher concentration of substrate will be found in that section of space in which the initial fluctuation occurred.

Turing developed this idea to include two or more open cells, each containing two "morphogens", perhaps hormones. These hormones are supplied from outside the cell, are destroyed inside, and can diffuse between cells. Such a system can become unstable if the diffusion rates take certain values, a random difference in concentration between the cells resulting in hormone accumulating in one cell. If the presence or absence of these hormones cause differential induction and repression of genes, then divergent development of the cells is possible.

Rosen (1977) gives a lucid description of the difficulties of identifying the components of these generalized dynamic descriptions with experimentally observable parts of particular real systems.

2.7 Finite Level Modelling

Finite level modelling appears particularly suited to the description and modelling of endocrinological and physiological systems at their present level of understanding. It provides relatively clear-cut answers to problems of structural organization familiar to endocrinologists which cannot yet be derived as easily by modelling with continuous equations. Many questions in endocrinology are not concerned with quantitative and temporal details of the non-linear responses produced by interconnected subsystems but, more basically, with determining which connections are made, and which of these are of critical importance to system performance. Continuous models describing the detailed mechanisms of interactions within an endocrine system often contain so many hypotheses, and so many "free" parameters for fitting to the data, that it is not possible to rule out any particular structural model (Chap. 8). The simplifying approach of finite level modelling may enable such rejection to be made.

The major application of this approach so far has been in discriminating between models describing areas where stimuli influence neural pathways in adrenocortical control (Gann et al., 1968; 1973: Gann and Cryer, 1973; Bush and Gann, 1975). The logical consequences of models proposing connections between components were determined and comparison with experimental results allowed some models to be eliminated. Application of finite level modelling has made several predictions about control of the release of ACTH which have been confirmed experimentally (Gann et al., 1968; Gann, 1969; Grizzle et al., 1974). The approach appears particularly suited to investigating interactions in neural systems where the usual technique of tissue ablation for investigating function can lead to confusing results.

Ashby (1956) describes in simple terms some of the fundamental ideas of finite level modelling. The concepts and advantages of the technique are described very briefly here; our meagre experience of its use prevents us from giving this approach the prominence it appears to deserve.

In finite level modelling the values of all variables are quantized. This means that the continuous range of values which a variable can take is divided into a few levels only. Each experimental result is described by assigning to it the value of its

Finite Level Modelling

appropriate level (Sect. 1.2.4). Finite levels can be designed to discriminate only between those values which are statistically distinguishable.

A description of experimental data by finite levels is a list of quantized values of input variables and their related outputs, rather than a continuous graph. Empirical equations can be written using Boolean notation to describe these relationships. Non-linearities are no more difficult to deal with than linear behaviour.

A model of a system proposes a structure describing the connections between the subsystems suspected to be active in transforming input into output; this may be written like a block diagram. The structure will usually include some "internal" variables which have not, or cannot, be measured (such as c in Fig. 2.17). Identification of the values of these variables is equivalent to parameter estimation. In addition to satisfying the values of input and output data, the parameters will have other constraints placed on them. Some constraints will arise from known properties of the system, but the most important one is the requirement of functionality. *Functionality* is related to causality; it means that if two sets of inputs to a subsystem are equal then the related outputs are also equal. There is thus only one output possible for each input set. More than one output would mean that the system was not deterministic. An additional constraint of cardinality requires that the number of levels taken by the input set and internal variables must be sufficient to provide the variety of behaviour observed in the output set.

If parameters cannot be found satisfying data and constraints, the model structure is incorrect. If a unique solution is found then critical experiments may be carried out to further confirm this structure, unmeasured outputs may be predicted, and the behaviour of the internal variables indicated. If several sets of parameter values satisfy the data and constraints, there is insufficient data to characterize the system fully, and additional experiments must be carried out to distinguish between the possibilities. Several structures may, of course, yield satisfactory parameters and critical experiments must then be designed to distinguish between them. Apart from providing a guide to efficient experimentation, the major advantage of the method is that at least some models may be discarded.

As an example of the perhaps unexpected usefulness of these very simple concepts, consider the following. Three types of stimuli are known to influence the production of a particular hormone. All three stimuli could act directly on the organ which produces the hormone, or alternatively, some may act on a different organ which produces another, intermediate hormone. The latter may then influence production of the hormone of interest, which is measured as output. The following mechanism is proposed to test the second hypothesis (Fig. 2.17). Stimuli x_1 and x_2 act at G_1 to produce hormone c. This output, together with stimulus x_3, influences the output of hormone y. Data from four experiments in which the input levels were varied sufficed to test this structure. The input x_1 was constant in all experiments, while x_2 and x_3 were each either absent or present (designated 0 or 1). The resulting three distinguishable values of y are shown in Table 2.1.

Fig. 2.17. Proposed structure for interactions in a finite level model. The symbols, and the application of the model in elucidating the mechanism of cortisol feedback, are explained in the text

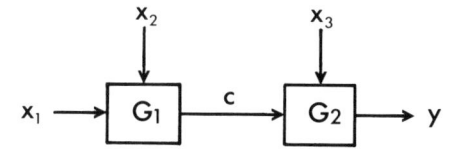

Table 2.1. Experimental data, in finite level form, used to test the model of Fig. 2.17

Experiment	Variables				
	x_1	x_2	c	x_3	y_1
1	1	1	c_1	0	2
2	1	0	c_2	0	2
3	1	1	c_3	1	1
4	1	0	c_4	1	0

To test the proposed structure it is necessary to show that values of c can be identified that are consistent with the input–output relationships, and the constraint of functionality. The test of functionality is applied to each subsystem. It can be seen that in Experiments 1 and 3 the outputs c_1 and c_3 are determined by the same values of the input set x_1 and x_2. Therefore $c_1 = c_3$, and by the same reasoning $c_2 = c_4$ in Experiments 2 and 4. In Experiments 1 and 2, however, equal values of y are determined by c alone because there is no influence from $x_3 = 0$; therefore $c_1 = c_2$. It follows that $c_1 = c_2 = c_3 = c_4$.

In Experiments 3 and 4 the inputs to G_2, x_3 and c are therefore equal, but the outputs of y are clearly distinguishable. This contradicts the constraint of functionality where equal inputs sets produce equal outputs. Therefore, values of c cannot be identified which are consistent with the proposed structure, and another model must be devised.

The model described above is one of several proposed by Gann and Cryer (1973) when investigating the feedback effect of cortisol on the production of adrenocorticotrophic hormone (ACTH) in dogs. The production of ACTH (y) was measured in response to the stimuli of haemorrhage on the neural system (x_1), renin levels in blood from the renin–angiotensin system (x_2), and infusion of the synthetic corticosteroid dexamethasone (x_3). The unmeasured variable c represents corticotrophin-releasing factor secreted by the median eminence, G_1, and acting on the anterior pituitary, G_2, to produce ACTH. By the use of finite level models, a number of proposed structures were rejected. Further experimental testing could be reserved for more feasible models.

In the above example a minimum data set was selected from a larger one for the purpose of illustration. Proposed mechanisms in biological systems must frequently be consistent with very large data sets. Searching for consistent values of internal variables without the aid of a computer can be very tedious. Schoeffler et al (1968), Gann et al (1972, 1973) and Ostrander (1968) describe how to carry out such a search using binary Boolean algebra which is readily dealt with by computer. In using these methods each model variable has only two levels, with values 1 or 0. Experimental variables requiring more than two levels to describe the range of data are assigned additional model variables, two binary digits allowing four levels (00, 01, 10, 11) and three giving eight (000, 001, and so on). Note that many experimental variables are binary in character; nerves are intact or severed, kidneys present or excised, drugs added or not, ovulation occurs or it does not. In continuous equation modelling two equations are written to describe the different behaviours produced by the participation or absence of a variable. In finite level modelling such variables producing alternative models of behaviour are an integral part of the model.

For any proposed structure of a system, tables are constructed giving all possible relationships between inputs and outputs of each subsystem, as well as the experimental data showing input and output for the system as a whole. Experimental data is converted to finite levels and the results are entered into the tables. These relationships, the constraints imposed by functionality, and any others known are written as a set of simultaneous Boolean equations. Trial values are substituted for the unknown internal variables and their consistency with these equations is checked. A search is carried out on these parameter values to find which, if any, satisfy the equations.

The model used as an example above is static, but the technique can also be applied to dynamic systems where relationships between input and output are measured and calculated at discrete time intervals. The feedback of cortisol on the release of ACTH has been studied in this way (Bush and Gann, 1975), as has the secretion of cortisol in response to the stimulus of ACTH (Gann et al., 1972). A continuous equation model of the latter has also been presented (Urquhart and Li, 1969). A finite level approach to menstrual cycle is discussed in Sect. 8.8 in which the events of the cycle delimit discrete intervals of time. In many biological systems, it is more rational to define intervals of time by using the occurrence of events causing changes in the system behaviour, than it is to divide time into equal increments; many systems are adapted to respond to favourable external or internal conditions rather than changing solely as a function of elapsed time (compare Sects. 8.6 and 8.8).

When investigating the adrenocortical system a number of experimental problems were encountered which are common to many other biological systems. The finite level approach was particularly useful in dealing with these, in comparison with continuous equation modelling. The problems were (1) the difficulty of supplying a continuous input, (2) the difficulty of sampling outputs more than a few times from any one animal, (3) the variable magnitude of the response to the same input from animal to animal, (4) the range of time constants of interest in the system, varying from milliseconds to hours, (5) the internal mechanisms of interaction being unknown and untestable, (6) the many non-linearities of interactions and (7) experiments being costly in terms of animals and time.

2.8 The Need for Statistics

While we cannot avoid introducing errors when we make measurements it is essential to ensure that they are random, and as small as possible. If they are not random they will cause *biased* or *inaccurate* results. If they are large the results will be *imprecise*, though not necessarily inaccurate; it will also be impossible to tell whether models give good representations of the data, or to distinguish between similar models.

The comparison of models with data involves estimating values for the parameters of the equations that ensure the best fit of the model, and which are compatible with the properties of the real system (Chap. 3). (A simple example is the estimation of the rate constant of a removal process.) Because experimental measurements contain random, unknown errors the true parameter values of the underlying physical model cannot be determined, even assuming that the form of the model is known. Instead, the parameters are estimated, and the role of statistical method is to provide the most accurate estimates, together with measures of uncertainties in each.

For a parameter estimate to have any validity uncertainties must be calculated and quoted. If different laboratories report different parameter values without providing measures of their precision, it is impossible to know whether previous findings have been confirmed or challenged. Elaborate theories may be built on the basis of such dubious information. In every area of endocrinology, and indeed biology, it is essential to place some measure of reliability on measurements. Quantitative questions cannot be argued when no estimate of reliability is available.

Uncertainties calculated by statistical methods probably represent no more than lower limits to true uncertainty in the match of model to real system behaviour. This is partly explained by the simplification required in biological modelling (Sect. 1.2.7). For other aspects see Colquhoun (1971, p. 102).

Several helpful discussions of the use of statistics in endocrinological research are given by McArthur and Colton (1970).

2.8.1 Transformation and Weighting

When the response of a system varies with the value of the independent variable, so almost always does the degree of precision with which it can be measured. Therefore it is essential to assign more weight or importance to those measurements that are more precise. The need for this is shown clearly by the following example, which is both impressive and extremely well documented.

The double reciprocal or Lineweaver-Burk model of enzyme kinetics has been affirmed repeatedly to yield parameter estimates that are badly biased – see Wilkinson (1961), Dowd and Riggs (1965), Walter (1965, Chap. 5; 1974; 1977) and Colquhoun (1971). The reason for this is very simple, and the conclusions have important implications.

The Michaelis-Menten equation is expressed as

$$v = Vs/(K+s) \tag{2.25}$$

where v is the observed initial velocity of an enzyme-catalysed reaction, s is the substrate concentration, and V is the maximum velocity of the reaction attained when the enzyme active site is saturated with substrate. K, the Michaelis constant, is a measure of the affinity of the active site for the substrate. The theoretical basis of this model equation stems from the view that the interaction between an enzyme and substrate is a reversible association preceding the chemical reaction in which the substrate is converted to product.

The Lineweaver-Burk method of estimating the two parameters V and K involves the transformation of Eq. (2.25) and the experimental data. When transformed, the equation looks like this

$$1/v = 1/V + K/(Vs) \tag{2.26}$$

which implies that a graph of $1/v$ against $1/s$ is a straight line with intercept $1/V$ and slope K/V. This is, of course, the reason for the transformation: a straight line is easy to draw by eye, and the intercept and slope define the parameter values directly. However, when the data are transformed for plotting, small values of v become large, large ones become small, and the relative magnitudes of the uncertainties are altered. If the uncertainty in each of the original v measurements was approximately constant, then it is clear that it will not be so after taking reciprocals. When a straight line is drawn through the points it will lead to estimates of the two parameters that are, generally, quite different from the values obtained if another transformation and plot had been used. The way in which the relative magnitudes of the uncertainties in measurements change as a result of this kind of transformation is illustrated graphically in Figs. 6.4 and 6.3, in which the same data are shown both before and after transformation.

The correct approach is to weight the points before fitting the line. This means that transformed points which have the least uncertainty are taken relatively more into consideration when drawing the line. It is easy to show that if the variance in v is constant with s the correct weight for a value of $1/s$ is approximately proportional to the fourth power of s (Sect. 10.2).

Correctly weighted plots yield unbiased parameter estimates, but variances are often not measured and so the correct weights cannot be assigned. Inevitably, estimates of V and K from an unweighted reciprocal plot are biased, i.e. incorrect. Although this conclusion was pointed out in the biochemical literature as long ago as 1961, reports continue to appear in which the double reciprocal plot is used to determine the parameters.

There are two difficulties in estimating the parameters correctly. The variances, and hence the weights for the data, may not have been measured, although it is probable that the variances in the data as collected are nearly constant. Also, the untransformed Michaelis–Menten equation is non-linear in the sense described in Sect. 3.4.1, and is much more difficult to fit systematically to data than is a linear model. Most of Chap. 3 is concerned with the fitting of non-linear models to data.

2.8.2 Parameter Uncertainty

The second important role of statistics in parameter estimation is in calculating the uncertainty in a parameter. This uncertainty may be expressed as either a standard deviation or a confidence interval (Sects. 10.1 and 10.12).

Standard deviations are themselves parameters, and their application carries the assumption that the scatter in the data values are distributed in a particular way, known as a normal distribution (Colquhoun, 1971, pp. 69–75). Statistical methods using standard deviations are called parametric methods; a summary of relevant definitions and tests is given in Appendix A. Most of the methods we shall describe for fitting models to data, or calculating parameter uncertainties, require the use of parametric statistics (Chap. 3). Non-parametric statistical methods, which do not require restrictive assumptions, are not generally useful when estimating the parameters of models; their use is illustrated in Chap. 9.

2.8.2.1 Monte Carlo Simulation

In Chap. 3 we shall show how to fit models to data when parametric methods can be proved, or justifiably assumed, to be applicable. It will also be shown that application of the methods to model equations non-linear in their parameters may lead to unavoidable bias in the parameter estimates, and inaccurate values of uncertainty.

Accurate measures of parameter uncertainties can always be found by replicating experiments to produce many samples of data; these are used to calculate many sets of parameter estimates, and from these means and uncertainties. This may, however, be time-consuming and wasteful of materials. An alternative approach is the exceedingly useful method known as *Monte Carlo simulation* which is used to investigate the statistical properties only of the model equations, rather than their ability to describe the real system.

This is done as follows. Parameter values, estimated from an initial laboratory experiment, are used to *simulate* or artificially generate output from the model equations. Appropriate errors, chosen to resemble the measurement uncertainties of the experiment, are added to this output. The model is then fitted to the simulated data and new parameter estimates are made. Repetition of this process (using the parameter values from the laboratory data for each simulation) generates a series of parameter estimates from which a mean and standard deviation can be calculated. To determine whether the original, calculated values of parameter uncertainties are plausible, they are compared with the estimates obtained from simulation.

It is possible at the same time to determine whether the method of estimating the parameters has introduced bias by comparing their values with those used to generate the data. This test of the estimation method cannot be done in the laboratory, but is possible only when using Monte Carlo simulation where "true" values of the parameters are pre-selected (Sect. 3.7.1.1). Monte Carlo simulation cannot prove whether or not a model is "true". Performance of experiments under controlled conditions is the only way in which estimates can be obtained of the parameter values of a real, physical system. The purpose of simulation is solely to gain information about the way in which a model will behave under varying conditions, and its response to the magnitude and distribution of measurement uncertainty. The power of the Monte Carlo method lies in its ability to investigate the way in which measurement uncertainties will influence the outcome of experiments.

Returning to the example of enzyme kinetics, Monte Carlo methods have been used to demonstrate why it is impossible to derive correct, unbiased parameter values from unweighted double reciprocal plots (Wilkinson, 1961; Dowd and Riggs, 1965). Model output values were generated using the Michaelis–Menten equation and appropriate values of V and K. Various kinds of error were then introduced to represent measurement uncertainties, the data were transformed by taking reciprocals, and the parameter values were estimated by fitting a straight line to the unweighted points, as is done visually. It was found that the estimates were very different from the known parameter values, thus demonstrating that double reciprocal plots introduce bias into the evaluation of V and K.

Examples of the use of Monte Carlo methods will be found in Sects. 3.7.1.1 and 6.2.2.2. A full description of the technique is given by Hammersley and Handscomb (1964).

2.8.3 Testing Hypotheses

Statistical methods are needed to test hypotheses such as whether or not (1) a certain model provides an adequate description of a sample of data, (2) two or more parameter estimates are indistinguishable within the limits of their uncertainties or (3) two or more samples of individuals have, on the basis of the level of some common property, been selected from a homogeneous population. Tests suitable for all these cases are described in Appendix A and Chap. 9.

Unfortunately, most of the hypotheses we will wish to differentiate between in connection with fitting non-linear models to data can be tested only by parametric methods, because no comparable non-parametric tests exist. Clear accounts of the dangers of the indiscriminate use of parametric tests are given by Colquhoun (1971).

2.8.4 Normal Distributions in Biology

A normal distribution of measurements facilitates statistical analysis but it cannot be assumed that biological data take this form. Measurement errors alone can usually be justifiably assumed to be normally distributed. In fact, on the regrettably rare occasions that the distributions of results of biological experiments have been investigated, they have often been found to be log-normal. The log-normal distribution has been described by Gaddum (1945) who puts the normal distribution in its place, quoting Poincaré as saying

> Everybody firmly believes in it because the mathematicians imagine it is a fact of observation, and observers that it is a theory of mathematics.

Gaddum emphasizes:

> Even if one method of measurement gives normal distributions, it necessarily follows that most others will not; and since it is unlikely that the appropriate method will often be chosen first, it is only to be expected that most distributions will not be normal unless care is taken to select the appropriate method of measurement.

The plea for making no assumptions regarding the normality of distributions is reiterated by Colquhoun (1971).

The *log-normal* distribution is skewed, so that there are more high values than expected in comparison with the normal distribution. A log-normal distribution can be transformed into a normal one by taking logarithms – hence the name. The need for a transformation can only be discovered by trial and error based on observation, and tested by one of the methods outlined in Sect. 10.8. Gaddum has contended that there is probably more justification for transforming scientific observations than for not doing so, and has also noted that when observations have large uncertainties in comparison with the values of the measurements themselves, then the log-normal transformation will probably be appropriate. In order, therefore, that the uncertaintes calculated from data that are log-normally distributed be correct, both data and model should be transformed before beginning the fitting process.

2.8.5 Statistics and Experimental Design

Statistical considerations also influence the whole framework of experimental design. Chapter 4 describes statistical criteria used to select the best model from a group of possible models. This is done by predicting the experimental conditions which will discriminate most efficiently between the models, or which will determine their parameters most precisely.

3 Comparing Models with Experimental Results

The subject of this chapter is parameter estimation, an essential part of any analytical experimentation. Such experimentation involves the following steps. Data is collected describing the variation of one component with another. A model is devised showing the proposed form of the interaction between the components, and an equation is written to describe it. Values of the parameters in the equation must then be estimated which are compatible with the data and its precision. For a model based on theory, the parameters have physical meaning. In the case of empirical models the equations are non-unique and can be modified in any way until suitable parameters are found; furthermore, the parameters have no physical meaning. In either case the equations representing the model become tenable only with the evaluation of feasible parameter values.

Because experimental measurements contain error, the underlying "true" parameter values can only be estimated. An analysis of the reliability of these estimates is an essential, but often neglected part of the evaluation of a model.

Parameter estimation is central to the application of almost all the concepts mentioned in the previous two chapters, and is equally important to the methods described in the succeeding one.

It is introduced in the following sections by a brief description of approximate, rapid analyses. Attention is then concentrated on more precise and informative techniques. Explanations are descriptive, fortified where necessary with minimal mathematical and statistical detail; a comprehensive and rigorous mathematical treatment is provided by Bard (1974). A computer program is introduced which is suitable for fitting most models to data, including the examples in this book. Finally, sample parameter estimations for biological models are presented which provide specific illustrations of the concepts given here, and contain many practical details. Other examples will be found in later chapters.

3.1 Analogue Simulation

An *analogue simulation* is a representation of a system by a physical device, usually mechanical or electrical, which is suited to rapid and semi-quantitative investigation. A slide rule is a simple analogue computer in which numbers are represented as lengths. The clearance of a substance from the blood stream, the rate of which depends on the concentration of the substance, might be modelled mechanically by a container of liquid with a small hole at the bottom, or electrically by a charged capacitor shorted out by a resistance. In these analogues the speed with which liquid or electricity escapes is related to the level remaining in the container, and this determines the pressure or voltage, respectively.

The most convenient analogue devices are electrical, and are known as *analogue computers*. In these the process to be simulated is described in terms of a continuously varying electrical voltage generated by connecting together elements capable of adding, subtracting, multiplying, dividing, differentiating and integrating. There are also components for simulating delays, switches and regularly varying processes. Modern analogue computers are stable and accurate, and their convenience and ease of operation are a great advantage. A model of blood clearance, for example, is easy to set up and use. A real appreciation for how changes in parameter values and equations affect the behaviour of a model is quickly formed. The data points corresponding to experimental observations are displayed on a screen together with a curve representing the model. The parameters are adjusted by manipulating potentiometers until the model is matched as closely as possible to the data. The final parameter estimates are simply read from the potentiometer dials. Most non-linear relationships can be adequately represented.

But there are disadvantages. The "best" fit depends on a subjective decision by the user. It is not possible to calculate uncertainties in the parameter estimates. Scaling may be awkward because the range of variables able to be represented as voltages is limited to about three orders of magnitude. Parameters varying with time are particularly difficult to deal with, as are partial differential equations.

In summary, analogue computers are valuable for gaining preliminary insight into the way in which a new model will behave. They resemble a delicate and sophisticated combination of paper, pencil and French curve. It is easy and instructive to try the effect of altering the value of a parameter by turning a knob and watching the immediate response of a line on a screen. So powerful and useful is the analogue approach that the qualities characteristic of it have been copied in methods used in digital computers.

3.2 Approximate Simulation by Digital Computer

Digital computers can be used in the same way as analogue computers to simulate models of physical systems by evaluating their equations and comparing them approximately with data. In contrast to analogue machines, in which values are represented by continuously varying voltages, digital computers can deal only with discrete numbers, formed by sequences of electrical "on or off" binary patterns. Changing the value of a parameter is done not by turning a knob, but instead by supplying a sequence of numbers each of which is evaluated in the model. Digital computers obey sets of instructions called programs supplied by the user. Because the instructions can be very complex in their effect and yet are easily changed, these machines are exceptionally versatile tools.

Digital computers can be programmed to simulate physical systems modelled in terms of continuous, discrete, stochastic and other equations. Here we shall deal almost exclusively with continuous systems, the nature of which are discussed in Sect. 2.1.1.3. Programs for simulating models on digital computers, while adopting the best characteristics of analogue machines, also exploit the superior flexibility and precision of digital devices. These programs are relatively easy to use and no thought need be given to details of mathematics or machine operation. Very simple instructions are used to activate the complex machine processes of multiplication, integration and so on. Typical modern programs for continuous system modelling such as CSMP for IBM machines, or the language MIMIC used on computers made by the Control Data Corporation, operate in this way. The fitting of models to data is similar to that using an analogue computer; the investigator changes the values of parameters until a "best" fit of the model to the data is obtained, as judged visually. Other, more accurate methods, are discussed below.

Examples of the use of the program CSMP mentioned above in modelling endocrinological processes will be found in the work of Yates and his associates (Yates et al., 1968) concerning the adrenocortical system, and Schwartz and Waltz (1970) on the regulation of the oestrous cycle in rats, as discussed in Chap. 8. Rather than using elaborate pre-existing programs, it is also possible to simulate systems by means of simpler, specifically designed programs. An illustrative example was the investigation of the effects of changing the values of a range of parameters on the population dynamics of the African elephant, reported by Hanks and McIntosh (1973).

Most widely used simulation programs are so large and flexible that they can be used only on large and elaborate computers (CSMP can be used under the control of a light-pen on a display screen, for example) but similar, more compact program packages have been designed that are specifically for use on small laboratory computers (Benham, 1971). We provide details (Sect. 11.2) of a simple and convenient program known as SIMUL which is suitable for simulating any of the models described in this book. SIMUL illustrates the behaviour of a model by calculating values of the dependent variable when provided with a short FORTRAN subprogram defining the equations of the model, values of the parameters, and a range of the independent variable.

3.3 Suitable Digital Computers

All computers consist of a few basic operational units. As the size of the machine increases so does the number of units, the versatility, and the price. All computers have an input unit for reading both instructions and data. Once read, information is either held in the central memory unit for processing, or transferred to a supplementary unit known as disc storage. When required, instructions or data are retrieved rapidly from disc storage which, unlike central memory, has great capacity. Calculations are done in an arithmetic unit and intermediate workings are held in central memory. Results are printed or plotted on one or more output units. The computer is managed by a control unit which carries out either the instructions of a human operator or those of a program. Large scientific computers usually have very flexible control programs known as operating systems which prepare each job and allocate resources.

Computers are instructed to perform calculations or other tasks by means of programs provided by the user. Programs are written in languages such as FORTRAN, the widely used scientific programming language employed in this book, BASIC, ALGOL or PASCAL. The computer has a special program called a compiler for translating the user's program into commands intelligible to the machine. This is an essential step because the many different computers available today are built differently, and each must have a special translation code to convert generally defined languages, such as FORTRAN, to machine-dependent instructions known as machine code. Finally, the machine code is broken down to simple binary pulses which the computer can deal with.

A special, specific program is sometimes written to carry out the calculations required in fitting a model to data. However, it is usually more convenient and faster to use an existing, generally applicable program, together with a few extra instructions defining the particular equations of the model. This is because existing programs have usually been used extensively and errors eliminated.

The programs supplied in this book can be run on any so-called mini-computer, now available in many laboratories, or from a terminal connected to a large machine administered by computing centres at most universities and research establishments. A large computer will usually have several different programs running concurrently, some of which are in direct communication with users at electronic typewriters, known as terminals. At the same time the machine will be working on large, time-consuming jobs which are given a lower priority. The greatest efficiency is obtained by keeping the computer continuously busy, so large jobs are queued awaiting their turn. The operating system which manages the computer is understandably very complex.

The programs provided in this book are short and fast. They will work, after minor modification, on any mini-computer equipped with a FORTRAN compiler and 16,000 to 32,000 words of central memory (depending on the make). The slowest programs are those involving numerical integration. A Nova 2 mini-computer made by the Data General Corporation took 270 s to do the calculations that gave the results in Table 5.4, while a Control Data Corporation Cyber 173 computer, a large machine typical of the sort found in universities, required only 3.5 s. However, most examples were completed much more quickly, taking about 10 s on the small machine and 0.01 to 0.2 s on the large one.

Summaries of the basic principles of analogue and digital computers, and computers which are hybrids of both, will be found in Chaps. 1, 2 and 15 of the book edited by Whitby and Lutz (1971), which also contains an extensive glossary of computer terms. Roberts (1977, Chap. 10) gives a clear description of the use of analogue machines in the simulation of enzyme kinetics. Davies (1971) in a book on computer programming in biology, provides a synopsis of the FORTRAN language and an introduction to computing concepts.

3.4 Estimation of Parameters

In contrast to the qualitative methods described above, the remainder of this chapter is concerned with techniques for the systematic fitting of mathematical models to experimental data. Logical rules called *algorithms* take the place of subjective adjustment of parameter values. In addition, these algorithms allow calculation of the reliability of each parameter estimate, which is essential to the proper evaluation of a model.

For simplicity, we shall consider model equations or functions in which only a single independent variable x is varied to influence a dependent variable y, where y is a function of x; $y=f(x)$. If more than one equation is required to describe the model there will be a corresponding number of dependent variables. The general approach, after extension, is also applicable to equations in which two or more independent variables are altered simultaneously.

3.4.1 Linearity and Non-Linearity in Parameter Estimation

Linearity and non-linearity were defined in Sect. 2.2 in terms of the variables of equations. The difference is equally important here, but now refers to parameters rather than variables. This is because in parameter estimation we vary the parameter values, having already fixed the independent and dependent variables at values determined by the results of the experiment. Whether an equation is linear or non-linear in its parameters can be decided by inspection. It is linear if the dependent variable y is a *linear function of the parameters*, the value of x being regarded as constant. An alternative definition is that a function is linear in its parameters if none of the sensitivity coefficients are functions of any parameter(s) (Beck and Arnold, 1977, Sect. 1.4). The *sensitivity coefficients* are the first derivatives of the model equation with respect to each parameter. Sensitivity coefficients are important measures, which are calculated and used in the computer programs introduced in later sections of this book. Thus a function consisting of a sum of terms in x to any power, such as Eq. (2.6), is linear in its parameters even though its graph is a curve. On the other hand, most models of biological systems with a theoretical basis are non-linear in their parameters. For example, inspection of the Michaelis-Menten equation of enzyme kinetics [Eq. (2.25)] shows that the response, v, is not a linear sum of the parameters.

It is very much easier to estimate parameter values producing the best fit of a model to data if the parameters are related linearly. If a non-linear relationship exists between them, simple calculation is no longer possible. Instead, it is necessary to search for the required values by trial and error methods (see below).

3.4.2 Defining the "Best" Fit of a Model to Data

The most obvious criterion of the goodness of fit of a model to data is that the differences between them should be as small as possible. A simple and well-established technique for ensuring this, and which is usually appropriate, is the method of least squares. It is a special case of a more general approach known as the method of maximum likelihood. Bevington (1969) gives a simple account of maximum likelihood analysis; a more rigorous one is provided by Bard (1974).

In the *method of least squares*, the *objective function* is defined as the sum of the squares of the differences between each experimental determination and the response of the model $f(x)$ at the same value of x. That is

$$\text{objective function} = \sum_{i=1}^{N} [y_i - f(x_i, A_1, A_2, ..., A_p)]^2 \qquad (3.1)$$

where the nomenclature means that the contents of the square brackets are to be squared and summed over all values of i, from 1 to the number of data points N. The measured response of the system is y_i, and $f(x_i, A_1, A_2, ..., A_p)$ represents the value of the equation of the model at point x_i. The parameters are A_1 to A_p. *Parameter optimization* is the adjustment of the parameter values until the objective function is minimized. The remaining differences between model and data are known as the *residuals*. These terms are illustrated in Fig. 3.1.

Estimation of Parameters

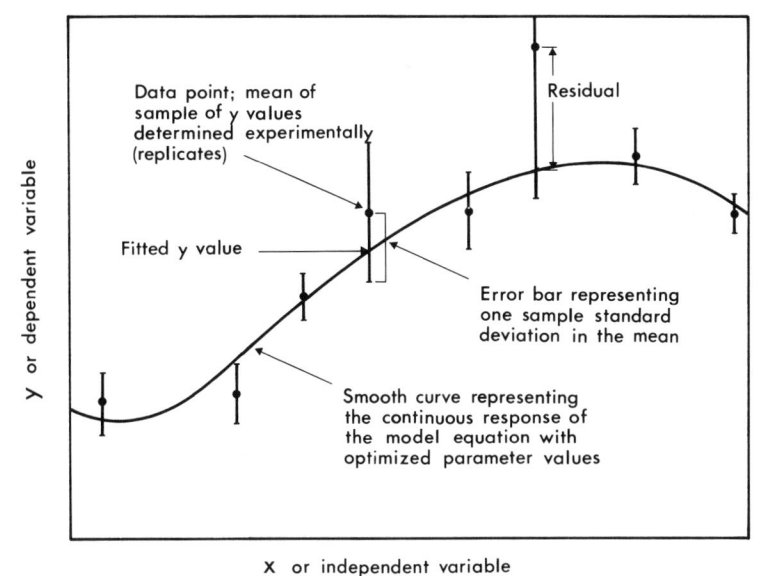

Fig. 3.1. Pictorial representation of the terms used in describing the fitting of equations of models to experimental data

Several important assumptions underly the method of least squares. These are (1) that the *correct* form of the model has been chosen, (2) that the data are *typical*, (3) that the values of y are *uncorrelated* in the statistical sense and (4) that there is *no error* in the values of x. The most difficult of these to satisfy is (1); (4) can be allowed for if grossly untrue, and minor deviations from (2) and (3) are tolerable. An example of a common occurrence of correlation is when measurements have been made over an extended period of time during which an uncontrolled, progressive change has taken place in the experimental conditions, or the properties of the system. If these requirements are not met the statistical basis of the method is weakened and correct results will not be obtained. Beck and Arnold (1977, pp. 185–199) describe the consequences of violating each requirement.

It is not necessary to assume normality in the distribution of experimental errors (Sect. 2.8.4) in order to apply the method of least squares. However, a normal distribution is essential for the accurate calculation of parameter uncertainties.

Minimization of the objective function is done using the methods of the differential calculus for determining minima, namely setting the differential of the function with respect to each parameter to zero and solving for the parameters. The solutions of these simultaneous equations are the required parameter estimates. When the equations are linear with respect to the parameters, the solution is easy to obtain as an algebraic equation. This is the case, for example, in the common least squares estimation of the slope and intercept (parameters) of a straight line.

However, when the model equation is non-linear in its parameters, the derivatives of the objective function are no longer linear and the problem becomes one of locating the minimum of a non-linear function. Algorithms for doing this have been known since the time of Newton but it is only with the development of computers that they have become practicable. General approaches are described next and then a more detailed account of a particularly successful method is given. Details of a computer program incorporating this method, and suitable for use on any computer, are given in Sect. 11.1.

3.4.3 Methods of Parameter Search in Non-Linear Models

Finding the combination of parameter values that minimizes the objective function of a model equation non-linear in its parameters, entails a sequential search of all combinations of parameter values. These combinations define *parameter space* which may be visualized as a kind of landscape of many dimensions where the valleys represent minima in the objective function (see Fig. 3.2).

The search is conducted in a series of steps or *iterations* controlled by a *search algorithm*. These algorithms may be classified according to whether they are direct or gradient methods (see below). Direct methods are easier to implement computationally, but gradient techniques usually find the minimum more quickly. A practical problem arises when a search ends in a false or *local* minimum. Local minima occur unpredictably in the parameter space of non-linear models. It is essential that they be identified and discarded in favour of the lowest minimum. It is, however, impossible to prove that any minimum found is not a local one. One good practical test is to re-start the search several times from new initial parameter values. If the same minimum is found, confidence increases progressively. Search methods vary in their ability to extricate themselves from local minima; those that "look ahead" are relatively effective (Bremermann, 1970; Swartz and Bremermann, 1975).

3.4.3.1 Direct Search Methods

The simplest form of *direct search* is to divide the feasible range of parameter space into a grid of values, and to evaluate the objective function at each point. The combination of parameter values yielding the minimum sum of differences is then selected.

The simplex approach, originated by Spendley et al. (1962), in which the objective function is evaluated at $p+1$ mutually equidistant points in the space of p parameters, is more efficient. The principle of the method requires that in a model in which there are two parameters the response of the equation is evaluated at three combinations of parameter values at the vertices of an equilateral triangle, known as

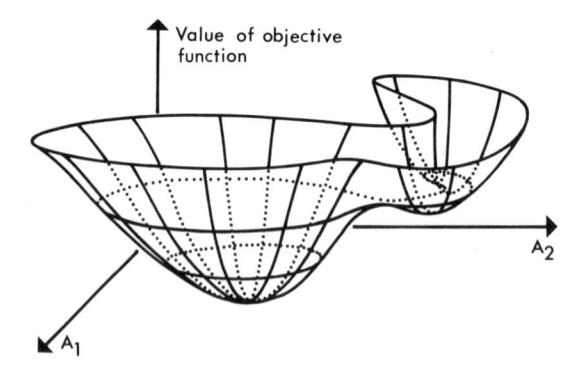

Fig. 3.2. Geometric representation of parameter space about the lowest minimum, for a hypothetical non-linear model with two parameters A_1 and A_2. The value of the objective function is illustrated at different combinations of the parameter values. A false, or local minimum, is shown on the right

the *simplex*. The vertex at which the objective function is *maximum* is noted, and the simplex is reflected about the two other vertices to define a new point, where a new evaluation is made. This process is repeated until a minimum is located. The simplex method replaces "trial and error" techniques, and is greatly superior to the common practice of varying one parameter at a time, especially when the parameters are not independent of one another but interact.

The basic method has been improved (Nelder and Mead, 1965) by incorporating an expansion and contraction of the simplex that is controlled by the progress of the search. This improved version has been applied successfully to many problems where the equations are deterministic and measurement error is small. Other improvements have been described by Routh et al. (1977), and a general discussion is given by Ross (1972).

Simplex methods have wider application than the minimization of objective functions. They can be used directly to *maximize* the response of a system having a large number of independent variables. Simplex maximization could be used, for example, to find the best combination of constituents of a culture medium in order to produce the highest production of steroid by a tissue in culture. The simplex method has often been applied in this form to maximize responses in chemical and biochemical analyses (Krause and Lott, 1974). The well-known practical optimization method known as "evolutionary operation" or EVOP (Box and Draper, 1969), applied originally in chemical engineering and production, is a simplex algorithm.

On the whole, direct search methods are less efficient than gradient ones and we shall not consider them further. However, the simplex is easy to understand, requires no elaborate calculation, is capable of following an optimum which moves with time and is readily applied in the laboratory to stochastic or deterministic problems. In fact, many investigators incorporate such procedures subconsciously when designing their experiments.

3.4.3.2 Gradient Search Methods

Gradient search methods select the search direction using information about the response of the model equation to changes in its parameters. This information is contained in the values of the partial derivatives (sensitivity coefficients) which show how fast the objective function is diminishing with changes in each parameter, and also in the results of previous steps in the search. The direction of parameter space providing the most rapid diminution in the value of the objective function is known as the *direction of steepest descent*. One very important advantage of gradient methods is that the derivatives can, at the minimum, be used to calculate the all-important precision of each parameter estimate.

Methods which follow the path of steepest descent fail as the minimum is approached, tending to "hunt" inefficiently. Techniques relying on linearization of the fitting function are more effective in the vicinity of the minimum. (Many versions of these have been described, most being roughly exemplified by the Gauss-Newton method. This seeks the minimum in a single step by attempting to calculate its position analytically as if the objective function were really linear, but falls short of this goal in proportion to the degree of non-linearity. However, relatively close to the minimum even a non-linear equation becomes fairly linear; the objective function can be recast without serious distortion as a linear approximation by using a Taylor series expansion and omitting all but the linear terms. An almost direct approach to the minimum can then be calculated analytically, further iterations being required only to adjust for error caused by the assumption of linearity. Serious error may be introduced by the arbitrary linearization and convergence to the minimum prevented, even after a number of iterations. Successful use of the Gauss technique therefore requires guessed initial estimates of the parameters which are close to the optimum values.)

One of the most generally useful and widely applied techniques combines steepest descent and linearization methods, and is due to Levenberg (1944), and Marquardt (1963). In this algorithm, the steepest descent approach is automatically applied when it is most effective at points relatively far from the minimum, while linearization of the fitting function is made dominant as the minimum is approached. Bard (1970) has shown that for a range of problems both the Gauss and Marquardt-Levenberg approaches were superior to the other gradient methods he tested. We will base our detailed description of practical model fitting on the Marquardt-Levenberg algorithm.

A number of books and reviews deal with methods of searching for the minimum of the objective function and discuss parameter estimation. Especially recommended are those by Box et al. (1969), Swann (1969), Beveridge and Schechter (1970) and Johnson (1974). General introductions to the fitting of linear and non-linear models are given by Draper and Smith (1966), Bevington (1969) and Daniel and Wood (1971). For a complete, detailed and rigorous account of non-linear methods, see Bard (1974).

3.5 Practical Details of Fitting Non-Linear Models to Data

This section describes how to go about fitting any model, whether linear in its parameters or not, to experimental data. The description is embodied in the computer program MODFIT (Sect. 11.1).

3.5.1 Weighting by Variance in the Data

The testing of a model is begun by collecting experimental measurements. These measurements usually consist of pairs of values, one each for the independent and dependent variables. The independent variable is often time, and the dependent one the response of the experimental system at that time.

An additional, extremely important piece of information is always potentially available. This is the estimate of reliability or uncertainty in each measured value of the dependent variable. The most useful estimate of uncertainty is the standard deviation, or its square the variance, because this has a precise statistical meaning. Fortunately, it is usually possible to be much more certain of the value of the independent, or x variable, which greatly simplifies the analysis.

Standard deviations are easily calculated from replicate measurements made under constant conditions. The estimated errors are then entirely random. The uncertainty in the mean of replicates is found by dividing the standard deviation by the square root of the number of replications, and is known as the sample mean standard deviation, or standard error of the mean (Sect. 10.1). The term sample is used because the replicates form a sample of the entire population of replicates that might ever be observed.

The standard error of the mean, when squared, provides a good measure of the precision of the mean relative to other means. The process of assigning this precision to a mean is known as weighting, and the weight used is the reciprocal of the variance. In this way, the weight of a mean grows as its variance decreases; the more precisely a value is known, so is its weight increased. It is thus possible to associate a numerical confidence with each mean value of the dependent variable and the fitting procedure will effectively "take more notice" of variable values that have a high confidence. One of the most important statistical manipulations carried out during the fitting process is an analysis of how this uncertainty in the dependent variable is transmitted to uncertainties in the parameters of the model equation.

3.5.2 Measurement Error Estimated from the Fitting Process

It can happen that the standard deviations of the y values cannot be determined because only single measurements are available. This means a serious loss of information. No longer is there any way of testing quantitatively whether a model provides a plausible description of data (Sect. 3.5.7), because it is then impossible to say whether an experimental point lies further from the fitted model than is reasonable to expect in view of the precision with which it was measured. Every effort must be made to estimate precision by direct experimental replication, and to use this information to weight each mean value, as described above.

When replication of data has been neglected, an estimate of experimental precision may yet be calculated at the time of fitting the model to the data. It is then necessary, however, to assume that the model describes the data perfectly so that the residuals measure random experimental error only. The squares of the residuals are summed, divided by the number of degrees of freedom (the number of experimental measurements less the number of parameters) and the square root is taken. The result is known as the *root mean square;* it equals the mean residual error which, provided the model accurately represented reality and therefore introduced no bias or error, is an estimate of the mean random error in the measurements. The effect of this procedure is to assign equal weights to all points.

3.5.3 Constraining the Search

It is sometimes necessary to restrict the range of values that a parameter may take. There are two reasons for this: (1) the nature of the model demands restrictions, or (2) certain parameter values make calculation difficult or impossible. An example of the first would be when the physical meaning of a parameter in the system required it to be positive. For example, if a parameter representing an association constant was calculated as the root of a quadratic equation, the positive root would always be chosen.

The second kind of constraint is imposed only during the search for the minimum. For example, it might be known that a certain parameter could not be zero, and that if the search algorithm assigned such a value in the process of seeking the minimum, some insuperable difficulty, such as division by zero, would occur. In order to steer the search away from impossible parameter values such as these, it is convenient to apply constants known as penalty functions. *Penalty functions* modify the objective function so as to reduce almost to zero the probability of a parameter value as it approaches the value of the constraint. Their use is fully described by Bard (1974, Chap. 6).

3.5.4 Terminating the Search and Examining the Residuals

The search is best terminated when the parameters attain relatively constant values. An upper limit should be imposed on the number of iterations in order to conserve computing resources because some searches approach the minimum very slowly. While a simple linear model such as a straight line will be fitted in one or two iterations from any initial parameter values, good initial guesses must be provided for non-linear models.

When the parameter values have been optimized a smooth curve representing the fitted model should be superimposed on the experimental data. An examination of the residuals is vitally important. Preferably, they should be plotted against both experimental x and y values to facilitate a search for trends caused by neglecting to include terms in the equation of the model. A plot of the residuals against the time at which the observations were made may reveal a consistent trend, indicative of change in the experimental system with time. A cumulative frequency histogram of the residuals can be informative. The residuals are ordered from lowest to highest, each is expressed as a fraction of their sum, and these fractional values are plotted on normal probability graph paper. The points should all lie reasonably close to a straight line. If one or two at the high end deviate clearly from this line, they may be outliers (see below). Clusters of points rather than a straight line with the points evenly distributed suggests that more than one source of error occurred in different subsets of the observations.

In addition, a runs-test (Sect. 10.6) should be carried out on the signs of the residuals. Too few or too many changes between positive and negative residuals, expressed in terms of this statistical test, are evidence of an inadequate model. A good discussion of the need for careful examination of residuals is given by Draper and Smith (1966, Chap. 3).

3.5.5 Outliers

It is essential to detect and eliminate measurements that fall far from the fitted model and are clearly in error, because their presence can seriously bias or distort the parameter estimates. Such points, known as *outliers*, arise from transient malfunctioning of the experimental apparatus, or human error in, say, pipetting or recording results. Equally important, of course, is the need for appropriate checks to detect and eliminate permanently faulty apparatus or poor experimental technique, before they introduce disastrous bias into the experimental results.

If a point is grossly in error its presence will be obvious in a list or plot of the residuals. The standard deviation of a mean will be abnormally high if the sample contains an outlier. Outliers are particularly noticeable if each residual is normalized to the mean residual standard deviation, that is, converted to a z-score (Sect. 10.4).

It is equally important not to eliminate arbitrarily points that deviate considerably from the fitted model. Such points may contain valid information, namely that the model is inadequate. Outliers should be rejected only if they can be traced to errors in recording the results or setting up the apparatus. The important property

Practical Details of Fitting Non-Linear Models to Data

of an outlier is that it stands alone from its immediate neighbours. There is really no good statistical test for showing up such points. They are best detected by the experienced judgement of someone thoroughly familiar with the measuring technique. Anscombe (1960) gives useful extra information.

3.5.6 Interpretation of Parameter Estimates

The most valuable results of fitting a theoretical model to experimental observations are the parameter estimates. (The parameters of an empirical model, fitted to data for purposes of interpolation only, are usually of lesser interest.) The parameter values obtained are merely estimates because of unavoidable experimental uncertainty, but it is essential to know how precise each estimate is. For a linear model, accurate, statistically meaningful standard deviations in each parameter can be calculated from the uncertainty in the data. Such is not the case for non-linear models. However, approximate uncertainties can be calculated by a method which yields accurate results when applied to linear models. What is more, when independent estimates of the precision of the parameters of most non-linear models are made by simply repeating the whole experiment several times, good agreement is usually found with the approximate values.

It is unnecessary to carry out real experiments in order to prove this important conclusion. All that is required is to simulate, from the equations of the model, experimental results having the statistical characteristics of the real data. The simulated data is used to explore the effect of the error it contains on the uncertainties in the fitted parameters. This clever technique, known as "Monte Carlo" simulation, is introduced in Sect. 2.8.2.1 and examples with practical details are given in Sects. 3.7.1.1, 6.1.1.1 and 6.2.2.2. Monte Carlo simulation may be carried out conveniently using program SIMUL (Sect. 11.2).

Because of the approximations in the calculations used to determine parameter uncertainties from experimental data discussed above, any error is likely to be on the generous side, leading to falsely high uncertainties in the parameters. This ensures that wrong conclusions will not be made on account of misleadingly precise estimates. If there is evidence of parameter interaction (Sect. 3.5.8.1), then uncertainties must be interpreted very cautiously.

3.5.7 Goodness of Fit of the Model

A very useful test of the worth of a model can be made when uncertainties in the experimental data have been determined by replication. This consists simply of comparing the estimates of the experimental error with the residuals from fitting the model to the data. If the model adequately describes the experimental points the ratio of the two estimates, known as reduced chi-square, will be close to 1; if not, the ratio will be too large (Sect. 10.7). The fact that a model performs well with a given set of data does not mean that it will do so with other sets or, in particular, with more precise measurements. A model that passes this test can be said to agree with the sample of experimental observations, but it has not been proved to accurately represent the physical processes underlying the data. Nevertheless, this test is a useful way of eliminating an unsatisfactory model or giving an estimate of its suitability.

3.5.8 Difficulties in Parameter Optimization

Any procedure for minimizing the objective function can fail to find the minimum because of poor initial guesses for the parameters, or because the equation of the model becomes unbounded, or both. An example of unboundedness occurs in the following equation

$$y = (A_1 + A_2 x)/(A_3 + A_4 x). \tag{3.2}$$

Here, y is unbounded when $A_3 = -A_4 x$. Penalty functions applied during the search, or judicious recasting of the equation, will help to resolve the difficulty.

Scaling problems are indicated when change in a parameter value produces little change in the response. For example, in the equation of a model with two independent variables

$$y = x_1 A_1 - x_2 A_2 \tag{3.3}$$

the value of y would be unaffected by changes in A_2 if the values of the parameters are comparable when x_1 and x_2 have different magnitudes, such as 100 and 0.1, respectively. This situation is easily corrected (if recognized) by introducing into the equation arbitrary multiplying constants.

3.5.8.1 Parameter Interaction and Sums of Exponentials

Sometimes one finds that a search is slow to converge and that the estimated error in one or more parameters is much larger than would be expected from the uncertainty in the data. When this occurs the parameters are said to be "poorly determined" and the cause, a linking of the influences of the parameters, is known as *parameter interaction*. Interaction occurs in proportion to the linear interdependence of the sensitivity coefficients of the model equation.

The cause of interaction is a restricted range of the independent variable or, equivalently, an excess of parameters. The equation of a model is well-behaved and stable if its response, y, in each region of x is dominated by the influence of mainly one parameter. Thus, if the range of x is too short some or all of the parameters may be imprecisely estimated. For example, in fitting the equation of a straight line

$$y = A_1 + A_2 x \tag{3.4}$$

to data, the intercept A_1 will be clearly defined when x approaches zero, while the term $A_2 x$ containing the slope will dominate the value of y at high values of x. If the data is collected over a narrow, intermediate range, both slope and intercept will be inadequately estimated. It is important to be aware that interaction can occur purely as a result of badly chosen x values, that is, poorly designed experiments.

Looking at it another way, interaction is caused by redundant parameters. As Box and Lucas (1959, p. 89) have pointed out, parameter estimates in many non-linear models are highly correlated and poorly estimated, and the common reason for this is that there are too many parameters.

Parameter interaction sometimes occurs as the result of a mistake in formulating the equation of a model. For example, in the equation

$$y = A_1 A_2 + A_3 x \tag{3.5}$$

two parameters are multiplied together. Gross interaction occurs because no matter what value is chosen for either A_1 or A_2, compensation can be achieved by altering the other.

More subtle semi-redundancy leading to strong interaction is a feature of models like Eq. (3.6) containing exponential terms. It is clear from an analysis of the sort outlined by Magar (1972, pp. 162–163) that parameter interaction is inherent in this kind of model. The problem is exacerbated when several exponential terms are added together, as occurs in the analysis of many physiological experiments concerned with compartmental systems, or the clearance of substances from the blood stream (Chap. 5). The difficulty is increased when the exponential parameters in a function represented by the sum of two terms of the form of Eq. (3.6) are similar. Thus, if two decay processes are described in terms of two decreasing exponential functions with similar decay constants, they are very difficult to separate mathematically. Many pairs of parameters will produce indistinguishably good (or bad) fits of the model to the data. It is unwise, therefore, to attach physical meaning to the parameters of exponential terms in a theoretical model. Experience of fitting exponentials makes one suspicious of reports describing the resolution of a decay curve into as many as four components, when each is identified with a particular physical process (see, for example, Sandor et al., 1978).

It is enlightening to sample the large literature on the hazards of fitting exponential models with a view to putting physical interpretations on the parameters. This problem is entirely due to parameter interaction, the effects of which are to amplify the tiny errors of painstaking experiments up to parameter uncertainties of hundreds of percent. Monte Carlo simulation is suitable for analysing the way in which error is propagated in any particular exponential model with which one is experimenting, and the program SIMUL provided here is ideal for that purpose. See also Riggs (1963, pp. 139–161), Myhill (1968), Glass and de Garreta (1971) and Julius (1972).

It may be possible to recast a model so as to minimize parameter interaction. Himmelblau (1970, pp. 194–195) shows how to do this for a troublesome single exponential model. Jennrich and Sampson (1968) suggest using stepwise regression, a linear technique in which parameters are altered one at a time in the search for the minimum, so as to avoid having to rearrange the model. Beck and Arnold (1977, Sect. 1.5) describe a criterion based on the sensitivity coefficients for determining whether the parameters of a given model can in fact be estimated from the range of the data available; they also provide (pp. 350–351) graphs of linearly interdependent sensitivity coefficients as functions of the independent variable, and give an account of the usefulness of such graphs when investigating parameter interactions.

In summary, parameter interaction can be reduced by expanding the range of x values, eliminating redundant parameters, or recasting the equations of the model.

There are three convenient measures of parameter interaction, in addition to slow convergence and the appearance of unexpectedly large parameter uncertainties. One is *dependence*, which shows the degree to which changes in the value of each parameter is related to changes in the others. Dependence is defined precisely in Sect. 11.1. A dependence of more than about 0.95 (out of a possible maximum of 1) means that significant interaction occurs between the affected parameter and one or more other parameters. Note that dependence is not a linear measure; a value of 0.95 does not mean "95% dependent". Another measure is the correlation between pairs of parameters. The *correlation* equals the covariance divided by the product of the standard deviations of the two parameters; its sign indicates whether the relationship is direct or inverse. A third measure is the condition number, which is particularly sensitive to the inclusion of too many parameters in the equation. The *condition number* is the ratio of the maximum to the minimum eigenvalues of the latent roots of the matrix of sensitivity coefficients or *curvature matrix* so-named because it measures the curvature of parameter space. See Wilkinson (1965) for an explanation of these terms.

A condition number greater than about 1,000 indicates parameter interaction caused by having too many parameters for the data to support. This means that the model is suspect and requires careful inspection — the parameter uncertainties may be worthless. As will be seen from several examples below, it is sometimes necessary to tolerate an empirical model with too many parameters giving rise to a large condition number in order to achieve a satisfactory fit to data over a narrow range of x.

3.6 Models Containing Differential Equations

Before models containing differential equations can be compared with experimental data, it is necessary to integrate the equations (Sect. 2.1.1.2). The integrated forms of some differential equations are known, but it is often necessary to integrate them numerically.

Special methods must be used to integrate systems of stiff differential equations or serious errors will be introduced. Two very successful approaches are summarized in the algorithms of Treanor (1966) and Gear (1971). Illustrations, and a discussion of the relative merits of the two algorithms, are given by Chandler et al. (1972), and Kropholler and Senior (1976). It is best to routinely use one of these special methods for integration, rather than worry whether or not any particular system is stiff.

When integrating differential equations it is necessary to supply a value of y known as the initial condition, usually where x is taken as being equal to zero. Parameters to be optimized may appear also in these initial conditions, as well as in the differential equations. Thus the initial conditions may be known theoretically, be measured or be unknown parameters.

Differential equations of order greater than one cannot be integrated directly by most computer methods. They can, however, be transformed into a number of first order equations suitable for numerical integration (see Bard, 1974, pp. 223–225).

The dynamic behaviour of equations describing non-linear systems depends on the values of the parameters (Sect. 2.4.2). If the parameter values chosen for the model happen to give the wrong type of behaviour, such as instability when the system is stable, optimization will fail. There is thus often a need to use penalty functions in order to prevent divergence of the objective function from the minimum, and contain the optimization within feasible regions of parameter space. Good initial guesses of the parameter values are particularly important.

The stability during optimization of parameters in negative exponential terms sometimes appears to be too great. The usual explanation of this insensitivity of the response of the model to the values of certain parameters is that they have become too large; being coefficients of negative exponential terms, such terms then have negligible effect in comparison with others. The remedy is to supply very small initial estimates for any parameter that is, for example, a rate constant.

Many of these points are illustrated in the numerical integration of the equations of compartmental systems described in Sects. 5.2.4 and 5.2.5.

3.7 Using the Computer to Fit Models to Data

In Sect. 11.1 details are given of a complete computer program, known as MODFIT, for fitting any model, linear or non-linear in its parameters, to experimental data.

We have developed MODFIT over seven years, inspired originally by algorithms published by Bevington (1969). The program will fit models of great variety simply by changing a single subprogram that provides a mathematical description of the model. MODFIT can be used to fit all the examples of model equations given in this book, including those consisting of systems of differential equations.

The program has performed equally well on four large time-sharing computers and a small laboratory machine. Conversion for use on different computers is easy because the program is written in standard FORTRAN, the most common scientific programming language. MODFIT is short, simple, fast and versatile. It is not unique; many computing centres provide similar programs. In our experience these are large and cumbersome in comparison with MODFIT, although some are extremely flexible and provide additional features. A short list of alternative programs will be found in Sect. 11.17.4. MODFIT has the advantage, however, that it can be put into operation easily by anyone having a small computer equipped with a FORTRAN compiler.

Also provided (Sect. 11.2) are instructions for using another program known as SIMUL which is used for either of two purposes. The first, option (1), is to calculate the responses of model equations given parameter values and a range of the x variable. The second, option (2), is to introduce random errors with known characteristics into these responses and then to re-estimate the parameters thus carrying out a Monte Carlo simulation (Sect. 2.8.2.1).

SIMUL performs the same operations as MODFIT, but rather than fit the model to a single sample of experimental observations, it produces up to 100 sets of simulated data. This replication enables a statistical evaluation to be made of the fitting process. The way in which this program can be used is best understood by studying the examples provided in Sects. 3.7.1.1, 6.1.1.1 and 6.2.2.2.

A brief introduction has been given in Sect. 3.3 to the kinds of computers required for using MODFIT and the other programs provided in Appendix B. The following examples are intended to introduce the details of fitting models to data using MODFIT. These will also clarify the concepts dicussed above and show a little of their practical significance. Other examples will be found in Chaps. 5, 6 and 7.

3.7.1 Exponential Decay: Clearance of PMSG

Many physical models can be described by an equation having an exponential term, or sum of exponential terms. Such functions are also often useful for empirical curve-fitting. However, it may be extremely difficult to determine a unique set of parameter values for these models (Sect. 3.5.8.1). The following example illustrates the fitting of an empirical exponential model to data.

Any number of exponential decay terms can be fitted to data using the FUNCTN subprogram RESERVR listed in Table 11.7. The number of exponentials used is controlled by the value of NTERMS. When NTERMS is 2, one exponential decay is modelled; when NTERMS is 4, two terms are summed, and so on. Details of using MODFIT in conjunction with subprogram RESERVR will be found in Sects. 11.1 and 11.3.

The data, describing the disappearance of intravenously injected pregnant mare serum gonadotrophin (PMSG) from sheep plasma, were obtained from experiments outlined in Sect. 5.1.1. NTERMS was 4 defining an equation consisting of the sum of two exponential decays

$$y = A_1 \exp(-A_2 t) + A_3 \exp(-A_4 t) \tag{3.6}$$

and representing an empirical description of clearance (Sect. 5.1). Table 3.1 shows the progress of the fit; the data, fitted model, and residuals are illustrated graphically in Fig. 5.1.

The meanings of the results shown in Table 3.1 are described in detail here as a guide to interpreting the many similar Tables in Chaps. 5 and 6. Superscripts in the following text refer to the legend of Table 3.1.

Only one determination of PMSG was made at each time interval after injection. No uncertainties could therefore be assigned to measurements and MODE[j] was set to 0 causing the residual variance[e] to be calculated, rather than reduced chi-square (Sect. 10.7). The square root of this, 0.593 iu/ml, was the mean residual or root mean square difference between the fitted and experimental values. As shown by the calculated standard deviations and percent coefficients of variation[f], the estimates of parameters[b,d] A1, A3 and A4 were all well determined while A2, the exponential coefficient of the first term, was less precise. This, together with the low values of the dependencies[g] and correlation coefficients[i], gave little evidence of any parameter interaction — the parameter values appeared to be stable. However, the fairly high condition number[h] suggested that there were too many parameters for the range of the x variable, time. It would be necessary to increase the number or range of the x values, or both, to remedy this.

The correlation coefficients are arranged in a table so that the measures of correlation between any two parameters is found at the intersection of the appropriate row and column. Interpretation of the correlation coefficients is straightforward; no parameter was strongly correlated with any other. As expected, A1 and A3 were inversely related because their sum equalled the response at time zero and if one was increased, compensation was achieved by decreasing the other.

The data points[m] are reproduced for ease of comparison with the calculated responses[n] of the model equation using the optimized parameter values. The residuals[o] were reasonably small. A runs-test (Sect. 10.6) showed no significant trends at the 5 percent level, and there was no evidence of outliers[p]. (Had measured uncertainties in the y variable been available they also would have been reproduced[q].) We conclude, therefore, that the equation $[PMSG] = 6.1 e^{-0.6t} + 19 e^{-0.022t}$ represents an adequate description of the experimental observations.

Using the Computer to Fit Models to Data   91

In view of the condition number would a model with a single exponential term have sufficed? To answer this, optimization was performed on the same data but with NTERMS set to 2, thus defining a single exponential decay. The fitted model is shown in Fig. 5.1. The resulting residual variance of 1.86 was much greater, and it is clear from a plot of the residuals (Fig. 5.1) that there were trends in successive values. A runs-test on the residuals showed systematic divergence between model and data. So although the condition number was reduced from 1,302 to 333, indicative of less parameter interaction, the four-parameter model with large condition number provided a superior description of the data.

3.7.1.1 Application of Monte Carlo Simulation

The parameter optimization procedure requires a linearizing approximation of the model equation (Sect. 3.4.3.2). This approximation may introduce an unknown error into the parameter estimates (bias), and also into their calculated uncertainties. There are two unknown aspects to a parameter estimation problem. One is that the "true" model is unknown. The other is that the technique for estimating the parameters may, for the reasons given above, yield incorrect results. It is not possible to demonstrate the validity of both aspects simultaneously with the techniques used by MODFIT. However, Monte Carlo simulation enables the second aspect to be verified by defining a "correct" model, and then measuring the efficiency with which the known parameter values are estimated (Sect. 2.8.2.1).

The "correct" model is taken to be the one yielding the best description of the sample of experimental data. "Perfect" y values are calculated from the model using the optimized parameter estimates. Simulated data is generated having the same error characteristics as the real experimental data by adding to the perfect responses uncertainties selected randomly from a suitable population of values. The usual method of parameter optimization is then applied to this generated data. If the resulting parameter estimates are indistinguishable from the "true" ones (the ones used for generating the y values), and their uncertainties agree with those calculated during the fitting process, the linear approximation has been validated.

To illustrate this, let us return briefly to the more plausible model above containing two decay processes, and investigate the validity of the optimization process by means of Monte Carlo simulation. The program SIMUL was used, together with subprogram RESERVR; instructions will be found in Sect. 11.2. The input for this program was the same as that for MODFIT except that here the initial guesses of the parameter values were replaced by the optimized estimates taken from Table 3.1. From these, "perfect" responses of the model were generated. The second mode of operation of SIMUL [option (2)] was chosen by providing, on UNIT 1, requests for 100 simulations (NSETS) and no printing of parameter estimates (KEY=0). These were followed by an arbitrary seed for the pseudo-random number generator (ISEED) and a value of SDEV, the required mean standard deviation in the simulated data. This was taken to be constant and equal to $(0.3520)^{1/2}$, i.e. 0.5933, which was the root mean square residual found for the experimental data (Table 3.1). The assumption of constant experimental standard deviation estimated from the residuals of the model was unavoidable because the experimental data were not replicated.

SIMUL carried out the Monte Carlo simulation and printed the results shown in Table 3.2. The superscripts in the following text correspond to the labels in the

Table 3.1. Detailed interpretation of the output of program MODFIT[a]

RES VARIANCE	A 1	A 2	A 3	A 4
1.2548	5.0000	.50000	20.000	.20000E-01
.35622	6.1629	.57399	19.082	.21952E-01
.35212	6.1549	.54586	19.055	.22174E-01
.35204	6.1452	.55614	19.084	.22212E-01
.35204	6.1491	.55272	19.073	.22200E-01
.35203	6.1479	.55389	19.077	.22204E-01

STD DEVS	.64581	.13634	.55073	.93316E-03
	10.5%	24.6%	2.9%	4.2%

DEPENDENCIES	.72204	.76119	.89827	.63809

CONDITION NUMBER 1302.4

CORRELATION COEFFICIENTS

	A 1	A 2	A 3	A 4
A 1	1.0000			
A 2	-.22778	1.0000		
A 3	-.69762	.74462	1.0000	
A 4	-.54473	.51883	.75863	1.0000

MODE = 0, DEGREES OF FREEDOM = 19
FINAL LAMBDA = .00000010000000000

X	Y	YFIT	RESIDUAL	Z-RESIDUAL
0.	25.000	25.225	-.22480	-.37889
.41700	24.000	23.781	.21895	.36903
.53300	23.000	23.429	-.42874	-.72261
1.3300	23.000	21.465	1.5352	2.5875
1.8300	20.000	20.548	-.54836	-.92421
2.6700	19.000	19.380	-.37984	-.64019
3.5000	18.000	18.535	-.53518	-.90200
5.8300	17.000	17.004	-.39335E-02	-.66296E-02
7.6700	16.000	16.177	-.17742	-.29903
13.500	15.000	14.139	.86055	1.4504
21.670	12.000	11.791	.20920	.35259
30.000	10.000	9.7998	.20025	.33750
37.500	8.0000	8.2964	-.29645	-.49964
47.250	6.0000	6.6815	-.68148	-1.1486
53.750	5.0000	5.7835	-.78352	-1.3206
61.700	5.0000	4.8476	.15236	.25679
69.500	4.0000	4.0768	-.76752E-01	-.12936
77.500	4.0000	3.4133	.58674	.98890
85.500	3.0000	2.8578	.14224	.23974
94.000	2.5000	2.3662	.13376	.22544
102.00	2.0000	1.9811	.18861E-01	.31789E-01
110.00	2.5000	1.6587	.84129	1.4179
117.00	1.0000	1.4199	-.41994	-.70777

[a] Illustrated by the results of fitting a model consisting of a double exponential decay to the time course of the disappearance of an injection of PMSG from the blood plasma of a sheep. Fitting was done using program MODFIT and subprogram RESERVR, with NTERMS=4. The data and fitted model are illustrated in Fig. 5.1.
[b] Parameters of the model equation (Sect. 3.5.6).
[c] Progress of the optimization (Sects. 3.4.3.2, 3.5.3, 3.5.4).
[d] Optimized parameter estimates (Sect. 3.5.6).
[e] Residual variance: measure of difference between model and data (Sects. 3.4.2, 3.5.2). Where reduced chi-square is printed: comparison of error in fit with error in data (Sects. 3.4.2, 3.5.1, 3.5.7).
[f] Uncertainties in parameter estimates (Sect. 3.5.6).
[g] Measures parameter interaction (Sect. 3.5.8.1).
[h] Indicates over-parameterization (Sect. 3.5.8.1).
[i] Measures parameter interaction (Sect. 3.5.8.1).
[j] Code for error treatment and penalty functions (Sect. 11.1).

Table. First, the model and estimates of the parameter values[c] were used to calculate "perfect" y values[d], which are shown together with the corresponding values of x. [This output alone would have been obtained if option (1) had been selected.] Using the calculated y values as a basis, SIMUL added to each an error chosen randomly from a normally distributed population, the mean of which was zero and the standard deviation 0.5933[b]. (The mean root mean square residual from the 100 simulation runs, 0.5917[i], was very similar, proving that the random deviates were chosen correctly.) The model equation [Eq. (3.6)] was then fitted to this simulated data and estimates were made of the parameters and their uncertainties. This process was repeated 100 times to yield 100 sets of parameter estimates. The mean and sample standard deviation in the mean of the 100 estimates of each parameter were then calculated[e]. The key point about Monte Carlo simulation is that, unlike a real experiment, the true values of the model parameters being sought are already known, and are used to generate the data. The smaller the bias, or difference between each mean parameter estimate and the true value, the more successful is the estimation process. The magnitude of each bias[f] was examined by means of the t-test (Sect. 10.9), using the corresponding standard deviation in the mean parameter estimate. In no case was the bias significant. This may not have been true for other values of the parameters, another range of the x variable, or with greater experimental error.

Let us now consider the uncertainties in the parameter estimates. There are two approaches to obtaining these uncertainties. One is to calculate a standard deviation from the distribution of the 100 replicate estimates of each parameter[g]. This is the average uncertainty in any one estimate; where there is no bias, it is the "correct" standard deviation in a parameter because it has been established from a large sample by replication. The other is to use the values of standard deviations calculated by the linear approximation employed in the algorithm used to fit the model to the data set in each simulation run (a typical example is shown[d] in Table 3.1). The means of these 100 estimates[h] are compared with the "correct" values[g]; if there is no significant difference (t-test) between each pair, then the linearization method of the fitting algorithm is giving valid results.

This was found to be the case for the present example. Thus the parameter estimates and their uncertainties, calculated from a single set of real experimental data reported in Table 3.1, were not influenced by the assumptions of the fitting method.

A description of the use of Monte Carlo simulation to investigate the properties of an empirical model of protein–ligand interaction is given in Sect. 6.2.2.2, where additional information was obtained by comparing the results with those from replication of genuine laboratory experiments.

Table 3.1 (continued)

[k] Number of data points minus number of parameters (Sect. 10.10).
[l] Measures degree of linearization of the function at the minimum (Sects. 3.4.3.2, 11.1).
[m] Experimental data.
[n] Calculated y from model with optimized parameter estimates.
[o] Residual at each point; shows trends in data (Sect. 3.5.4).
[p] Normalized residuals; detects outliers (Sects. 3.5.5, 10.4).
[q] Standard deviations in data (SIGMAY): used when available to weight the fit (Sect. 3.5.1).

Table 3.2. Monte Carlo simulation of the clearance of injected PMSG from the blood plasma of a sheep[a]

```
NUMBER OF SIMULATION RUNS = 100
DEGREES OF FREEDOM =  19
MODE = 0
CONSTANT EXPERIMENTAL STANDARD DEVIATION =   .59332   (b)
```

PARAMETERS	A 1	A 2	A 3	A 4
(c)	6.1479	.55389	19.077	.22204E-01

X	YFIT
0.	25.225
.41700	23.781
.53300	23.429
1.3300	21.465
1.8300	20.548
2.6700	19.380
3.5000	18.535
5.8300	17.004
7.6700	16.178
13.500	14.140
21.670	11.791
30.000	9.7998
37.500	8.2965
47.250	6.6815
53.750	5.7836
61.700	4.8477
69.500	4.0768
77.500	3.4133
85.500	2.8578
94.000	2.3663
102.00	1.9811
110.00	1.6587
117.00	1.4199

(d)

MEAN VALUES OF PARAMETER ESTIMATES

	A 1	A 2	A 3	A 4
	6.2089	.56722	18.994	.22127E-01	(e)
STD DEVS	.63509E-01	.14792E-01	.58116E-01	.86383E-04

| MEAN BIAS | -.60981E-01 | -.13334E-01 | .83229E-01 | .76636E-04 | (f)

STANDARD DEVIATIONS OF PARAMETER ESTIMATES

| | .63509 | .14792 | .58116 | .86383E-03 | (g)

MEAN VALUES OF CALCULATED STANDARD DEVIATIONS

| | .65861 | .14018 | .56270 | .94270E-03 | (h)
| STD DEVS | .11768E-01 | .43165E-02 | .12936E-01 | .17058E-04 |

| DEPENDENCIES | .79027 | .78850 | .92477 | .69091 |

CONDITION NUMBER   1515.2

CORRELATION COEFFICIENTS
```
A 1   1.0000
A 2  -.35129    1.0000
A 3  -.77728     .77151    1.0000
A 4  -.63459     .56757     .79729    1.0000
```

MEAN RES VARIANCE   .35942
STD DEV   .11556E-01
MEAN ROOT MEAN SQR   .59172 (i)

[a] SIMUL together with FUNCTN subprogram RESERVR was used, with NTERMS = 4. The labels are explained in the text.

Using the Computer to Fit Models to Data 95

Monte Carlo simulation has other important applications. One of these is to show how variation in the precision of the experimental measurements is reflected in the precision of the parameter estimates. What uncertainty in the measurements can be tolerated if reasonable uncertainties are to be retained in the parameters? Conversely, is it realistic to attempt to increase the experimental precision in the hope of attaining a given level of precision in a parameter estimate? These questions are readily answered by performing a series of Monte Carlo simulations over a range of values of the experimental uncertainty. The following example illustrates this approach. In particular, a level of experimental uncertainty is sought which will yield a percentage coefficient of variation of 10 percent in parameter A2 of the above example.

Monte Carlo simulations of 25 replicates each were carried out at six values of SDEV, the experimental standard deviation. The results, together with the values from the previous simulation, are shown graphically in Fig. 3.3. It can be seen that the uncertainties in the four parameters rose in an approximately linear way with increasing experimental error. The mean values plotted were only estimates of the uncertainties and could not, therefore, be expected to lie on perfectly smooth lines or curves. (Approximate errors in the mean estimated uncertainties are shown for parameter A2 only, as an indication of this scatter.)

The answers to the questions posed above are now clear. In particular, in order to attain a relative error (percentage coefficient of variation) of 10 percent in parameter A2 it would be necessary to reduce the experimental standard deviation to about 0.25. This is less than half the value attained in the experiments, and to achieve it would require many more determinations of PMSG.

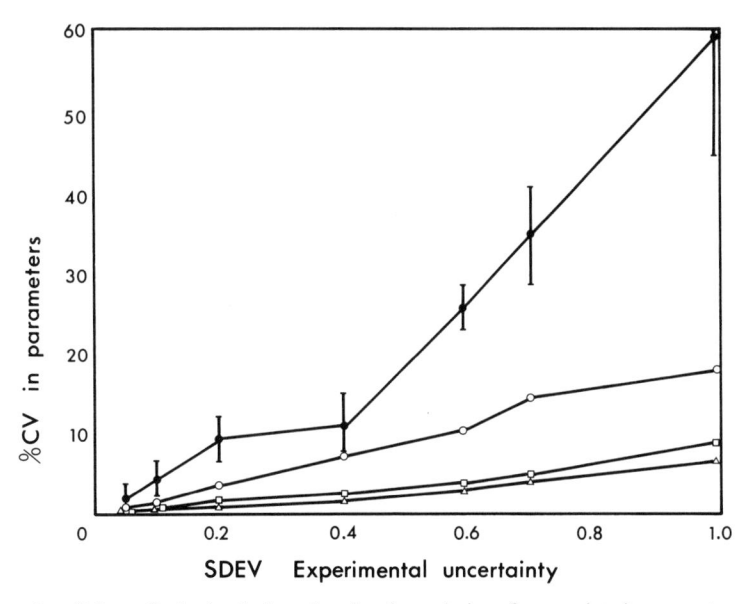

Fig. 3.3. Results of a series of Monte Carlo simulations showing the variation of uncertainty in parameter estimates (expressed as percentage coefficients of variation) as a function of experimental uncertainty. The model was represented by Eq. (3.6) and the experimental conditions are described in the text. The error bars, equal to one standard deviation in the mean, are shown for the uncertainties in the estimates of parameter A2 only. ○, Parameter A1; ●, A2; △, A3; □, A4

3.7.2 Growth of Elephants

This example illustrates a model which, although couched in theoretical terms, should only be used empirically. We conclude from the results of applying MODFIT to experimental data that, in this case, only one of the parameters has possible physiological significance.

Increase in the size and weight of animals with advancing age has been described by a variety of models. While it does not seem possible to derive a universal representation of growth in a mathematical form, it is clear that functions can be determined that are adequate for particular purposes. The growth of many animals as a function of time is markedly sigmoidal. Regarding an organism as analogous to a reacting chemical system obeying the law of mass action, von Bertalanffy (1938) expressed the rate of change of its mass as the sum of physiological processes of anabolism and catabolism. This theoretical, differential equation model, developed in detail by Beverton and Holt (1957) in relation to the growth of fish in the North Sea, and von Bertalanffy (1973), can be integrated to yield the equation

$$w(t) = A_1 \{(1 - \exp[-A_2(t - A_3)]\}^3 \tag{3.7}$$

where $w(t)$, the dependent variable, is the mass of the organism at any age t, A_1 is the asymptotic mass or maximum mass that it can attain under given conditions, A_2 is a coefficient of catabolism of body materials per unit mass and time, and A_3 is the theoretical age at which the organism would have zero mass with the same growth pattern as observed in later life. The parameter A_3 is artificial because the adult growth pattern is never found at the earliest age. Hanks (1972) has successfully used the model of Eq. (3.7) to describe the growth of African elephants.

MODFIT and the FUNCTN subprogram EXPCUBE, which embodies Eq. (3.7) and is listed in Table 11.8, were together used to fit the von Bertalanffy growth function to measurements of the weights of female elephants as a function of age. We are grateful to J. Hanks for permitting us to make use of unpublished data for illustrative purposes. The progress of the fit is shown in Table 3.3, and the mean weights and standard deviations, as well as the data and fitted model, are depicted in Fig. 3.4.

The table illustrates the slightly different format of the results when estimates of the precision in the experimental measurements are available. Thus reduced chi-square rather than the residual variance was printed, and the estimated standard deviations in the y values, used to weight the fit, are reproduced in the last column (labelled SIGMAY).

According to a table of reduced chi-square the value obtained here, with 36 degrees of freedom, indicated that the residuals of the data about the fitted equation were significantly greater ($p = 0.02$) than would be expected from the measured uncertainty in the data. In other words, this test suggests that the model is an inadequate description of the measurements. Nevertheless, there does not appear to be any systematic discrepancy between model and data, and a runs-test confirmed this. The several mean responses at some distance from the fitted curve were responsible for the elevated value of reduced chi-square. They may have occurred because of errors of measurement, either in misreading the weighing scales or improperly estimating the ages of the animals. However, it is probable that they go beyond expected statistical variation and represent instead genuine biological

Using the Computer to Fit Models to Data 97

Table 3.3. The model of Eq. (3.7) fitted to data on the growth of African elephants[a]

R CHI SQUARE	A 1	A 2	A 3
111.88	1500.0	.10000	-6.0000
34.123	2551.8	.58941E-01	-9.7479
1.9812	2550.1	.73810E-01	-9.2535
1.5492	2614.4	.75006E-01	-8.8628
1.5488	2614.6	.74962E-01	-8.8807
1.5488	2614.6	.74963E-01	-8.8804
STD DEVS	37.279	.24784E-02	.37886
	1.4%	3.3%	-4.3%
DEPENDENCIES	.83510	.97108	.94938

CONDITION NUMBER   86087.8

CORRELATION COEFFICIENTS
```
    A 1   1.0000
    A 2  -.82648    1.0000
    A 3  -.66736     .95012    1.0000
```

MODE = 1, DEGREES OF FREEDOM = 36
FINAL LAMBDA = .0000001000000000

X	Y	YFIT	RESIDUAL	Z-RESIDUAL	SIGMAY
1.0000	356.00	374.47	-18.469	-1.3192	14.000
3.0000	536.00	535.85	.14530	.60541E-02	24.000
4.0000	687.00	620.80	66.196	1.5045	44.000
5.0000	725.00	707.24	17.758	1.3660	13.000
6.0000	792.00	794.29	-2.2911	-.81824E-01	28.000
.					
.					

[a] MODFIT together with FUNCTN subprogram EXPCUBE was used. The fitted model is shown in Fig. 3.4.

variants, animals which were abnormally large or small for their ages because of effects which were not included in the model, or controlled for in the sampling of animals. For instance, certain individuals or groups of animals may have experienced transient or prolonged growth spurts as a result of some local environmental effect, perhaps several years before.

In this case, therefore, the value of reduced chi-square should not be regarded as ruling out a model which provides a good description of the growth pattern. The unavoidably gross simplification of many biological models often leads to this type of problem. Some of the animals may have had important additional factors influencing their rates of growth which have not been included in the equation. The mistake in this particular example lies in assuming that a measure of "experimental uncertainty" (indicated by the error bars in Fig. 3.4) could be obtained by combining the masses of animals of the same age. It would, in this case, have been preferable to have entered the mass of each animal individually and assessed an overall error from the residual variances.

From Table 3.3 it can be seen that the parameter uncertainties were all low, particularly the uncertainty in A1, the asymptotic mass. This was especially well-determined because information from the whole range of ages contributed to it. The relatively greater uncertainties in the other two parameters, and their fairly high dependencies, were indicative of interaction. It is clear by inspection of Eq. (3.7) that A2 and A3 will be related to soem extent — a change in one can probably be

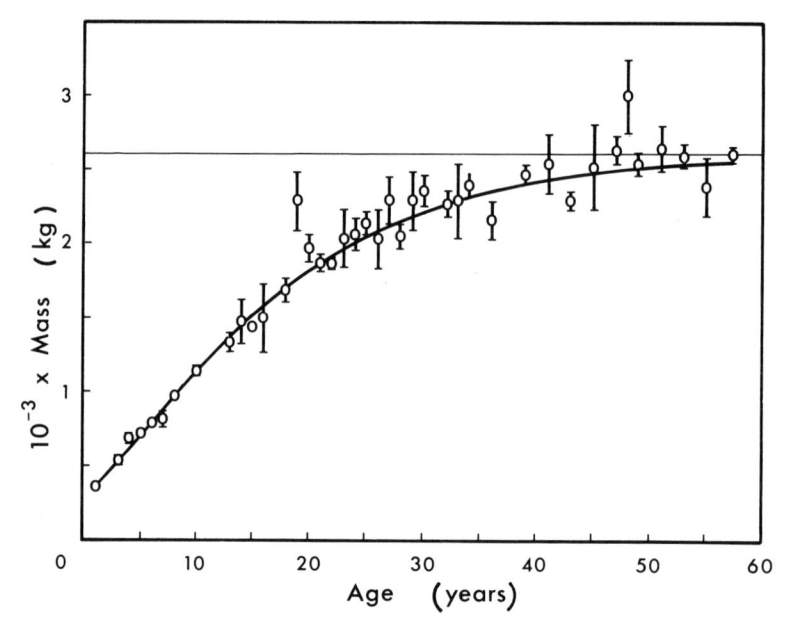

Fig. 3.4. Increase in weight of African elephants as a function of age. Each *point* represents the mean mass of several animals. The *error bars* show one sample standard deviation of the mean. The *smooth curve* is the result of fitting Eq.(3.7) to the data, as described in the text. The *thin horizontal line* represents the optimized estimate of parameter A 3, the asymptotic or maximum mass attainable by the population of elephants of which this is a sample. The progress of the fit is shown in Table 3.3

partially compensated for in the other. Also, information for the estimation of A3 comes mainly from the low end of the age range. Biological constraints prevent one from obtaining more information by extending the age range to lower values!

The correlation coefficients showed that most of the dependence of A2 and A3 was positive, and that some negative correlation occurred between A1 and A2.

The condition number was very large, clearly indicating an excess of parameters. This gave extra weight to the previous conclusion that either A2 or A3 was largely redundant, and meant that almost as good a fit would be obtained with a much simpler exponential function containing two parameters only. Thus, although the model is based on theoretical concepts of protein turnover, the final equation represents too great a simplification of the processes involved to be anything but empirical. While some credence can be given to parameter A1, the asymptotic mass, as a measure with physiological relevance, the other two parameters can only be regarded as empirical coefficients, at least as regards the range of this experimental data.

Nevertheless, the model is useful for comparing different populations of animals, such as different genetic types, or similar groups which have experienced dissimilar environments. In these cases, the *t*-test (Sect. 10.9) could be used to examine estimates of asymptotic mass from two populations of animals to see whether they differed significantly.

This example also clearly illustrates the advantages of applying non-linear parameter estimation to untransformed data, rather than using linearizing transformations (Sect. 2.8.1). When Hanks (1972) carried out several hand calculations requiring linearizing transformations to fit Eq. (3.7) to data, he was unable to apply weighting and obtained misleading estimates of the asymptotic weight, the parameter of interest to him. This underlines the danger of attempting to fit a model to data transformed into terms of new co-ordinates without proper weighting.

3.7.3 How Thick is the Wall of an Ovarian Follicle?

Now let us examine the process of forming a simple theoretical model of a system. The parameter of the equation evolved has physical interpretation and also could be estimated by direct measurement, thus allowing comparison with the results of parameter optimization.

In experiments on the effects of gonadotrophin on steroid production by sheep ovarian follicles, Moor et al. (1973) compared groups of treated follicles with control groups. The follicles in each group were matched as closely as possible with respect to size but there was still a range of about 2 mm diameter in each group. In order to reduce variance within each group caused by differences in tissue mass it was necessary to normalize the data by expressing the results in terms of steroid production per unit mass. Thus it was essential to know the mass of the steroid-producing tissue in each follicle. An ovarian follicle is a thin-walled sphere of tissue containing fluid. It was impossible to weigh the cellular material in the wall prior to culture because this would have meant collapsing the follicle to release the fluid. Instead, the relationship was investigated between the mass of tissue and the overall diameter in order to find a way of predicting mass from measurements of diameter, which are easy to make.

A total of 242 follicles between 1 and 7.2 mm diameter were dissected from the ovaries of sheep. Stromal tissue was peeled away to reveal the intact follicles. After recording the diameter of each follicle, fluid was drained with gentle blotting and the remaining theca and granulosa tissues were weighed. Follicles were divided into 49 groups differing by 0.1 mm in diameter. The mean and sample standard deviation of the mean of each group was then calculated. These values are shown in Fig. 3.5.

It can be seen that the relationship between the mass of tissue and the diameter of an intact follicle was not linear. As the diameter expanded the mass of the tissue increased more than proportionally.

Let us first consider an empirical model for relating mass to diameter, using a polynomial equation. The simplest polynomial with a curved response is a quadratic $y = A_1 + A_2x + A_3x^2$. Fitting was done using program MODFIT together with the FUNCTN subprogram POLYNOM (Sect. 11.5) and NTERMS set to 3. The next more elaborate polynomial, a cubic $y = A_1 + A_2x + A_3x^2 + A_4x^3$, was also fitted, again using POLYNOM but with NTERMS equal to 4. Both versions of the model described the data fairly well. The fitted cubic is shown by the broken line in Fig. 3.5.

The values of reduced chi-square obtained were 4.93 and 4.28, respectively, much higher than would be expected to occur by chance in an experiment with over 40 degrees of freedom. As in the elephant weight example, the reason for this was probably not inadequacy of the model but instead poor estimates of experimental uncertainty. It can be seen from the lengths of the error bars in Fig. 3.5 that variance was extremely heterogeneous, suggesting the presence of outliers in the samples

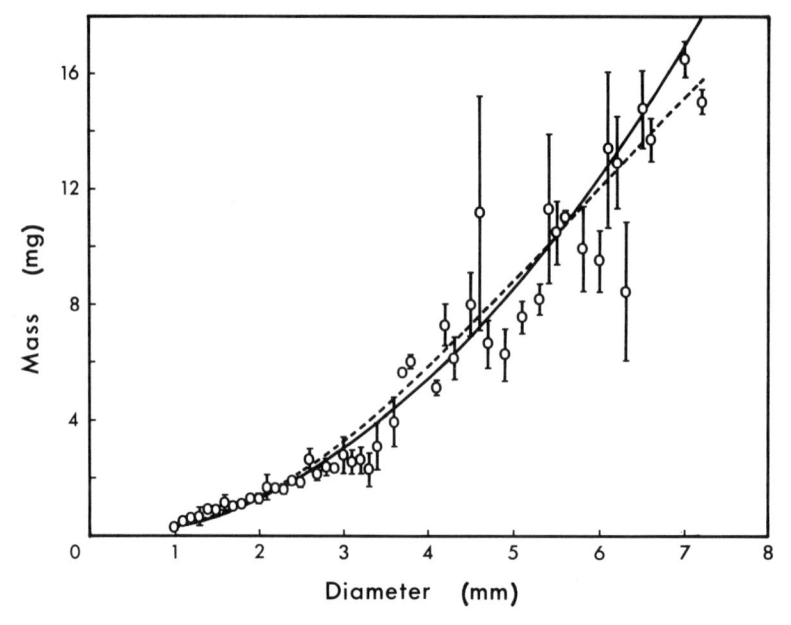

Fig. 3.5. Relationship between the mass of tissue in the wall of a sheep ovarian follicle and its diameter. Each point represents the mean of results from between 2 and 14 follicles. The *error bars* show one sample standard deviation of the mean. The result of fitting a general cubic polynomial to the data is shown by the *broken line*. The *solid line* represents the theoretical model of Eq. (3.9); the progress of the fit is shown in Table 3.4

with high variance. Most of the data points lying far from the fitted line represented the means of two measurements only, and it was these that inflated the value of reduced chi-square.

In the case of the cubic, for example, there were four parameters estimated, each with a coefficient of variation of almost 100%, and dependencies of from 0.986 (A1) to 0.999 (A3). Thus a reasonable description of the data was obtained, but with the need for at least three highly interactive parameters having no physiological significance.

Let us now formulate a theoretical model to describe the relationship between the mass of cellular material and the diameter of the follicle. We shall assume for simplicity that the theca and granulosa cell layers form a perfectly spherical shell within which is contained the follicular fluid. Fig. 3.6 represents this idealization.

The volume of the shell of tissue, or wall, is equal to the difference between the volumes of two spheres of diameters $2R_o$ and $2R_i$. That is

$$\text{wall volume} = (4/3)\pi(R_o^3 - R_i^3). \tag{3.8}$$

Assuming that the density of tissue was 1, and expressing the equation in terms of the external diameter D we have

$$\text{mass of wall tissue} = (\pi/6)[D^3 - (D - 2A_1)^3] \tag{3.9}$$

where A_1 is a parameter equal to the thickness of the wall. We thus have a theoretical model with which we can calculate the mass of tissue (the dependent

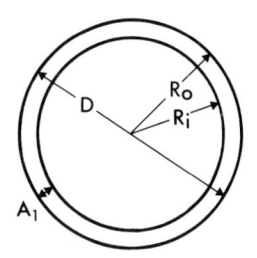

Fig. 3.6. Physical model of an idealized ovarian follicle of diameter D showing a cross-section through the centre. The distance $R_o - R_i$, or thickness of the follicle wall, is represented by the parameter A_1 in Eq. (3.9)

variable) in any follicle as a function of its diameter (the independent variable), and a single parameter A_1. This equation is embodied in FUNCTN subprogram FOLL, described in Sect. 11.6.

Before we can make use of this model it is necessary to estimate the value of A_1. To do this the model must be fitted to as large a sample of data as possible. Program MODFIT together with FUNCTN subprogram FOLL were used for this purpose. The progress of the fit is shown in Table 3.4, and the fitted model is represented by the continuous curve in Fig. 3.5.

The theoretical model represented by Eq. (3.9) is a cubic, but unlike the second of the empirical equations considered earlier it has no squared, linear or constant terms, and its single parameter has physiological meaning. Thus from measure-

Table 3.4. The theoretical model of (Eq. 3.9) fitted to data relating the mass of tissue and the diameter of sheep ovarian follicles[a]

```
R CHI SQUARE        A 1
   8444.5        1.0000
   5554.2        -.28809
   121.36         .45784E-01
   5.8539         .11181
   5.7701         .11370
   5.7701         .11370
   5.7701         .11370

STD DEVS           .94240E-03
                   .8%

DEPENDENCIES    0.

CONDITION NUMBER        0.0

CORRELATION COEFFICIENTS
        A 1    1.0000

MODE =   1, DEGREES OF FREEDOM =   48
FINAL LAMBDA =    .0000000100000000
```

X	Y	YFIT	RESIDUAL	Z-RESIDUAL	SIGMAY
1.0000	.30000	.28212	.17880E-01	.68770	.26000E-01
1.1000	.50000	.34901	.15099	3.6828	.41000E-01
1.2000	.60000	.42304	.17696	2.4924	.71000E-01
1.3000	.67000	.50421	.16579	.50239	.33000
1.4000	.92000	.59253	.32747	2.7289	.12000
.					
.					
.					

[a] MODFIT together with FUNCTN subprogram FOLL was used. The fitted model is shown in Fig. 3.5.

ments of follicular diameter and mass it was possible to estimate the mean wall thickness to be about 114 µm. It was difficult to gain an accurate measure of the uncertainty in this value from the calculated standard deviation (0.94 µm) because of the large value of reduced chi-square. When the value of reduced chi-square is larger than 1, indicating inadequacy of the model, the calculated uncertainties are erroneously low. A more accurate result is obtained by multiplying the uncertainty by the value of reduced chi-square. In the present case this yielded a final estimate of wall thickness of (114 ± 5.5) µm.

Although more elaborate models are not warranted it would be possible, for example, to write an equation in which the thickness of the wall varied with diameter rather than remaining constant. There was, in fact, no experimental evidence for such variation. When measurements were made of the thickness of the walls of 65 follicles of various diameters on fixed sections using a calibrated microscope, there was no consistent variation in wall thickness with changing diameter. The mean thickness by measurement was (165 ± 4) µm, which was higher than the value of A_1 estimated above. However, in the direct measurements no allowance was made for the effects of fixing, and when measuring the weights of the follicles it was impossible to prevent some loss of granulosa cells.

The lack of confidence in the estimate of wall thickness did not in any way detract from the empirical usefullness of this model for predicting tissue mass from measurements of diameter. When determinations of steroid production by follicles were normalized by tissue mass, the range of results within each group was reduced in comparison with data which was not normalized. Normalization thus permitted more clear-cut differences to be shown in comparative experiments where the stimulatory effects of gonadotrophin were measured.

4 Design of Analytical Experiments

The design of an experiment is vitally important to its success. An ill-conceived experiment is unlikely to yield any useful information no matter how ingeniously the data is analysed. Careful planning is therefore essential.

The first step is to decide on the purpose or goal of the proposed investigation; only then can effective experiments be designed. Experiments must be devised that will realize this goal as efficiently as possible. The most important aspect of design is the delineation of the experimental frame (Sect. 1.2.1). While this is partly dictated by considerations outside the direct control of the experimenter there remains considerable scope for intelligent choice.

There are two types of experiments. Common in endocrinology is the *comparative* kind, in which the effect of treatment is compared with untreated controls. The other sort is *analytical*, in which the parameters of a model (either theoretical or empirical) are estimated by fitting it to experimental data. We are concerned with analytical experiments here. In practice the distinction between the comparative and analytical approaches is not clear-cut. It is often of interest, for example, to compare the parameters of a model applied to experimental material from different sources.

There is a considerable literature on the design of comparative biological experiments. We shall concentrate instead on modern methods for designing analytical experiments where the aim is to choose between models with the maximum efficiency, and to estimate the values of parameters as precisely as possible with the minimum number of experiments.

4.1 Principles of Design

The principles of the design of comparative biological experiments are described lucidly and non-mathematically by Finney (1955), and Fisher (1971). Concepts common to the design of both kinds of experiments are summarized below.

4.1.1 Randomization

R.A. Fisher was the first to emphasize the importance of dealing with the effects of extraneous variables. These variables cannot themselves be controlled but their influence, often referred to as uncontrolled *biological variation*, can be cancelled. This makes experimentation in the biological sciences especially difficult, because the variation can seldom be summarized in convenient and statistically well defined frameworks such as normality. The implications of this have been discussed in Sects. 2.8.4 and 1.2.7.

Efficient *randomization* was shown by Fisher to be the best way of managing variation of this kind. For example, in an experiment to determine the effect of a drug on a certain kind of animal it is possible to recognize in advance the major variables such as sex, age and weight, and to match individuals between control and treatment groups with respect to these variables. But there will remain many variables that are unrecognized and therefore uncontrolled. The only way to ensure that these will not affect the results is to distribute them randomly between treatment and control groups. The effect of the variables will not be eliminated, but instead distributed without bias.

Experimental units should be numbered and then randomized by assigning them to groups using tables of random numbers. It is important that this be done efficiently, as all statistical methods used to analyse experimental results depend absolutely on the samples having been drawn randomly from the parent population. It is not good enough, for instance, to divide a cageful of animals into two groups by catching and removing half of them. It is quite likely that the act of capture will separate them on the basis of weight or tameness (Emmens, 1948, pp. 56–59).

4.1.2 Replication

It is necessary always to *replicate* measurements in order to determine their precision. Replication enables the basic residual error or variance to be calculated. This is a composite sum of the measurement errors, which depend upon both the precision of the observations and instruments, and the uncontrolled biological variation. The more replication there is, the more precisely can a sample mean be determined. Restriction of sampling to subgroups with less variation will improve precision, but narrow the scope of the conclusions.

In simple comparative experiments it is easy to calculate how many experimental units will be required to achieve a given level of precision in a mean result, if some measure of random variation is available. This is not, however, true for analytical experiments, where it may be very difficult to estimate the uncertainty in the precision of a parameter before doing the experiment. Monte Carlo simulation, rather than laboratory experiments, offers an efficient way of examining the relationship between experimental error and the resulting uncertainty in the parameter estimates (Sects. 2.8.2.1 and 3.7.1.1).

4.1.3 Reduction of Random Variation

In comparative experiments precision is enhanced by pairing groups. Individual experimental units (e.g. an animal or sample of tissue) are matched in pairs for as many attributes as the experimenter is aware of. One unit from each pair is assigned randomly to the treatment or control group, while its pair is added to the other group. At the end of the experiment, the effect of treatment is examined by comparing results between each pair. Rather than restrict the experiment to pairs, several relatively homogeneous groups or blocks may be compared in a *randomized block* design. It is sometimes possible to employ a unit as its own control, because there is usually less variation in the behaviour of a single unit than there is between them. A block can thus consist of replications upon an individual. Alternatively, heterogeneity of experimental material can be allowed for during calculation of the results by means of the statistical method known as analysis of covariance

(Snedecor and Cochran, 1967). In analytical modelling, individual variation may be reduced by making the model more complex (Sect. 1.2.7).

4.1.4 Factorial Experiments

Early in the development of his ideas concerning the design of comparative experiments in agriculture, Fisher emphasized the advantages of varying many *factors* (independent variables) simultaneously in a single experiment. In those sciences where experiments are completed rapidly there is often less need for complex designs. However, it is still necessary to determine the extent to which factors interact, that is, the non-linearity of the system, and in order to measure this, factorial experiments are essential. In a typical comparative factorial experiment it is usual to test two or more factors at several doses or intensities in all possible combinations. A well-designed experiment, though complex, will provide conclusions with little calculation. Factorial comparative experimentation is essential in many areas of endocrinology where there is a need to untangle complex webs of interaction and variability. The statistical technique of analysis of variance is used to analyse factorial experiments by determining the significance of dominant effects and interactions by means of Fisher's F-test (Sect. 10.11 and Colquhoun, 1971).

By contrast, the design of most analytical experiments is usually less complex. This is because the experimental frame has been deliberately restricted by limiting the number of factors investigated. The aim is to estimate precisely the parameters of a model in a well-defined area of the problem. Often only one independent variable is used, although this restriction is entirely unnecessary.

4.2 Sequential Design

Sequential experimental designs are those in which information from previous experiments is used to guide later ones. This approach is common in the long term, where the outcome of a series of experiments will determine the future path of a research effort (Fisher, 1952). Here, we are concerned with ways in which sequential methods can be used to improve the effectiveness of a group of experiments.

The principles of sequential design were first applied in production engineering to maximize output. The same ideas have also been used in analytical chemistry (Sect. 3.4.3.1). Clinical trials are often conducted in a sequential manner, testing being terminated for ethical reasons immediately a predetermined level of statistical significance has been attained (Bross, 1952). Wald (1947) showed that a smaller number of sequential experiments is generally required to determine a parameter with a given precision than if they are performed simultaneously. There are two reasons for this. Not only is information available from early experiments to help in the design of later ones, but experimentation can cease as soon as sufficient precision has been attained.

The methods of sequential design described here appear to have been little used as yet for the design of analytical experiments in the biological sciences. This is probably because they are based on techniques for fitting models to data (Chap. 3) which are themselves unfamiliar to biologists, and may also be in part due to doubts expressed regarding their application to biological problems (Finney, 1955, pp. 116–

117). However, Finney (1960, p. 153) later says about early ideas of sequential methods that they are:

> perhaps the most exciting developments in experimental design since the period of Fisher's first major contributions.

It is clear from recent comments (Rodbard and Munson, 1978) that a need exists for a simple, practical process for discriminating between competing models. The methods outlined below are intended to do just that, as rapidly and effectively as possible.

The development of methods of sequential design are due mostly to Box and his associates, originating from an article by Box and Lucas (1959). A clear review of the subject is given by Bard (1974), and recent work is summarized by Atkinson (1978).

4.2.1 Design Criterion for Parameter Estimation

Our aim is to use sequential methods to optimize the design of experiments. In this context, design means choosing values of the independent variable x at which the dependent variable y is to be measured. Although the following approaches are equally applicable to systems in which there are several independent variables we shall, for simplicity, restrict our discussion to those with only one. We require to estimate parameters with the maximum precision and the least number of experiments, and to differentiate as efficiently as possible between rival models.

Choice of experimental conditions is limited by the physical constraints of time, temperature, concentration and so on. Box and Lucas (1959), and Box and Hill (1967) have shown how the efficiency of designs for both estimating parameters and distinguishing between models depend on the sensitivity coefficients, i.e. the values of the partial derivatives of the model equation with respect to each parameter. These are, not surprisingly, the same quantities involved in calculating the uncertainties in parameter estimates. To gain the maximum increase in precision of the parameters the next experiment in a series must be carried out at a value of x at which least is known about the response of the model: to obtain the maximum amount of information we must do the experiment for which the outcome is most uncertain. This is equivalent to choosing the next x value at which T is maximized, where

$$T(x) = V(\bar{y}) + V(A) \, [\delta f/\delta A]. \tag{4.1}$$

$V(\bar{y})$ is the variance of $\bar{y}$ at the point x, $\delta f/\delta A$ is the vector of values of the partial derivatives of the model with respect to the vector of parameter estimates A, and $V(A)$ is the vector of variances of the parameter estimates. In the case of a non-linear model this is an approximation only. If $V(\bar{y})$ is constant, variation in $T(x)$ is caused only by the second term of Eq. (4.1).

Eq. (4.1), which can be generalized so as to apply to models with several independent variables (Bard, 1974, pp. 262–265), may be derived in several ways (Bard, 1974, Sects. 10.2 and 10.3; Box and Hill, 1967; Atkinson and Hunter, 1968).

4.2.2 Design Criterion for Model Discrimination

The preceding section considers one model only. Often, however, several similar models have been devised and we attempt by experimentation to differentiate

Sequential Design

between them. It is easy to devise experiments capable of choosing between models that are distinctly different. For instance, suppose it is unclear whether a straight line or a parabola is the better model to describe a physical relationship. In order to distinguish between these two models it is sufficient to make measurements at three points, because if the three results do not lie on a straight line the first model must be unsuitable.

This assumes, of course, that the data are sufficiently precise to allow the distinction to be made. When the choice between models is not obvious we can obtain very useful information about the best experimental design to adopt by applying the following approach, in which any number of models can be examined, each containing different numbers of parameters.

Using the principles of information theory, it is possible to derive a measure of *divergence* or *information for discrimination* (Box and Hill, 1967; Bard, 1974, pp. 266–267). When comparing two models in the form of single equations, each with a single independent variable, the measure of divergence is given by

$$D0_{1,2}(x) = -1 + 0.5 \left[(T_2+1)/T_1 + (T_1+1)/T_2 \right] (y^{(2)} - y^{(1)})^2 \qquad (4.2)$$

where $D0_{1,2}(x)$ is the measure of divergence between models 1 and 2, T_1 and T_2 are the values of T [Eq. (4.1)] for models 1 and 2, respectively, and $|y^{(2)} - y^{(1)}|$ is the magnitude of the difference between the responses of the models, all at a given value of x. It is possible to generalize this approach for more than two models by calculating the likelihood (L) of each model and weighting the divergence measure by the likelihoods, so as to obtain the point of maximum divergence between the current two most likely models.

The meaning of the measure $D0$ is clear if one assumes that the T values for the two models are almost constant, as is sometimes the case. $D0$ is then solely a function of $|y^{(2)} - y^{(1)}|$. It is obvious that the best value of x at which to do the next experiment is the one at which $D0$ is maximal, because this is most likely to distinguish the models. Conversely, if the experiment were to be carried out at a value of x for which the responses of the two models happened to be the same, no useful information would be gained.

4.2.3 Combined Model Discrimination and Parameter Estimation

It is possible to combine the criteria of Sects. 4.2.1 and 4.2.2 to give a *joint design criterion* $C(x)$ for model discrimination and parameter estimation. One method is to emphasize the criterion for model discrimination when there is considerable doubt as to which model is best, and then, after the best model has emerged, change to the criterion for parameter estimation in further experiments (Hill et al., 1968).

The design criteria can also be used to determine the best times at which to record results in kinetic runs or other dynamic experiments (Box and Lucas, 1959; Heineken et al., 1967; Atkinson and Hunter, 1968).

4.2.4 Termination Criteria

Experimentation can cease when one model has been selected as being superior to the others at a given level of probability, or the estimation of its parameters has attained a sufficient degree of precision, or both. Wald (1947) has proposed a likelihood ratio test suitable for determining the superiority of one model relative to another (Bard 1974, pp. 270–271). The *likelihood L* of model i is defined as

$$L^{(i)} = (2\pi V^{(i)})^{-(N/2)} \exp(-N/2) \qquad (4.3)$$

where $V^{(i)}$ is the residual variance of model i and N is the number of experiments that have been performed. The *likelihood ratio* is

$$L^{(1)}/L^{(2)} = (V^{(2)}/V^{(1)})^{N/2}. \qquad (4.4)$$

If H_1 is a hypothesis stating that model 1 is correct, H_2 is the alternative, and a and b are two constants such that

$$0 < b < 1 < a \qquad (4.5)$$

then the *likelihood ratio test* states that if $L^{(1)}/L^{(2)} > a$ accept H_1, if $L^{(1)}/L^{(2)} \leq b$ accept H_2, and if $b < L^{(1)}/L^{(2)} \leq a$ continue experimentation. The values of a and b are related to the familiar probability value α; if one wants to be 95 percent certain of accepting H_1 or H_2 only if they are true, $\alpha = 0.05$, $a = (1-\alpha)/\alpha = 19$, and $b = \alpha/(1-\alpha) = 0.0526$. When there are more than two competing models the test is applied to the two currently most likely ones.

The *confidence in the model* with the maximum likelihood is given by

$$C_N^{(l)} = L_N^{(l)} \Big/ \left(\sum_{i=1}^{m} L_N^{(i)} \right) \qquad (4.6)$$

where $C_N^{(l)}$ is the confidence after N experiments in model l with the maximum likelihood, $L_N^{(l)}$, and m is the number of models.

4.2.5 Implementation

For each experiment, that value of x is chosen which maximizes the value of the desired criterion. There are always several local maxima within the experimental frame, approximately equal in number to the largest number of parameters in any of the contending models. The value of x corresponding to the position of the highest maximum varies from one experiment to the next, but the locations for the maxima are fairly constant. Some are always on the boundaries of the experimental frame. In the case of models with a single independent variable the search for the current maximum value is straightforward; the x range is divided into small increments and each model is estimated at every increment, using the current values of its parameters. The maximum value of $T(x)$, $D0(x)$ or the combined criterion $C(x)$ is then noted, and the next experiment performed at the corresponding value of x. Locating the highest maximum is more difficult in models with more than one independent variable, being often a non-linear search problem (Bard, 1974, p. 274).

For models non-linear in their parameters, the design criteria cannot be evaluated unless initial estimates are available for the parameters. It is usual therefore to carry out several traditional, undirected experiments to initiate or prime the process.

It must be appreciated that these design methods are capable only of selecting between models presented for comparison; there may be a better model which has not been defined. Neither can the method be used to construct models. An absolute measure of the suitability of a model for describing a given sample of data is the value of reduced chi-square (Sect. 10.7).

4.2.6 A Computer Algorithm for Combined Design Criteria

A diagrammatic representation of a sequential experimental procedure is shown in Fig. 4.1. Our computer program called DESIGN, which is suitable for designing a series of experiments based on the criteria for model discrimination and parameter estimation, is reproduced in Table 11.4. An outline of the working of this program is given here; details appear in Sect. 11.3. We are unaware of any other published computer program performing this function.

The first step is to carry out a series of random, undirected experiments in the usual way within a given experimental frame. An experiment consists of obtaining a single value of y (preferably together with an associated uncertainty for weighting) at a particular value of x. The uncertainty is best estimated by replication. The number of priming experiments required is equal to at least one more than the maximum number of parameters in any of the models considered.

At this stage the program DESIGN is loaded into the computer together with up to five FUNCTN subprograms, each describing a different model. Input to the program consists of the experimental data together with the estimates of variance at each point (if available), and initial estimates of the parameters for each model. DESIGN then fits the models to the data by the methods described in Chap. 3. The likelihood of each model is calculated, as well as the criteria $T(x)$, $D0(x)$ and $C(x)$.

Output consists of the residual variance or reduced chi-square, the current parameter estimates and uncertainties for each model, and the values of the design criteria. The most important result is the value of x at which the next experiment should be performed. When this has been carried out, the new result is added to the data and the fitting and design processes are repeated. This cycle continues until one

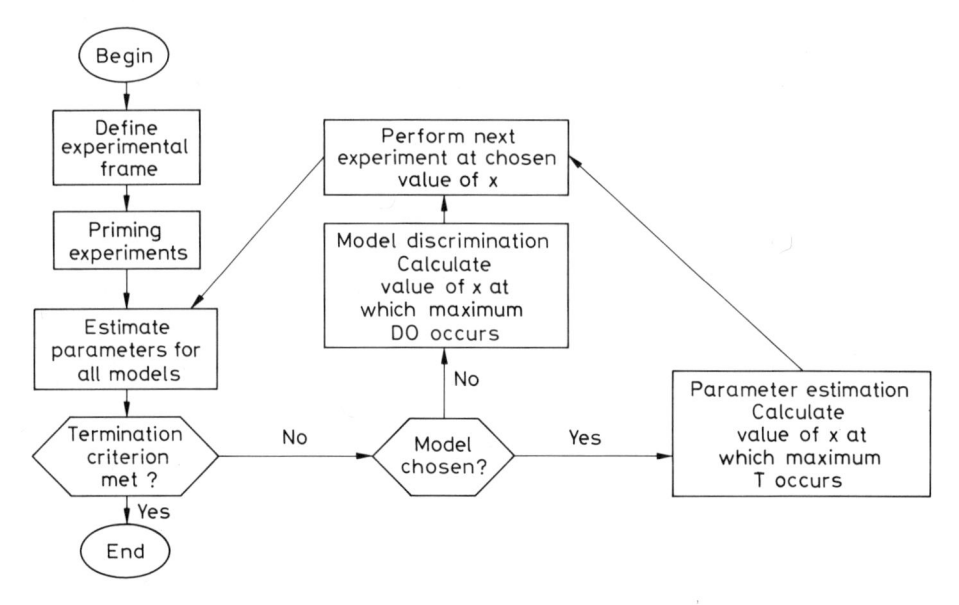

Fig. 4.1. Strategy for model discrimination and parameter estimation. Representation of the action of program DESIGN in differentiating between models and minimizing parameter uncertainty

of the models emerges as being the best among those tried, and its parameters have been estimated with sufficient precision.

4.2.7 Does Sequential Experimentation Work?

What evidence is there that sequential experiments, directed by the design criteria described, have any advantage in comparison with traditional, undirected methods? Very little work has been done to test the strategy so far and its possible contributions to the biological sciences have yet to be explored.

The most convincing case for the effectiveness of sequential design can probably be made using simulation, because by this means it is possible to compare easily the results of sequential experimentation with those from undirected designs. Bard (1974, Sect. 10.9) presents evidence obtained by simulation to show that sequentially designed experiments were capable of rapidly differentiating between two very similar models; in comparison, undirected designs were incapable of achieving any significant differentiation.

A similar approach is used in the following example in which Monte Carlo simulation is used to demonstrate that a properly designed series of experiments is capable of rapidly choosing the correct model. By contrast, a traditional, undirected design failed to differentiate between the models in the same number of experiments.

4.2.8 Testing the Design Criteria by Monte Carlo Simulation

In this example, "experimental observations" were generated using a particular model to which were added random "uncertainties", normally distributed with a known standard deviation and a mean of zero (Sect. 3.7.1.1). In this way it was possible to test which approach, sequential or undirected, most rapidly picked out the "true" model. In a real series of experiments the model is not, of course, known in advance; finding it is the object of the experimentation.

The example is concerned with investigating the interactions between testosterone and sex steroid binding globulin (SBG), under difficult experimental conditions. This protein is important for transporting steroids in the blood of pregnant women. In late pregnancy large amounts of SBG augment the role of another plasma protein capable of binding steroids, corticosteroid binding globulin (CBG). At this time it is easy, using equilibrium dialysis and a suitable model, to estimate the properties and concentrations of both binding proteins (Sect. 6.1.1.1). Early in pregnancy, however, the concentration of SBG is low, and the protein is much more difficult to detect. Sequential design methods are shown here to permit the identification of SBG early in pregnancy, when its level is still low, and to estimate its properties and concentration as precisely as possible within the constraints of the experimental frame and uncertainty in the data.

A sample of early pregnancy plasma was prepared, and its ability to bind various concentrations of testosterone measured by equilibrium dialysis. The method is described in Sect. 6.1.1.1, except that single determinations only were performed at eight concentrations of ligand. The results, expressed in terms of the ratio of bound to total ligand, $R_{B/T}$, are shown in Fig. 4.2. This way of presenting the results is explained in Sect. 6.1.1, where models of the interaction between ligands and macromolecules having independent binding sites are also described. Three models might be suitable for describing the observations: (1) a single class of high affinity

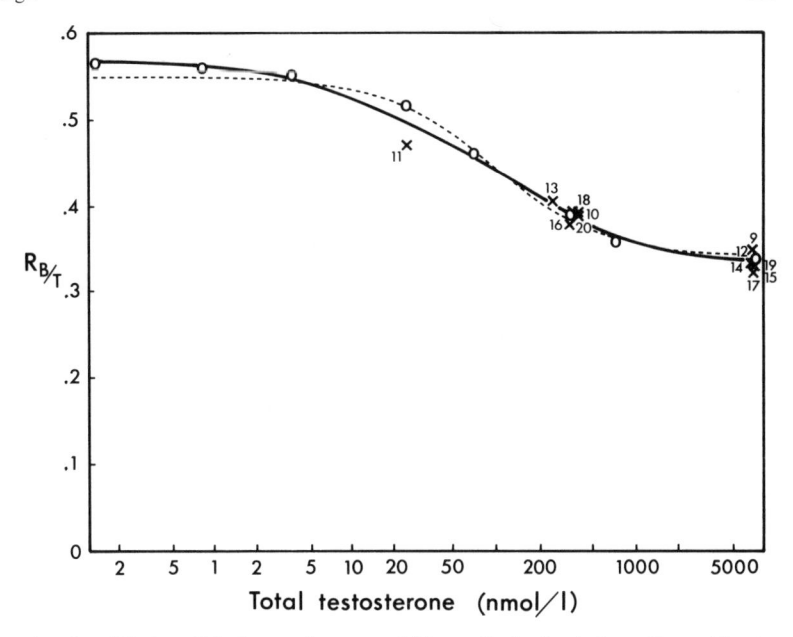

Fig. 4.2. The results of equilibrium dialysis experiments and Monte Carlo simulations, directed by the principles of sequential experimental design, for distinguishing between rival models. Details are given in the text. Eight *points* (○) were measured in the laboratory. The order in which the simulated results(×) were obtained is indicated by numbers. The *solid line* represents model (3) and the *broken line* model (1). Values of the independent variable were plotted on a logarithmic scale to allow display of the wide range of values. (This distortion of the x range makes intuitive assessment of the results very difficult)

binding sites plus low affinity, non-specific ones, (2) two classes of high affinity sites with different properties or (3) two classes of high affinity sites plus a low affinity one. These models are selected by using FUNCTN subprogram MASSACT with NTERMS set to 3, 4 or 5, respectively (Sect. 11.12).

From the experience of the experiments described in Sect. 6.1.1.1, model (3) provides the most appropriate description of the binding properties of late pregnancy plasma. The two specific binding sites correspond to the proteins SBG and CBG discussed above, and the non-specific, low affinity interaction represents binding by albumin. It is possible that, early in pregnancy, when the level of SBG is low, model (1) may be more appropriate.

However, for the purposes of this test of the design procedure, we shall assume that model (3) represents the "real" system, and use it to generate additional "data" as requested by DESIGN. Each new "data" point will consist of the response of model (3) to which is added a random uncertainty, taken from a set of errors with a mean of zero and standard deviations equal to the known experimental uncertainty at that point. Do sequentially directed experiments distinguish the "correct" model from this "data" more effectively than experiments designed in the conventional manner?

Program DESIGN, the necessary subprograms, and three copies of FUNCTN subprogram MASSACT, were loaded into the computer. Initial estimates of the three sets of parameters together with the experimental data were supplied as input, as described in Sect. 11.7.

Table 4.1. Results of applying DESIGN to the initial data from an equilibrium binding dialysis experiment in which the binding of testosterone to blood plasma proteins was measured[a]

```
EXPERIMENTS  1 -   8
******************

RESID VAR 1      PARAMETERS FOR MODEL 1
   .12040E-04    .32204E-01    23.532           .51425
STD. DEVS. =    .20379E-02     1.4547           .61282E-02
                     6.3%           6.2%             1.2%
DEPENDENCIES    .97126          .97706          .71989
FINAL LAMBDA =     .0000100000  DEGREES OF FREEDOM =  5   ITERATIONS =  2

RESID VAR 2      PARAMETERS FOR MODEL 2
   .32788E-03    .31322E-01    20.304           .49826E-04    11325.
STD. DEVS. =    .15537E-01    12.430            .23792E-04    5525.9
                    49.6%          61.2%            47.8%          48.8%
DEPENDENCIES    .99088          .99168          .99673          .99619
FINAL LAMBDA =     .0100000000  DEGREES OF FREEDOM =  4   ITERATIONS =  4

RESID VAR 3      PARAMETERS FOR MODEL 3
   .11393E-04    1.1931         .50099E-01    .28564E-01    25.256          .51131
STD. DEVS. =    3.0443          .15172         .41168E-02    2.2989          .66648E-02
                   255.2%        302.8%           14.4%           9.1%            1.3%
DEPENDENCIES    .99414          .99730          .99665          .99363          .86567
FINAL LAMBDA =     .0000001000  DEGREES OF FREEDOM =  3   ITERATIONS =  4

FIT DETAILS FOR CURRENT BEST MODEL: MODEL 3 (NEXT BEST IS MODEL 1)
      X              Y             YFIT           RESIDUAL       Z-RESIDUAL
   .15400         .56300         .56267         .32538E-03      .96402E-01
   .86300         .55800         .55870        -.70073E-03     -.20761
  3.7000          .55000         .54953         .46644E-03      .13819
 23.800           .51500         .51399         .10057E-02      .29797
 71.000           .45900         .46163        -.26285E-02     -.77875
331.00            .38600         .38153         .44654E-02     1.3230
709.00            .35800         .36025        -.22491E-02     -.66633
7086.0            .34000         .34067        -.66678E-03     -.19755

      LIKELIHOODS:    MODEL 1         MODEL 2         MODEL 3
                      .444976         .000001         .555024

L(3)/L(1)                        =      1.247
LN(L(3)/L(1))                    =       .2210
CONFIDENCE IN MODEL 3  =              55.5%                        PERFORM NEXT EXPERIMENT AT X
T(MAX) MODEL 3 =                 .2225E-02   AT X =   .1540        VALUE INDICATED BELOW FOR:
T(MAX) MODEL 1 =                 .1817E-03   AT X =   .1540
D0(MAX)          =                810.8      AT X =  7086.         -- MODEL DISCRIMINATION
E(MAX)           =                  1.000    AT X =   .1540        -- PARAMETER ESTIMATION
W1 = .9223   W2 =    .0777
C(MAX)           =                   .9264   AT X =  7086.         -- COMBINED REQUIREMENT
```

[a] Three different models were compared, obtained by setting NTERMS to 3, 4 and 5. Details are given in the text.

The results of the intial run are shown in Table 4.1. The final parameter estimates of the three models are summarized in the first half of the table. Values of residual variance are printed because standard deviations in the values of $R_{B/T}$ were not entered with the data (MODE = 0). It is immediately clear from the values of residual variance that at this stage models (1) and (3) provided almost equally satisfactory descriptions of the data, while model (2) was much inferior. The last few lines in the table give the results of the criteria calculations. The criterion for model discrimination, $D0$, shows that in order to maximize the chance of distinguishing between the two best models, the next experimental point should be measured at a total ligand concentration of 7086 nmol/litre, which is on the upper limit of the experimental frame. If the best model had already been found, and it was desired to reduce parameter uncertainty as rapidly as possible, the next experiment should have been done at a testosterone concentration of only 0.154 nmol/litre, which is at the other extreme of the experimental frame.

The new "experimental" point was generated from model (3) using the estimates of its parameters obtained in the initial run, to which was added a randomly selected error chosen from a normally distributed population of values with a mean of zero and a standard deviation of 0.008. This standard deviation was typical of the experimental uncertainty observed in values of $R_{B/T}$ of about 0.5, and was used rather than the imprecise estimate (with only three degrees of freedom) derived from the residual variance shown in Table 4.1.

DESIGN then re-analysed the data, including the new point, to produce a recommendation for a further experiment, this time at a total ligand concentration of 334 nmol/litre. This process was repeated until a total of twenty points was collected. These are shown in Fig. 4.2, together with curves representing the final, fitted models.

Before comparing the sequential procedure with the conventional one, confidence in the likelihood ratios obtained on the addition of each "experimental" point were increased by replication. Thus, the whole process was repeated four times to give a total of five sets of simulations. The five likelihood ratios at each experimental point were meaned, and the sample standard deviations of the means were calculated. Then, five more series of simulations were made in which each new point was added at randomly selected, rather than designed, levels of ligand concentration, and means were calculated as before. The selections were made from the list of original concentrations, just as experiments are usually replicated in the laboratory. All ratios, expressed as logarithms for convenience, are shown in Fig. 4.3 as a function of experiment number.

It can be seen clearly that while the sequential procedure chose the correct model with a confidence of 95 percent after adding nine extra "experimental" points to the original data, random replication failed to do so. This was because determinations were not made in the crucial parts of the experimental frame, but distributed ineffectively over the whole range of x. Thus, by carrying out sequences of experiments suggested by the design procedure, it should be possible to determine low concentrations of the pregnancy-specific transport protein in the presence of an excess of CBG, with the minimum of time, materials and effort.

Having demonstrated the ability of the sequential approach to select the correct model, "experimentation" was continued under the direction of the $T(x)$ criterion to increase the precision of the parameter estimates. At the beginning of this stage of the process, with a total of twenty points already "measured", the percentage coefficients of variance (%CV) in the five parameters were 124, 165, 61, 20 and 2.1, respectively. Because the SBG was present in very small amounts relative to the CBG, the two parameters associated with it were estimated with the least precision. After a further ten points were added under the direction of the sequential design for parameter estimation, with the same constant "experimental" error rate of 0.008, the %CV for each parameter was 85, 79, 29, 22 and 2.8, respectively. When ten extra points were "measured" at testosterone concentrations chosen randomly, values of 97, 108, 33, 25 and 3.0 were obtained.

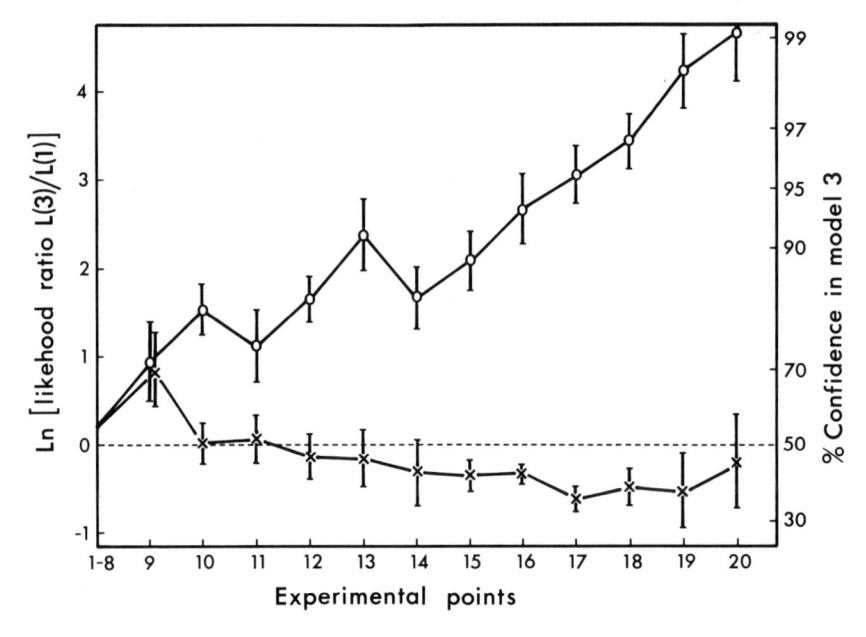

Fig. 4.3. The logarithms of the likelihood ratios of the two most likely models fitted to data from Monte Carlo simulations of equilibrium dialysis experiments. The results of sequentially designed (○) and randomly replicated (×) simulated experiments are expressed as a function of the increasing number of experiments. The *error bars* represent sample standard deviations of the means of five values

Thus, it was possible to show by Monte Carlo simulation that SBG early in pregnancy could only be determined by equilibrium dialysis with testosterone if sequentially designed experiments were performed. It is hoped that this technique will be seriously investigated and evaluated in the future because it appears to be capable of contributing greatly to many investigations in the biological sciences.

It may sometimes be impossible to perform a series of experiments on biological samples over an extended period of time because of deterioration. In this case, sequential design can be used in a preliminary investigation to indicate those parts of the experimental frame in which experimentation should subsequently be concentrated, so as to obtain the best results.

5 Dynamic Systems: Clearance and Compartmental Analysis

This chapter deals with methods of using tracers to analyse the dynamic behaviours of systems in terms of compartments. Modelling the response of a system to the administration of a drug can be done in the same way. We stress the advantages of the computer in comparing models composed of differential equations, and in estimating their parameters. The approach is practical rather than theoretical.

The theory of the subject is presented by many authors; especially recommended are the books by Sheppard (1962), Atkins (1969), Shipley and Clark (1972), Jacquez (1972) and, for a specifically endocrinological point of view, that by Gurpide (1975). The review by Rescigno and Beck (1972) is also interesting. However none of these texts makes more than passing reference to computer methods. Instead, the Laplace transform approach is used to integrate analytically the differential equations of dynamic models.

Here we wish to emphasize the value of the computer in fitting models and carrying out numerical integration by illustrating the methods developed in Chap. 3 and 4. The ability of the computer to integrate differential equations numerically removes many restrictions on the forms of models imposed by analytical integration.

Our examples begin with the subject of clearance and continue with the more comprehensive technique of compartmental analysis. Because it is impossible in the space available to deal with every model of potential interest we have concentrated on several which illustrate the numerical approach, and thus should prove useful to others embarking on similar studies.

5.1 Clearance

The clearance rate, or speed with which a substance is removed from a tissue such as the blood, was introduced into endocrinology as a practical measure of the rate of metabolism of hormones by Tait et al. (1962), and developed further by Tait and Burstein (1964). Gurpide and Mann (1970) provide a short introductory review. DiStefano (1976) has drawn attention to some common misconceptions and summarized current concepts.

A quantitative measure of clearance rates is important in helping to understand the time course (dynamics) of the effects of hormones or drugs on biological tissues. The clearance rate is an important factor in determining the biological potency of a hormone. Without a measure of clearance it would be difficult to interpret the results of most bio-assays.

The irreversible *clearance rate* of a substance from a compartment (defined in Sect. 5.2) is the size (in terms of either volume or mass) of the compartment from which the substance would be *completely* cleared in unit time. In reality, of course, material is lost evently from the whole of the compartment. An equivalent definition of clearance is the rate of removal of the substance from the compartment per unit of its concentration in the compartment. That is

$$\text{clearance} = (dQ_t/dt)/c_t \tag{5.1}$$

where dQ_t/dt is the rate of removal, and c_t the concentration of the substance at time t. A convenient measure of the irreversible loss from the blood plasma of a hormone or drug is the *plasma clearance rate*. This is an especially appropriate definition in endocrinological experimentation.

In the steady state (Sect. 2.1.2 and introduction to Sect. 5.2), the *secretion* or *production rate* of a hormone equals the clearance rate. That is

$$SR_s = (PCR_s)c_s \tag{5.2}$$

where SR_s is the secretion rate in units of (mass/time), PCR_s is the plasma clearance rate with units of (vol/time) (sometimes known as *metabolic clearance rate*) and c_s is the concentration of the substance (e. g. a hormone) (mass/vol), all under the steady state condition.

Plasma clearance rates can be measured experimentally either by infusing a known amount of tracer at a constant rate, or, less reliably, by giving a bolus injection (impulse dose) of tracer. The material infused or injected may be a tracer for an endogenous hormone or a drug.

The simplest way in which to estimate the plasma clearance rate after a bolus injection of tracer is to use the *Stewart-Hamilton equation*, derivations of which will be found in the references already cited. This equation states that the plasma clearance rate equals the dose administered, divided by the area beneath the curve describing its subsequent concentration in the blood plasma. This area is calculated between the time of injection and infinite time. Regrettably, significant error may be introduced by truncating the curve even when the concentration has diminished to a small fraction of its original value. A critical survey of the concepts of both production and clearance rates is given at the end of the article by DiStefano (1976). He also emphasizes that analysis by means of this equation assumes that hormone is secreted *directly* into the plasma, and does not enter the plasma from compartments outisde it.

5.1.1 Clearance of PMSG from the Blood

Calculation of clearance rates will be illustrated by an experiment on the clearance of pregnant mare serum gonadotrophin (PMSG) from the blood plasma of sheep (McIntosh et al., 1974). This investigation was part of a study of the effect of PMSG on the development of sheep ovarian follicles (Moor et al., 1973).

Five ewes were injected intravenously with 19,000 or 38,000 iu of a commercial preparation of PMSG. Blood samples were withdrawn at a series of time intervals after injection and the concentration of PMSG in the serum of each sample was determined.

Results from one sheep are shown in Fig. 5.1. The relatively rapid initial decrease suggests more than one removal process. An empirical model has already been fitted to the data of this experiment as an example of the use of the program MODFIT

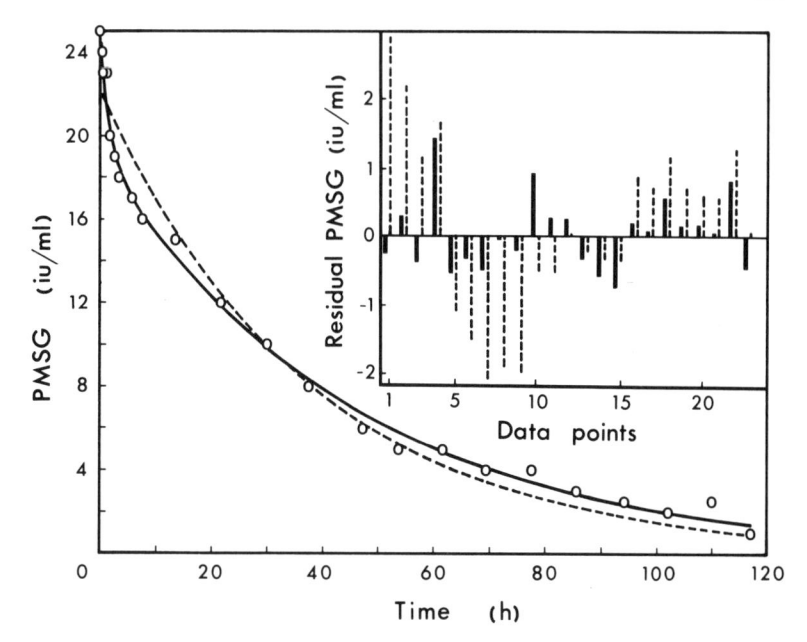

Fig. 5.1. Time course of the disappearance of an intravenous injection of PMSG from the blood plasma of a sheep. The *points*, representing concentrations of PMSG, are from a replicate assay of plasma samples taken from Sheep 2 of McIntosh et al. (1974). The *solid curve* represents a fitted double exponential decay model, the *broken* curve a single decay only; details are given in Sect. 3.7.1. The *insert* shows the residuals for both models at each data point. Trends are clearly visible in the residuals about the single decay model (*broken lines*), which provided an inferior description of the data. The progress of the fit is shown in Table 3.1

(Sect. 3.7.1). This model, consisting of the sum of two exponential terms, provided a satisfactory description of the data. It was

$$[PMSG]_t = A_1 \exp(-A_2 t) + A_3 \exp(-A_4 t) \tag{5.3}$$

where $[PMSG]_t$ is the concentration of PMSG (iu/ml serum) at time t (h) and A_1 to A_4 are parameters optimized so as to obtain the best fit to the data. The progress of the fit is shown in Table 3.1.

The aim of the experiments was to discover how long the PMSG remained in the blood because its presence there could influence the development of the ovarian follicles. The plasma clearance rate (referred to by McIntosh et al., 1974, as the metabolic clearance rate) was therefore estimated. The following form of the Stewart-Hamilton equation provided the required measure

$$PCR = D/(\int_0^\infty [PMSG]_t dt) \tag{5.4}$$

where PCR is the plasma clearance rate (ml/h), D is the dose of PMSG administered and $\int_0^\infty [PMSG]_t dt$ is the integral or area beneath the the concentration-time curve of Fig. 5.1, extended to infinite time.

This integral could be measured by cutting out and weighing a paper tracing of the area under the curve and comparing its mass with that of a sample of the same paper of known area. In this case, the error caused by truncating the curve at 120 h is probably minor. Preferably, however, the area is estimated by integrating Eq. (5.3) analytically. The integral, or area beneath the curve from times zero to infinity equals $A_1/A_2 + A_3/A_4$. This calculation includes an invisible portion beyond 120 h by assuming that the tail of the curve decays according to Eq. (5.3). This assumption might well introduce a significant error but does not, in the present example, invalidate the conclusions.

A prerequisite for obtaining reliable results is that the clearance rate be independent of the amount of drug injected. That is, the system must respond linearly. In the present example two doses of hormone yielded the same clearance rate, so that it is reasonable to assume that the behaviour of the system was linear over this range of concentrations. (For example, the physiological mechanism of clearance might have become less effective at higher doses owing to saturation effects.) Because of the linearity it was possible to combine results measured at different levels of injected PMSG.

The values of PCR for the five sheep gave a weighted mean of (37.8 ± 1.6) ml/h, where the uncertainty is expressed as the sample standard deviation in the mean. This PCR is very low in comparison with those of other hormones in sheep having similar actions, namely luteinizing hormone (LH; 2899 ml/h) and follicle stimulating hormone (FSH; 1440 ml/h) (Akbar et al., 1974). The difference is almost certainly due to the large content of sialic acid in PMSG.

This difference in clearance rates accounts for anomalous observations on the potencies of the gonadotrophins. The potency of PMSG is high relative to FSH in the rat prostate assay in which the response develops over three days. PMSG is present at effective levels in the circulation for most of this time whereas FSH is removed rapidly. Conversely, an equal amount of PMSG is relatively less potent in the ovarian ascorbic acid depletion assay which is complete in a few hours. This is because the slower clearance rate of the PMSG gives it no significant "advantage" over FSH in the short term.

More information about the characteristics of the processes governing the removal of PMSG from the circulation may be able to be derived from this kind of experiment. One, simple physical model yielding the mathematical relationship represented by Eq. (5.3), is illustrated in Fig. 5.2. The rate constants k_{21} and k_{12}

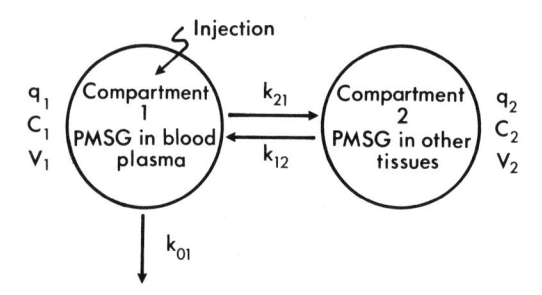

Fig. 5.2. A tentative physical model to describe the behaviour of PMSG after injection into the blood stream of a sheep. The symbols q represent the amounts, and c the concentrations, of PMSG in compartments with volumes V. The symbols k represent rate constants of transfer, k_{01} referring to the irreversible loss or disposal of PMSG from the system. PMSG is assumed to be injected into *compartment 1* at time zero. *Compartment 2* represents all pools with which PMSG exchanges lumped together

summarize the exchange of PMSG between blood and other tissues and k_{01} is the rate constant of disposal or irreversible loss from the system. In this model it is the value of k_{01} in which we are particularly interested when investigating the clearance of PMSG from the circulation.

This model makes several assumptions and grossly simplifies physiological conditions. For instance, PMSG probably passes into a number of tissues and we are assuming that these processes of exchange can be summarized by one pair of rate constants. One or more tissues (such as the liver) may contribute both to this exchange and to the irreversible loss by degradation of PMSG from the blood stream. These possibilities should be tested experimentally and several models advanced for comparison. The one suggested serves simply as a useful illustration.

The value of k_{01} can be calculated immediately. An estimate of the total volume of serum into which the PMSG was injected, V_{inj}, is equal to the dose administered divided by the sum of the parameters A_1 and A_3 (which together equal the concentration of PMSG in the serum at time zero). Then

$$k_{01} = PCR/V_{inj}. \tag{5.5}$$

The time taken for half the current quantity of PMSG in the blood stream to be cleared, the *half-time* of disposal, is given by

$$t_{1/2D} = \ln(2)/k_{01}. \tag{5.6}$$

The potential hazard in estimating V_{inj} by extrapolating the fitted curve to zero time in a system consisting of more than one compartment must be taken into account. If there were another unseen compartment, exchange with which was very rapid and partially completed before the first measurement, the calculated value of V_{inj} would be erroneously large. In the present example there is no evidence for such a compartment but its existence cannot be ruled out. For this reason it is very important to begin sampling as soon as possible after the complete mixing which is assumed to follow injection. Note that invisible, rapidly exchanging compartments are relevant particularly to the calculation of k_{01} (which depends on V_{inj}). Estimation of the PCR using the Stewart-Hamilton equation is less likely to be invalidated significantly because the presence of a compartment exchanging very rapidly will contribute a relatively small portion to the total area under the curve.

Values of V_{inj} for the five sheep ranged from 1.02 litre to 1.37 litre of serum and the weighted mean values of k_{01} and $t_{1/2D}$ were (0.0315 ± 0.0016) h^{-1} and (21.2 ± 1.1) h, respectively, where the uncertainty is expressed as the sample standard deviation in the mean.

In summary, a simple clearance curve usually provides enough information for estimating the clearance rate, the production rate, the volume of initial distribution, and the rate constant of irreversible loss. By extending the experiments, more details could be obtained. For example, if samples of another tissue were taken at various time intervals and the concentration of PMSG in these were determined, it would be possible by means of compartmental analysis to determine the rate constants of exchange of PMSG with this second tissue. Estimates of exchange rates with peripheral compartments can sometimes be obtained even in the absence of experimental observations on those compartments (Sect. 5.2.4).

5.2 Compartmental Analysis

Compartmental analysis is the description of a dynamic system by a simplified physical model consisting of a small number of separate *compartments* or "quantities of a substance having uniform and distinguishable kinetics of transformation or transport" (Atkins, 1969) "each of which is homogeneous and well mixed, and ... interacts by exchanging material" (Jacquez, 1972). The analysis consists of (1) determining the rates at which material moves between the compartments and often (2) the sizes of the compartments.

The term compartment can mean either of two things. It may be used to describe a distinguishable dynamic behaviour of a chemical species. Any species may exhibit more than one form of kinetic behaviour and so require more than one compartment for its description. In addition, compartments may (but not necessarily) correspond to physiologically distinct regions. While compartmental models satisfy in some respects the definition of analytical models, the mechanisms responsible for the dynamics are often not identifiable. A compartmental model is an elaborate, but essentially empirical representation of reality. In many cases the physical constraints which form the compartments cannot be established. Nevertheless, such models can be very useful for describing quantitatively in a simplified manner the inhomogeneous behaviour of substances diffusing linearly between tissues (Sect. 2.1.5).

Most analyses are done on systems that are in, or assumed to be in, the steady state. This means that the amount of a substance in the compartments of interest in a system is constant. At the same time, material enters and leaves each compartment — it is a dynamic, open system. But the inflow equals the outflow; there is no net change in concentration. A steady state is reached in an open system when input is constant. Alteration in the rate of input causes transient changes in the system, to which compartmental analysis cannot be applied simply. By contrast, a closed system is one in which there is no communication of material with the outside environment: a closed system exchanging no energy with the environment is expected to reach *dynamic equilibrium* and is not usually found in biology (Sects. 2.1.2 and 2.4).

Direct measurements of the concentrations of substances in unperturbed dynamic systems will yield constant values characteristic of the steady state. To visualize the continual movement and exchange which underlies this apparently tranquil exterior we must inject a tracer into the system at a suitable point. The ideal *tracer* cannot be distinguished by the system from the substance being traced; it is the kinetic behaviour of the tracer as it is distributed among compartments by the invisible flow of traced substance that reveals the characteristics of the system. The most generally useful tracers are radioactively labelled atoms or molecules.

Compartmental analysis is not limited to tracer experiments. The same approach can be applied to the movement of a drug or substance which is foreign to the body and for which a steady state does not exist. In this case, however, the system is perturbed and must be shown to respond linearly, as is explained above for clearance rates.

The particular advantage of a tracer, however, is that the kinetics of its distribution in a non-linear system *in the steady state* can be described by linear differential equations. This means that methods such as Laplace transforms are suitable for integrating these equations. The integration of tracer kinetic equations of non-linear systems not in the steady state can usually only be done by numerical computer methods. It is necessary to assume that both the substance of interest and its tracer are instantaneously and perfectly mixed throughout each compartment, and that the mass of tracer added is negligible in comparison with the amount of material being investigated.

Certain other terms must be defined. The rate constant characterizes the movement of a substance from one compartment to another. Rate constants appear in all differential equations involved in mathematical models of dynamic systems. The *rate constant* (with units of [time^{-1}]) of the movement of a substance from one compartment to another is the fractional loss from that compartment per unit time. A rate constant of 0.5 min^{-1} means that an amount of substance equal to half that contained in the compartment is transported every minute.

The *turnover time* (time) of a compartment is the reciprocal of the rate constant of transport *out* of that compartment. It is the time required for the passage of an amount of a substance equal to the total in the compartment to move in one direction across its boundaries.

The *flux* (mass/time) of a substance out of a compartment is the amount passing the boundary in unit time (as opposed to the fractional loss given by the rate constant). In the steady state the flux out of a compartment is matched by an equal flux into it.

The term *half-life* or *half-time* is not informative when applied to two-way exchange and is best confined to describing irreversible loss as in measurements of clearance. It means the time needed for half of the material to be lost from a compartment, but this information is already contained in the more general concept of turnover time. Half-lives are sometimes incorrectly calculated from the exponential parameters of models such as Eq. (5.3).

The above is merely an introduction to the terms of compartmental analysis. It is essential to become familiar with the concepts, methods and general conclusions of the subject before embarking on any dynamic experiments. The basic concepts are very simple but without the help of a computer the mathematical manipulations required to accurately and precisely estimate the underlying parameters are complicated and tedious.

The simple approaches described below, couched in terms of linear differential equations with constant coefficients (rate constants) and suitable for describing gross relationships in the short term, are inadequate when applied to lengthier experiments on more complex systems. Extensions in which rate constants are permitted to vary periodically, have stochastic elements, or be part of some control system are discussed by Jacquez (1972, Chaps. 9–12, 14). The greater complexity thus introduced inevitably adds extra parameters which require, for their estimation, the collection of many more data points.

Even when dealing with the simplest linear analyses, however, it can be very difficult to select a unique physical compartmental model to describe tracer measurements in the presence of even slight experimental uncertainty (see, for example, Brown and Godfrey, 1978). This is due in part to the problems of analysing processes of exponential decay discussed in Sect. 3.5.8.1.

Before experiments are begun, proposed physical compartmental models should be examined to determine whether the possibility logically exists of estimating all the unknown parameters from the planned tracer studies. This process is known as *identifiability analysis* (see, for example, Bellman and Åström, 1970; Corbelli and Romanin-Jacur, 1976; Corbelli et al., 1977).

5.2.1 Writing Equations to Describe Dynamic Systems

Rates of change should be expressed as differential equations rather than in terms of the absolute values of experimental data (Sect. 2.1.1). In fact, it is very much easier to describe a complex model in terms of differential equations than to carry out the integration necessary to make them compatible with experimental data.

Integration can be analytical, in which a generalized algebraic (integrated) equation is produced from a differential equation, or numerical, where real values (of parameters and independent variables) are first substituted in the differential equation and approximate (but arbitrarily precise) summing methods are then applied (Sect. 3.6). We shall illustrate both approaches. Analytical integration is the method of choice in most texts on compartmental analysis — our concern is to show the strengths of the numerical approach feasible only with the use of a computer.

To introduce the principles of writing differential equations to describe compartmental systems, we shall consider a simple model consisting of a single compartment (Fig. 5.3). The amount of the substance of interest in the compartment is Q_1, and that of the radioactive tracer injected is q_1. Thus the substance in the compartment has a specific radioactivity of $a_1 = q_1/Q_1$ at time zero, the instant of injection. Thereafter, the specific radioactivity decreases as both labelled and unlabelled material leaves the compartment and unlabelled substance enters.

It can usually be verified experimentally that the kinetics of tracer (or drug) loss from a compartment follows a first order law. (If the physiological mechanism of movement is related to simple diffusion then this result is predicted theoretically.) This implies that the *rate* of loss of tracer from a compartment is proportional to the *concentration* of tracer therein. The concentration may be expressed in terms of the amount of tracer per unit mass or volume of the compartment, but it is more convenient and illuminating to use the amount of tracer per unit mass of the substance being traced, i.e. the *specific activity*. This is because the specific activity of the traced material is the driving force behind the movement of tracer from one compartment to another: the system behaves as if it is seeking to equalize the specific activity throughout. It is sometimes appropriate to write equations in terms

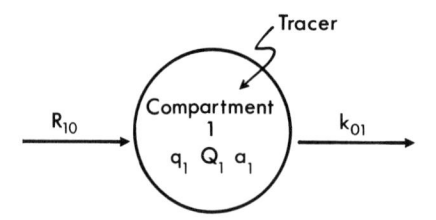

Fig. 5.3. A physical model representing a system consisting of a single compartment. R_{10} is the rate of flow of a substance into the compartment which, in the steady state, equals $k_{01}Q_1$, the rate of outflow. Q_1 is the total amount of the substance in the compartment, q_1 is the amount of tracer injected, and a_1 is the specific activity of the substance, which is equal to q_1/Q_1

of a fraction of the dose of tracer or drug rather than concentration; an example will be found in Sect. 5.2.4.

The rate law is always expressed as a differential equation of the form (with reference to Fig. 5.3)

$$dQ_1/dt = R_{10} - k_{01}Q_1 \tag{5.7}$$

where R_{10} is the flux into, and $k_{01}Q_1$ is the flux out of, the compartment. In the steady state the rate of change of Q_1 with time, dQ_1/dt, is zero so that $R_{10} = k_{01}Q_1$; input and output rates are equal. If tracer is administered to the compartment at time $t = 0$ then

$$dq_1/dt = k_{01}q_1 \tag{5.8}$$

where dq_1/dt is the instantaneous rate of change of q_1 and k_{01} is a proportionality constant which is, of course, the rate constant.

This equation is easily written in terms of specific activities (using the relation $a = q/Q$)

$$da_1/dt = k_{01}a_1. \tag{5.9}$$

Because Q_1 is a constant, it cannot be differentiated and is divided out.

This simple process is applicable to systems of interconnecting compartments of any complexity. One differential equation is written for each compartment in terms of all entries and exits. Examples will be found in Sects. 5.2.3 and 5.2.4.

5.2.2 Hormonal Influence on Zinc Transport in Rabbit Tissues

Now let us turn to a specific example which we shall use in the following sections to illustrate both analytical and numerical methods. Compartmental analysis is applied to measurements of the kinetics of zinc exchange between the blood plasma and certain tissues of the reproductive tract of female rabbits. Zinc is an important factor determining the success of pregnancy. Preliminary experiments showed that its uptake by certain tissues was under the influence of hormones. We wished to determine how the uptake of zinc varied at different stages of gestation (McIntosh and Lutwak-Mann, 1972 a).

This system is relatively simple to analyse, first because tissues must all derive zinc from the diet by way of the blood stream, and secondly because, unlike organic molecules, elements cannot be metabolized or otherwise transformed while in the body.

Non-pregnant and pregnant rabbits were injected with radioactively labelled zinc (^{65}Zn) and the following tissues, as available at a given reproductive stage, were analysed for the labelled zinc; blood plasma, endometrium, placental tissues, fetus, ovarian interstitial tissue, corpora lutea, liver, peritoneal fluid, oestrous uterine fluid, blastocyst fluid and fetal fluids. The animals were killed at 25 or 45 min, or 4, 16 or 48 h after injection and the tissues were removed. Measurements of radioactivity and total zinc were used to calculate specific activities, which were expressed as ratios by the method described in the report.

As examples, we shall analyse the way in which exchange of zinc occurred between (1) the blood plasma and endometrium of non-pregnant animals, and (2) the blood plasma and luteal tissue of five-day pregnant animals.

The abilities of three different physical models to fit the experimental data will be examined. These models are shown in Fig. 5.4. In model (a) a tissue (compartment 2) exchanges material reversibly with blood plasma (compartment 1). In models (b) and (c) a tissue is represented as having two compartments, both (or only one) of which independently exchange material with the plasma. Compartments 2 and 3 are in the same tissue and cannot be sampled separately. Instead, a combined specific activity is measured and the compartments are separated mathematically in the description of the model. Irreversible loss is assumed to occur only from the blood stream. Blood plasma represents a resevoir of labelled zinc, and is assumed to be the

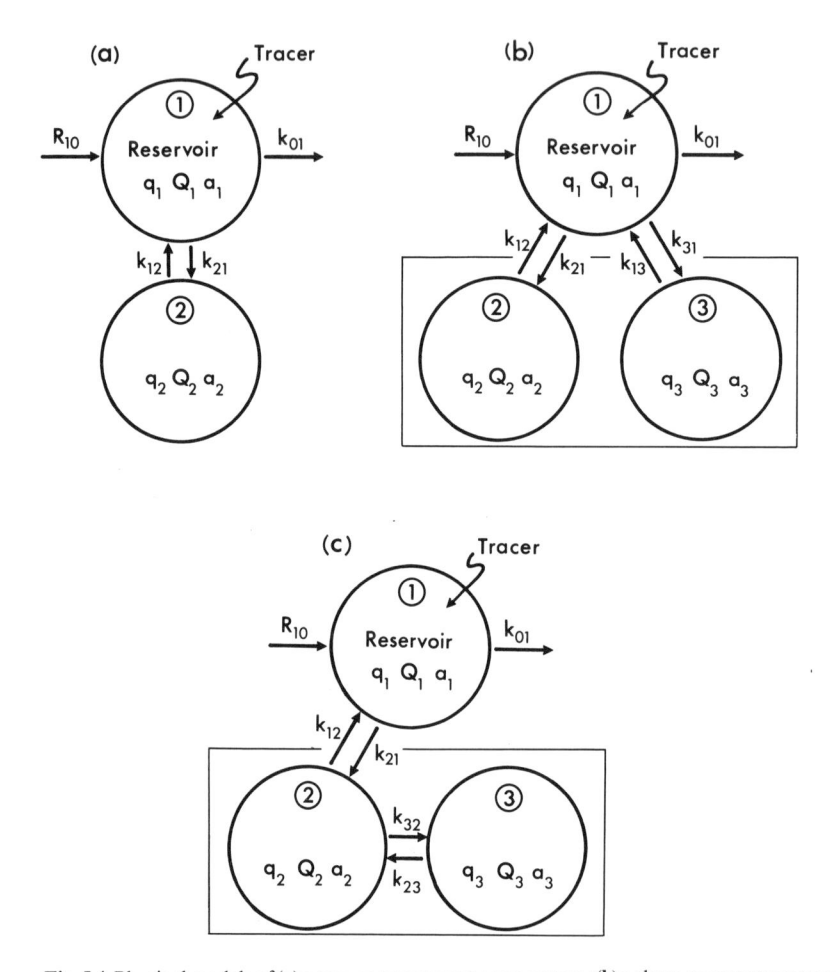

Fig. 5.4. Physical models of **(a)** a two-compartment open system; **(b)** a three-compartment open system in which two compartments each exchange a substance with the reservoir (parallel configuration); **(c)** a three-compartment open system in which *compartment 2* exchanges a substance with both the reservoir and *compartment 3* (serial configuration). There is no direct disposal from *compartments 2* or *3*. Tracer, q, is added to *compartment 1*. Q is the total amount of the substance in each compartment, and a is its specific activity at time t. The flux of the substance into the system is represented by R_{10}. Compartments 2 and 3 are enclosed to indicate that they are physically situated in the same tissue and are sampled together

only path by which zinc is transported to other tissues. Parameters Q_1 and either Q_2 [model (a)] or the sum of Q_2 and Q_3 [models (b) or (c)] were measured independently in other experiments. Thus the parameters to be determined from the tracer experiments were the rate constants governing the exchange processes between blood plasma and the tissue examined and, in models (b) and (c), the ratio of the sizes of the two peripheral compartments.

5.2.2.1 Analytical Integration: Two Compartments

The first experimental results to be analysed are shown in Fig. 5.5 as a graph of the specific radioactivity of zinc measured in blood plasma and endometrium at the five time intervals after injection of tracer. It can be seen that the specific radioactivity of zinc in the blood plasma was maximal soon after injection, declining fast as ^{65}Zn distributed throughout the tissues and then more slowly as it was excreted. The endometrium absorbed tracer zinc from the blood rapidly at first, and then more slowly until the specific radioactivities in the two tissues were comparable. Thereafter, the endometrial activity decreased slowly, lagging behind the level in the blood plasma. From the relative positions of the data points it was possible to predict, by means of the Zilversmit criterion (Zilversmit et al., 1943; Solomon, 1960; Atkins, 1969), that the two-compartment model was likely to yield a satisfactory fit to these measurements. Accordingly, equations were devised to represent model (a) of Fig. 5.4. This mathematical model also is described by Solomon (1960, pp. 132–137) with reference to an example on the uptake of phosphorus by phospholipids.

Because the specific radioactivity of the blood plasma is controlled mainly by many indeterminate exchange processes (the parameters of which are of no interest), its decrease with time cannot be described theoretically but is fitted instead by an empirical equation. This equation, known as a forcing function, is then used as input for modelling the endometrial exchange in terms of the physical parameter k_{12}, an estimate of which is the aim of the investigation. Thus the fitting is done in two stages. Use of forcing functions saves estimating too many parameters simultaneously, and is a common device (DiStefano et al., 1975). However, the uncertainties in the plasma parameter estimates cannot be transferred to the second stage and consequently must be ignored. This means that parameter uncertainties in the second stage are underestimated.

The function which is most convenient to fit to the plasma data, and which has some physical basis, consists of a sum of exponential decay terms [Eq. (5.3)]. This model is embodied in FUNCTN subprogram RESERVR (Sect. 11.3). A function composed of the sum of two exponential terms was found to be necessary and sufficient to describe the disappearance of labelled zinc from the blood plasma of rabbits between 25 min and 48 h after injection. The progress of the fit and the estimated values of the four parameters are shown in Table 5.1, and the fitted curve in Fig. 5.5. No attempt has been made to associate any physical process with the four parameters; the fitted function is nothing more than a mathematical description of the curve.

The next step is to fit the second part of the model to the data from the endometrial tissue of non-pregnant animals. An equation describing the variation with time of the specific activity of tracer in compartment 2 of model (a) (Fig. 5.4) is derived in Sect. 5.2.3.1 and integrated in Appendix C as an illustration of the application of Laplace transforms. This equation is in terms of the empirical

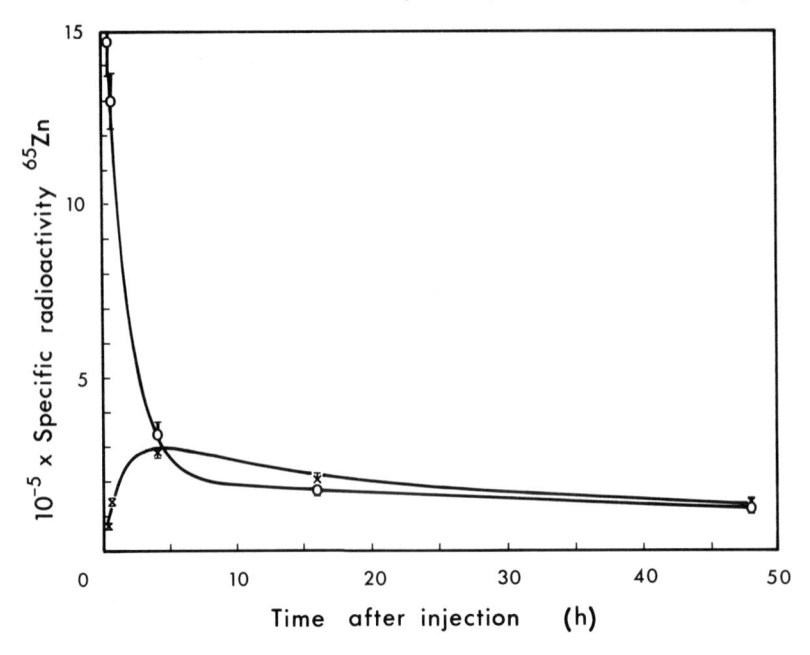

Fig. 5.5. The specific radioactivity of blood plasma (○) and endometrium (×) of rabbits as a function of time after injection of ^{65}Zn. The *bars* represent the sample standard deviations in the means of determinations made on samples from between five and eight animals. The *smooth curves* show the results of fitting the model equations described in the text. The progress of the fits are shown in Tables 5.1 and 5.2

coefficients describing the disappearance of tracer from the blood plasma, and k_{12}, the rate constant of transfer of zinc from the observed peripheral compartment to the reservoir. A generalized form of the integrated equation suitable for use with a forcing function having any number of exponential terms is embodied in FUNCTN subprogram CA1, a listing of which appears in Sect. 11.8. This model is thus the result of analytical integration of a differential equation. Unless an integrated form or solution is available or obtainable by the standard methods, this approach cannot be used.

It will be seen (Table 5.2) that the input to subprogram CA1 consisted of the experimental data and the four parameter estimates of the plasma disappearance curve shown in Table 5.1. The output was the estimate of the single parameter k_{12}, the rate constant of transfer of zinc from the endometrial tissue to the blood plasma.

The turnover time of zinc in the endometrium (compartment 2) was thus $1/0.122 = 8.20$ h and the uncertainty was $8.20 \times 0.00678 / 0.122 = 0.46$ h [Eq. (10.10)]. The flux of zinc from the endometrium to the blood plasma, which equalled the flux in the opposite direction (as a consequence of the steady state), was obtained by multiplying the rate constant by the size of the compartment (McIntosh and Lutwak-Mann, 1972 a). That is, flux $= (0.122 \pm 0.00678) \times (9.60 \pm 0.30) = 0.122 \times 9.6 \pm [(0.00678 / 0.122)^2 + (0.3 / 9.6)^2]^{1/2} \times 0.122 \times 9.6 = (1.17 \pm 0.07)$ µg zinc transported to or from the compartment/h g fresh wt tissue, where the uncertainty is expressed as the sample standard deviation of the mean. The results differ slightly

Compartmental Analysis

Table 5.1. An empirical exponential decay model[a]

R CHI SQUARE	A 1	A 2	A 3	A 4
15.677	1700.0	.63000	240.00	.10000E-01
.42000	1687.9	.62928	212.52	.12010E-01
.37936	1687.8	.62964	212.87	.12430E-01
.37935	1687.7	.62963	212.87	.12433E-01
.37935	1687.7	.62963	212.87	.12433E-01
STD DEVS	128.19	.80958E-01	22.904	.37569E-02
	7.6%	12.9%	10.8%	30.2%
DEPENDENCIES	.87594	.89907	.94513	.93780

CONDITION NUMBER   68407.0

CORRELATION COEFFICIENTS
```
         A 1   1.0000
         A 2    .64587     1.0000
         A 3    .12560E-01  .43050     1.0000
         A 4   -.54711E-03  .35248     .86639     1.0000
```

MODE = 1, DEGREES OF FREEDOM = 1
FINAL LAMBDA =   .0000010000000000

X	Y	YFIT	RESIDUAL	Z-RESIDUAL	SIGMAY
.41670	1470.0	1510.0	-40.025	-.40025	100.00
.75000	1300.0	1263.4	36.608	.44644	82.000
4.0000	334.00	338.54	-4.5405	-.13355	34.000
16.000	175.00	174.54	.45696	.41542E-01	11.000
48.000	117.00	117.20	-.20140	-.16783E-01	12.000

[a] Fitted to the disappearance of the specific radioactivity of zinc from the blood plasma of non-pregnant rabbits after injection of ^{65}Zn. FUNCTN subprogram RESERVR together with MODFIT was used, with NTERMS = 4. Compare the results with Table 1 of McIntosh and Lutwak-Mann (1972 a) where an unnecessary constant was included. Notice that although there was no evidence of parameter interaction from the dependencies or correlations, the high condition number showed that the data were insufficient to support four parameters.

from those in the original report because of the inclusion here of data from extra animals.

While this experiment could not have been done in any other way, it is, nevertheless, unwise to estimate parameters from the time-course of tracer distribution formed by joining points obtained from experiments on different animals. The better way is always, if possible, to follow the whole time-course in a single animal and to estimate the parameters from this, combining the estimates from replicate animals to examine the population distribution of values. Jacquez (1972, pp. 119–120) discusses the reasons for this.

5.2.2.2 Analytical Integration: Three Compartments

When the two-compartment model is insufficient to describe the experimental data it is necessary to use a more complex model. This was the case for the luteal tissue of six-day pregnant animals, the experimental results for which are shown in Fig. 5.6. Unlike the previous data the specific radioactivity in the luteal tissue reached a maximum value and began to decline before all its zinc had equilibrated with that of the plasma reservoir. This indicated that a relatively fast-exchanging compartment of zinc in the luteal tissue had reached equilibrium with the blood plasma but that

Table 5.2. Model (a) of Fig. 5.4 fitted to data on the exchange of zinc between blood plasma and endometrial tissue from non-pregnant rabbits[a]

```
R CHI SQUARE         A 1
-------------------------
CA1 - RESERVOIR PARAMETERS:
MULTIPLIER     EXPONENTIAL
  1687.7         .62963
   212.87        .12433E-01

-------------------------
  3.8740         .10000
  1.1600         .12037
  1.1483         .12181
  1.1483         .12185
  1.1483         .12185

STD DEVS         .67834E-02
                 5.6%

DEPENDENCIES   0.

CONDITION NUMBER      0.0

CORRELATION COEFFICIENTS
        A 1   1.0000

MODE =  1, DEGREES OF FREEDOM =   4
FINAL LAMBDA =    .0000010000000000

     X            Y          YFIT       RESIDUAL     Z-RESIDUAL      SIGMAY
   .41670       76.000       83.923      -7.9227       -.79227       10.000
   .75000      160.00       135.57       24.432       1.7451         14.000
  4.0000       285.00       296.07      -11.075        -.69217       16.000
 16.000        209.00       218.18       -9.1801       -.43715       21.000
 48.000        140.00       131.00        8.9966        .49981       18.000
```

[a] FUNCTN subprogram CA1 together with MODFIT was used, with NTERMS = 1. The fitted model is shown in Fig. 5.5. Both the dependency and condition number were zero because there was one parameter only. The value of reduced chi-square was close to 1, indicating that the model provided a plausible description of the experimental data.

there was also a "slow" compartment, containing little tracer at this stage, which lowered the specific radioactivity sampled from the whole tissue.

Integrated equations were derived from differential ones describing model (b) of Fig. 5.4 by a process of analytical integration similar to that described in Appendix C for the two-compartment case. Alternatively, the equivalent equations (42a) and (42b) provided by Solomon (1960) are suitable. These integrated equations are also embodied in FUNCTN subprogram CA1 (Sect. 11.8) and are invoked by setting NTERMS to 3. Two of the parameters to be estimated are the return rate constants (k_{12} and k_{13}) from the two luteal zinc compartments, while the third is the fractional size of compartment 2.

When MODFIT and CA1 were applied to the data for the luteal tissue the results in Table 5.3 were obtained. While clearly superior to the two-compartment model in describing these data, the three-compartment parallel configuration was not entirely adequate, as shown by the high value of reduced chi-square. Model (c) of Fig. 5.4 was no more satisfactory (as is described in Sect. 5.2.3.3). A possible explanation is that in this fast-developing tissue a steady state was not maintained.

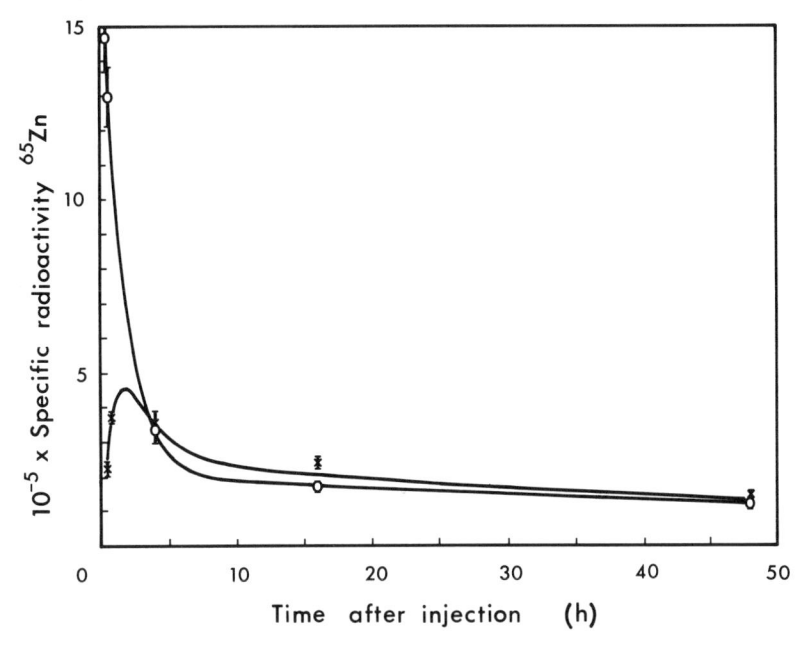

Fig. 5.6. The specific radioactivity of blood plasma (○) and luteal tissue (×) from six-day pregnant rabbits as a function of time after injection of ^{65}Zn. The *bars* represent the sample standard deviations in the means of determinations made on samples from between five and eight animals. The *smooth curves* show the results of fitting the model equations described in the text. The progress of the fits are shown in Tables 5.1 and 5.3

Very much more data would be required to extend the analysis to a more complex model incorporating transient (non-steady state) behaviour. In terms of model (b), therefore, the turnover time of compartment 2 was (1.08 ± 0.66) h, of compartment 3 (9.3 ± 6.2) h, and the fractional relative sizes of the two compartments were 0.37 ± 0.24 and 0.63 ± 0.24, respectively, where the uncertainties are expressed as sample standard deviations of the means. These latter fractional sizes, when multiplied by the total zinc concentration in the tissue (McIntosh and Lutwak-Mann, 1972a) yielded the sizes of the compartments as (4.3 ± 2.8) and (7.3 ± 2.8) μg zinc/g fresh wt tissue. The products of the estimated rate constants k_{12} and k_{13} (parameters A1 and A2 in Table 5.3) and the concentrations of zinc in the respective compartments were equal to the flux rates of zinc, namely (4.0 ± 3.5) and (0.79 ± 0.61) μg zinc transported to or from each compartment/h g fresh wt tissue.

Kinetic analysis cannot reveal the identities or locations of the two zinc compartments in luteal tissue. They may be cellular and extracellular or be in different cell types or intracellular organelles. Alternatively, they might be associated with different binding proteins or membrane structures.

The kinetics of zinc exchange in most of the rabbit tissues examined were adequately described by the three-compartment model in which total tissue zinc was distributed between a rapidly exchanging compartment, with a turnover time of about 1 h, and a slowly exchanging compartment, the turnover time of which was in liver 15 h, in peak-stage corpus luteum 8 h, and in other tissues 30–70 h. It was found

Table 5.3. Model (b) of Fig. 5.4 fitted to data on the exchange of zinc between blood plasma and luteal tissue of five-day pregnant rabbits[a]

R CHI SQUARE	A 1	A 2	A 3		
CA1 - RESERVOIR PARAMETERS:					
MULTIPLIER	EXPONENTIAL				
1687.7	.62963				
212.87	.12433E-01				
8.4321	1.0000	.10000	.30000		
4.8235	.94431	.11302	.35312		
4.8006	.92497	.10702	.36951		
4.7999	.93202	.10934	.36508		
4.7997	.92781	.10819	.36763		
4.7997	.92976	.10874	.36645		
4.7997	.92628	.10816	.36818		
STD DEVS	.56491	.72392E-01	.25241		
	61.0%	66.9%	68.6%		
DEPENDENCIES	.99276	.96950	.99609		
CONDITION NUMBER	43.8				
CORRELATION COEFFICIENTS					
A 1	1.0000				
A 2	.86226	1.0000			
A 3	-.98342	-.92814	1.0000		
MODE = 1, DEGREES OF FREEDOM = 2					
FINAL LAMBDA =	.0010000000000000				
X	Y	YFIT	RESIDUAL	Z-RESIDUAL	SIGMAY
.41670	222.00	245.78	-23.776	-1.1888	20.000
.75000	372.00	356.84	15.158	.89163	17.000
4.0000	355.00	353.92	1.0790	.28396E-01	38.000
16.000	242.00	202.00	40.004	1.8184	22.000
48.000	148.00	127.79	20.209	2.0209	10.000

[a] FUNCTN subprogram CA1 together with MODFIT was used, with NTERMS = 3. Notice the large value of reduced chi-square which, even with the few degrees of freedom, implies that the model is inadequate to describe the experimental data. The high dependencies reflect parameter interaction, which is seen from the correlation coefficients to occur as a negative relationship between A1 and A3. The condition number shows that this model is not over-parameterized.

that zinc transport to endometrial tissue varied with hormonal condition, being faster in tissues from non-pregnant than pregnant animals. Zinc transport to placental tissue varied with gestational stage, fetal tissue exchanging zinc with the maternal blood plasma four times more rapidly than did maternal placenta. Zinc uptake in erythrocytes, presumably during the synthesis of carbonic anhydrase, was the slowest of all examined.

An interesting hormonal response was shown by the luteal tissue. On days five to six of pregnancy the uptake of labelled zinc by corpora lutea was significantly faster than on other days (McIntosh and Lutwak-Mann, 1972 b). Compartmental analysis indicated that this transient increase was due not to a change in the relative sizes of the two luteal compartments but to a sevenfold increase in flux caused by a decrease in turnover time of zinc in the "slower" exchanging compartment. The total flux of zinc to the corpora lutea at this time was the highest recorded, exceeding even that of the liver.

5.2.2.3 Other Applications

The approach described above, in which exchange is measured between a peripheral tissue and a central reservoir of labelled material, has been most useful. The calculation goes smoothly because few parameters require optimization. This is the advantage of modelling the reservoir separately and using it as a forcing function.

Brooks and McIntosh (1975) have used this technique to investigate the distribution of carnitine, a compound important in fatty acid metabolism, throughout the body of the rat. Tissues were classified as having either one or two compartments of exchangeable carnitine. Turnover times of carnitine in each compartment and fluxes across compartment boundaries were estimated.

The same methods have been used to analyse the transport of calcium in the pre-implantation conceptus and associated maternal tissues of the rabbit (McIntosh and Lutwak-Mann, 1974). Exchange between oestrous endometrium and blood was extremely rapid having a turnover time of about 12 min and a flux of calcium equal to 500 µg Ca exchanged/h g fresh wt tissue. Hormonal and tissue-specific influences on calcium transport were clearly demonstrable.

5.2.3 Numerical Integration of Dynamic Model Equations

Frequently the differential equations describing compartmental models cannot be integrated analytically. Numerical integration is then required and indeed, with access to a computer, this is by far the easiest approach for any but the simplest system. The differential equations constituting a model are integrated (Sect. 3.6) after substituting the values of the independent variable and the current parameter estimates. The parameters are then adjusted in the usual way until the best fit is obtained.

5.2.3.1 A Two-Compartment System

As an illustration we shall develop a mathematical model of the two-compartment system shown in Fig. 5.4 (a) in terms of differential equations. Making the usual assumption that the rate of loss of tracer is proportional to its concentration in the compartment, we write a differential equation for compartment 2 in terms of tracer

$$dq_2/dt = k_{21}q_1 - k_{12}q_2. \tag{5.10}$$

Using the relationship $a = q/Q$ (specific radioactivity is the amount of tracer divided by the total amount of material)

$$d(a_2 Q_2)/dt = k_{21} a_1 Q_1 - k_{12} a_2 Q_2. \tag{5.11}$$

The total amount is constant and so can be removed from the differential and divided out

$$da_2/dt = k_{21} a_1 Q_1/Q_2 - k_{12} a_2. \tag{5.12}$$

Following the same procedure as before we shall assume that the disappearance curve in the plasma has been fitted by an empirical sum of exponentials – thus a_1 is known at any time.

There is a useful constraint that will allow us to eliminate the Qs. We have assumed that the system is in the steady state and so the exchange rates between the compartments must be equal. That is

$$k_{21}Q_1 = k_{12}Q_2,$$

or

$$k_{21} = k_{12}Q_2/Q_1. \tag{5.13}$$

Substituting into Eq. (5.12)

$$\begin{aligned}da_2/dt &= k_{12}Q_2 a_1 Q_1/(Q_1 Q_2) - k_{12}a_2 \\ &= k_{12}a_1 - k_{12}a_2 \\ &= k_{12}(a_1 - a_2).\end{aligned} \tag{5.14}$$

This means that the rate of change of specific radioactivity in the remote compartment is equal to the product of k_{12} and the difference between the specific radioactivities in the two compartments.

5.2.3.2 A Three-Compartment System

Numerical integration of Eq. (5.14) is straightforward. However, let us go on to model (b) which is more interesting. Writing the differential equation for the two remote compartments separately, we obtain Eq. (5.10) and

$$dq_3/dt = k_{31}q_1 - k_{13}q_3. \tag{5.15}$$

Substituting, dividing and applying the consequences of the steady state assumption as before, we have Eq. (5.14) and

$$da_3/dt = k_{13}(a_1 - a_3). \tag{5.16}$$

The specific radioactivities of compartments 2 and 3 cannot be measured separately, nor do we have any knowledge of Q_2 and Q_3 individually. Instead a mean value of specific radioactivity is calculated

$$\begin{aligned}a_m &= (a_2 Q_2 + a_3 Q_3)/(Q_2 + Q_3) \\ &= a_2 Q_2/(Q_2 + Q_3) + a_3 Q_3/(Q_2 + Q_3).\end{aligned} \tag{5.17}$$

If $Z = Q_2/(Q_2 + Q_3)$, $1 - Z = Q_3/(Q_2 + Q_3)$. That is,

$$a_m = Z a_2 + (1 - Z)a_3 \tag{5.18}$$

where a_m is the mean specific radioactivity of compartments 2 and 3, the value measured experimentally.

We have now constructed our dynamic mathematical model in terms of differential equations. The necessary integration can be done numerically using the FUNCTN subprogram embodying this model and known as CA2, which is listed in Sect. 11.9.

When we use MODFIT together with CA2 to fit the data of Sect. 5.2.2.2 the same results are obtained (compare Tables 5.4 and 5.3). That is, we have performed the integration numerically with the computer and arrived at the same result as when the integration was done analytically. In this case, where the analytical solutions were available, the numerical approach offered no advantage. However, while it is

Table 5.4. Model (b) of Fig. 5.4 fitted to the lutual data using numerical integration[a]

R CHI SQUARE	A 1	A 2	A 3
CA2 - RESERVOIR PARAMETERS:			
MULTIPLIER	EXPONENTIAL		
1687.7	.62963		
212.87	.12433E-01		
8.4319	1.0000	.10000	.30000
4.8187	.94156	.11263	.35419
4.8129	.88026	.10210	.38876
4.8001	.93531	.11206	.36003
4.7957	.92508	.10740	.36931
4.7950	.93260	.10959	.36466
4.7949	.92904	.10855	.36688
4.7950	.93559	.10963	.36363
STD DEVS	.56183	.72295E-01	.25163
	60.1%	65.9%	69.2%
DEPENDENCIES	.99271	.96940	.99606
CONDITION NUMBER	43.6		
CORRELATION COEFFICIENTS			
A 1	1.0000		
A 2	.86199	1.0000	
A 3	-.98333	-.92807	1.0000

MODE = 1, DEGREES OF FREEDOM = 2
FINAL LAMBDA = .0010000000000000

X	Y	YFIT	RESIDUAL	Z-RESIDUAL	SIGMAY
.41670	222.00	245.89	-23.886	-1.1943	20.000
.75000	372.00	356.77	15.230	.89589	17.000
4.0000	355.00	354.01	.98950	.26039E-01	38.000
16.000	242.00	202.35	39.649	1.8022	22.000
48.000	148.00	127.72	20.279	2.0279	10.000

[a] FUNCTN subprogram CA2 together with MODFIT was used. Notice the close similarity to the results of Table 5.3 where the equations of the model were integrated analytically (see also the comments there regarding parameter interaction).

usually easy to write the differential equations of a physical model and to solve them numerically with a computer, analytical integration is frequently not possible.

5.2.3.3 Comparison of Series and Parallel Models

The three-compartment model of Fig. 5.4 (b) is said to have a parallel configuration because both peripheral compartments exchange material independently with the reservoir. Model (c) of Fig. 5.4 differs in that the third compartment exchanges with the second, rather than directly with the reservoir; the peripheral compartments are in series. Following the process outlined in Sect. 5.2.3.2 we can write differential equations describing model (c) which are very similar to those for the parallel configuration.

An AUX subroutine defining the required differential equations (known as CA2A) appears in Sect. 11.10. Only AUX is reproduced because the FUNCTN subprogram (CA2A) which calls it is identical to FUNCTN CA2.

Using FUNCTN CA2A and MODFIT the series model was fitted to the data of Sect. 5.2.2.2 with the results shown in Table 5.5. The value of reduced chi-square was almost identical to that found with the parallel model (Table 5.3 or 5.4) showing that neither model was superior. The parameter estimates are, however, different. Parameter A1, while still representing the rate constant k_{12}, is diminished. Parameter A2, now equal to k_{23}, the rate constant of movement from compartment 3 to compartment 2, is greater than when compartment 3 exchanged zinc directly with the reservoir. Parameter A3, the size of compartment 2 as a fraction of the combined sizes of both luteal compartments, is increased. Therefore, although the rate constants and compartment sizes in the two models are different they predict the same overall behaviour. While it is clearly impossible with the present experimental data to choose between the parallel and series models, would it

Table 5.5. Model (c) of Fig. 5.4 fitted to the luteal data[a]

```
R CHI SQUARE         A 1             A 2             A 3
----------------------------------------------------------
CA2A - RESERVOIR PARAMETERS:
MULTIPLIER     EXPONENTIAL
  1687.7        .62963
   212.87       .12433E-01

----------------------------------------
  36.404       1.0000          .10000          .30000
  21.226        .54347         .12982          .53327
  12.616        .93168         .18217          .38134
   5.0149       .81514         .12162          .49398
   4.8025       .80814         .13465          .50888
   4.7981       .80475         .12642          .51103
   4.7957       .79814         .12957          .51407
   4.7954       .79700         .12753          .51475
   4.7951       .79388         .12800          .51626
   4.7952       .78941         .12669          .51852

STD DEVS        .37003         .10660          .18557
                46.9%          84.1%           35.8%

DEPENDENCIES   .99315          .82954          .99354

CONDITION NUMBER      22.3

CORRELATION COEFFICIENTS
         A 1   1.0000
         A 2    .79652         1.0000
         A 3   -.99305         -.80946         1.0000

MODE =  1, DEGREES OF FREEDOM =    2
FINAL LAMBDA =    .0010000000000000

    X              Y           YFIT      RESIDUAL    Z-RESIDUAL     SIGMAY
  .41670         222.00       245.76     -23.761      -1.1880       20.000
  .75000         372.00       356.83      15.168       .89223       17.000
 4.0000          355.00       354.09       .91128      .23981E-01   38.000
 16.000          242.00       201.97      40.030      1.8195        22.000
 48.000          148.00       127.82      20.178      2.0178        10.000
```

[a] FUNCTN subprogram CA2A together with MODFIT was used. Compare the results shown here for the series model with those for the parallel model given in Table 5.4. The fitted values are almost identical, but the parameters differ. The comments about parameter interaction in Table 5.3 apply here also.

be possible to obtain information about the degree of precision required to enable a firm choice to be made?

In order to attempt to answer this question Monte Carlo simulation experiments were carried out using the principles of sequential experimental design described in Chap. 4. Program DESIGN was used to determine the most efficient experiments for differentiating between the two models. The experiments were not done in the laboratory but instead were simulated mathematically, because it was necessary only to determine the maximum level of experimental error permitting reliable differentiation between the models.

Models CA1 (with NTERMS set to 3) and CA2A were each fitted to the experimental data from the luteal tissue. The program calculated the value of the independent variable (time) at which a further experiment, with the maximum likelihood of distinguishing between the models, should be done. In place of a genuine laboratory experiment, a simulated response was calculated by assuming that the series model was correct. An appropriate uncertainty, in the form of a standard deviation randomly selected from a set of normally distributed values, was added (Sect. 4.2.8). Thus the simulated result represented the response of the real system, assuming it to have the series configuration. The fitting of both models was then done again. As the process of simulation and analysis was repeated it was expected that if the "experimental" points were sufficiently precise, it might become possible to demonstrate the superiority of the series model in describing the data.

The result of applying DESIGN to the original data are shown in Table 5.6. In fact, when this process was repeated 50 times, there was no improvement in the likelihood of either model. Decreasing the uncertainty in the simulated data to levels unobtainable in genuine experiments still did not permit differentiation between the series and parallel models. It was thus possible by means of simulation, without needless loss of animals or time, to predict that experiments in which the reservoir compartment was labelled and the two luteal compartments sampled as one, could not differentiate between the two models. It should, however, be possible to gain extra, essential information by sampling the two luteal compartments separately, if that were physically possible. An identifiability analysis (see the end of Sect. 5.2), although not attempted here, might assist in defining the minimal experimental requirements for distinguishing between the parallel and series models.

5.2.4 A Generalized Mammillary System

It sometimes happens that only the reservior can be monitored and no sampling of peripheral compartments is possible. For example, this would mean that after injection of tracer (or drug) into an animal, measurements could be made only of its disappearance from the blood plasma.

Enough information is contained in the disappearance curve of the reservoir compartment to define the number of pheripheral compartments and their kinetic properties. However, unless the data is plentiful and precise there is bound to be ambiguity, particularly when the system is an open, biological one. Nevertheless, it is sometimes possible in favourable circumstances to extract useful information from observations on the reservoir compartment alone.

Table 5.6. Initial results of attempting to distinguish between the parallel and series models as descriptions of the luteal data[a]

```
------------------------------
CA1 - RESERVOIR PARAMETERS:
MULTIPLIER    EXPONENTIAL
  1687.7        .62963
   212.87       .12433E-01

------------------------------
------------------------------
CA2A - RESERVOIR PARAMETERS:
MULTIPLIER    EXPONENTIAL
  1687.7        .62963
   212.87       .12433E-01

------------------------------

EXPERIMENTS 1 -  5
*******************

R CHI SQ 1        PARAMETERS FOR MODEL 1
   4.7998         .92506        .10799        .36875
STD. DEVS. =      .56603        .72488E-01    .25275
                  61.2%         67.1%         68.5%
DEPENDENCIES      .99278        .96958        .99610
FINAL LAMBDA =    .0010000000   DEGREES OF FREEDOM =  2   ITERATIONS =  7

R CHI SQ 2        PARAMETERS FOR MODEL 2
   4.7953         .79596        .12871        .51520
STD. DEVS. =      .36385        .10585        .18382
                  45.7%         82.2%         35.7%
DEPENDENCIES      .99298        .82752        .99338
FINAL LAMBDA =    .0010000000   DEGREES OF FREEDOM =  2   ITERATIONS =  6

FIT DETAILS FOR CURRENT BEST MODEL: MODEL 2 (NEXT BEST IS MODEL 1)
     X            Y          YFIT       RESIDUAL    Z-RESIDUAL    SIGMAY
   .41670       222.00      245.91      -23.908      -1.1954      20.000
   .75000       372.00      356.76       15.240       .89646      17.000
  4.0000        355.00      354.07        .93202      .24527E-01  38.000
 16.000         242.00      202.32       39.683      1.8038       22.000
 48.000         148.00      127.74       20.257      2.0257       10.000

LIKELIHOODS:      MODEL 1       MODEL 2
                  .496196       .503804

L(2)/L(1)                     =    1.015
LN(L(2)/L(1))                 =    .1522E-01
CONFIDENCE IN MODEL 2 =            50.4%              PERFORM NEXT EXPERIMENT AT X
T(MAX) MODEL 2 =              .3461E+05  AT X = 1.140  VALUE INDICATED BELOW FOR:
T(MAX) MODEL 1 =              .4710E+05  AT X = 1.140
D0(MAX)        =              .7781E-01  AT X =  .4167   -- MODEL DISCRIMINATION
E(MAX)         =             1.000       AT X = 1.140    -- PARAMETER ESTIMATION
W1 = .9985   W2 = .0015
C(MAX)         =              .9992      AT X =  .4167   -- COMBINED REQUIREMENT
```

[a] FUNCTN subprograms CA1 and CA2A together with DESIGN were used. The first section of the output reproduces the parameters of the forcing function derived from the blood plasma data. This is followed by the results of the final iterations in fitting the two models and the fitted values of the current, marginally better-fitting model. Then follows the likelihoods and other relevent results, including the recommended values of the independent variable at which the next experiment should be carried out. A summary of the results of subsequent experiments is given in the text.

Compartmental Analysis

Consider the physical model shown in Fig. 5.7. Generally, the number of peripheral compartments is unknown. We shall attempt to determine this number from the experimental observations.

An analytical solution for a system consisting of any number of peripheral compartments can, in principle, be obtained. Shipley and Clark (1972, Appendix II) provide the general solution for an open four-compartment system in which there is exchange between each compartment and every other, as well as with the exterior. It is a simple matter to delete terms from this solution so as to obtain the description of the model depicted in Fig. 5.7. However, we shall deal with this problem more generally by means of numerical integration.

Following the principles outlined above, a differential equation is written to describe the rate of change of injected tracer or drug in each compartment. The solution to these equations, obtained by numerical integration, provides a numerical value for the concentration of tracer in each compartment at time t. This approach provides no estimates of the sizes of the peripheral compartments.

Fitting this model to the data entails matching the calculated value for the reservoir compartment to the experimental measurements on it. The calculated values for the peripheral compartments appear in the fitting process but are not compared with the data. If measurements on one or more of the other compartments were available, the present approach would become equivalent to that described in Sect. 5.2.3, with the added complexity of the simultaneous fitting of the reservoir.

Equation (5.19) has been used to derive a generalized FUNCTN subprogram suitable for fitting to data the model of Fig. 5.7, in which there are any number of peripheral compartments. This subprogram, referred to as CA3, is listed in Sect. 11.11 where details of its use will be found, together with outlines of the modifications required when fitting data collected simultaneously from the peripheral compartments.

5.2.4.1 Transport of Albumin

Subprogram CA3 can be used in either of two ways depending on whether the initial concentration of tracer in the reservoir compartment is known, or whether it must be estimated as a parameter. As an illustration of the first of these cases we shall use

Fig. 5.7. Generalized mammillary compartmental model which has a central reservoir (*compartment 1*) and up to n peripheral compartments, each exchanging a substance with the reservoir. The reservoir receives the substance at the rate R_{10} and discharges it by a process with rate constant k_{01}. The amount of the substance in the reservoir is Q_1. The system is in a steady state

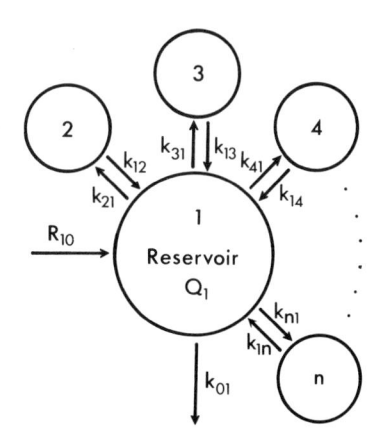

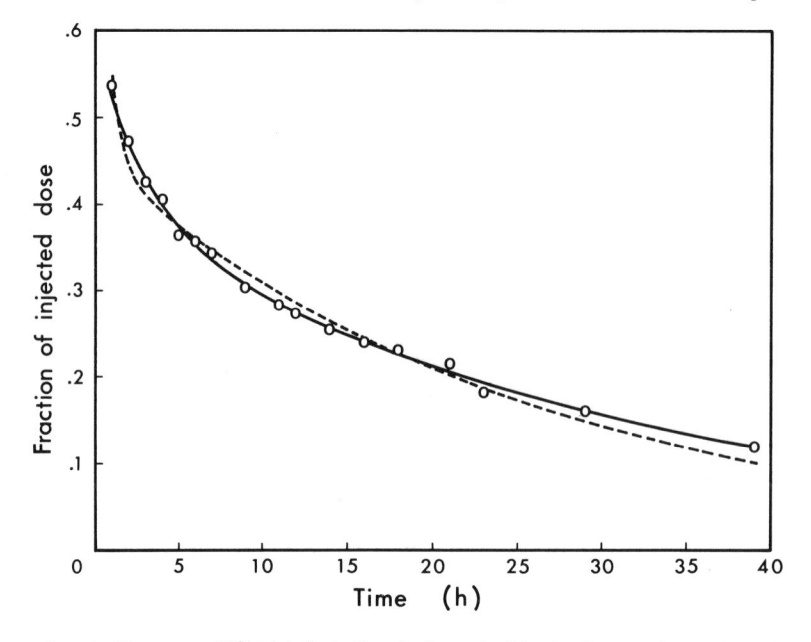

Fig. 5.8. Clearance of ^{131}I-labelled albumin from the blood. The experimental results, expressed as a fraction of the radioactivity in the blood at time zero, were input to MODFIT and FUNCTN subprogram CA3. With NTERMS = 5 a model consisting of three compartments, two peripheral and one central, was obtained (*solid curve*). When NTERMS = 3 the number of peripheral compartments was reduced to one (*broken curve*). The progress of the fits are shown in Tables 5.7 and 5.8. The data are from Matthews 1957. The theory of tracer experiments with ^{131}I-labelled plasma proteins. Phys. Med. Biol. 2: 36–53. With kind permission of the Institute of Physics, London, and the author

it to analyse the behaviour of ^{131}I-labelled albumin, using experimental observations reported by Matthews (1957). This provides a convenient example because the results can be compared with those reported by Feldman (1977) who fitted this model in a somewhat different way.

MODFIT and subprogram CA3 were used to fit a model of an open system consisting of a reservoir and two peripheral compartments to Matthews' data (as reported by Feldman, 1977, Table 3). NTERMS was set to 5 and the initial activity in compartment 1 was assumed to be 1.

The results of the fitting are shown in Table 5.7 and Fig. 5.8. The parameter estimates are similar to those found by Feldman (Table 2) with his method. Notice that the condition number is large, indicating severe parameter interaction caused by over-parameterization. The very high dependencies of parameters A4 and A5 and the almost perfect positive correlation between them are reflected in their large uncertainties. This shows that the experimental data do not define precisely the behaviour of the second peripheral compartment.

Table 5.8 and Fig. 5.8 give the results obtained if the existence of only one peripheral compartment is assumed. The residual variance is considerably greater showing that this model provides a poorer description of the data. On the other hand, the condition number is now very low and the parameter uncertainties can be relied upon. We conclude that the model with two peripheral compartments

Compartmental Analysis

Table 5.7. The model shown in Fig. 5.7 fitted to data on the clearance of labelled albumin from the blood[a]

RES VARIANCE	A 1	A 2	A 3	A 4	A 5
.13344E-02	.68000E-01	.23000	.14000	2.4000	1.2000
.45238E-04	.73641E-01	.21878	.14772	2.2571	1.4206
.42770E-04	.74182E-01	.21893	.14860	2.3365	1.4802
.42770E-04	.74156E-01	.21855	.14846	2.3252	1.4731
.53936E-04	.74208E-01	.21986	.14933	2.4559	1.5580
STD DEVS	.35899E-02	.72858E-01	.47796E-01	5.9803	3.8840
	4.8%	33.1%	32.0%	243.5%	249.3%
DEPENDENCIES	.92377	.99067	.99392	.99994	.99994

CONDITION NUMBER   6398.2

CORRELATION COEFFICIENTS
```
      A 1   1.0000
      A 2    .85874   1.0000
      A 3    .73645    .96587   1.0000
      A 4    .67031    .82827    .83299   1.0000
      A 5    .66175    .81511    .81711    .99954   1.0000
```

MODE = 0, DEGREES OF FREEDOM =   12
FINAL LAMBDA =   .0000100000000000

X	Y	YFIT	RESIDUAL	Z-RESIDUAL
1.0000	.53700	.52560	.11402E-01	1.5525
2.0000	.47300	.46918	.38244E-02	.52075
3.0000	.42500	.43007	-.50692E-02	-.69024
4.0000	.40500	.39897	.60289E-02	.82091
5.0000	.36400	.37378	-.97761E-02	-1.3312
6.0000	.35700	.35296	.40407E-02	.55020
7.0000	.34300	.33539	.76071E-02	1.0358
9.0000	.30300	.30694	-.39443E-02	-.53707
11.000	.28300	.28423	-.12280E-02	-.16721
12.000	.27300	.27428	-.12785E-02	-.17408
14.000	.25400	.25631	-.23122E-02	-.31484
16.000	.24000	.24023	-.22958E-03	-.31261E-01
18.000	.23100	.22553	.54712E-02	.74497
21.000	.21500	.20547	.95277E-02	1.2973
23.000	.18200	.19320	-.11203E-01	-1.5254
29.000	.16100	.16077	.23046E-03	.31380E-01
39.000	.11900	.11834	.65675E-03	.89426E-01

[a] FUNCTN subprogram CA3 together with MODFIT was used, with NTERMS=5. This produced a model consisting of a reservoir and two peripheral compartments. Notice the very high dependencies, and the almost perfect correlation between parameters A4 and A5 which are indicative of serious parameter interaction. These explain the excessive uncertainties in the estimates. of A4 and A5. The condition number is also high, indicating that there are too many parameters for the data to support.

provides a superior representation, but the range of the data is insufficient to allow precise estimates to be made of the parameters.

5.2.4.2 Transport of PMSG

Now let us return to the data of Sect. 5.1.1 on the clearance of PMSG from the blood plasma of sheep. It was noted that if information was required about the exchange of PMSG with compartments outside the blood a more sophisticated approach would be required. We are now in a position to illustrate this.

The model of Fig. 5.7 was fitted to the PMSG data using subprogram CA3 with NTERMS set to 4. This selected a single peripheral compartment and included the

Table 5.8. The model shown in Fig. 5.7 fitted to data on the clearance of labelled albumin from the blood[a].

RES VARIANCE	A 1	A 2	A 3
.26232E-01	.70000E-01	.26000	.10800
.81878E-02	.84976E-01	.65645	.35680
.91128E-03	.87110E-01	.87481	.73881
.24621E-03	.84324E-01	.73147	.78738
.23521E-03	.82787E-01	.73044	.78069
.23520E-03	.82748E-01	.72887	.77959
.23520E-03	.82741E-01	.72855	.77932
STD DEVS	.30578E-02	.76704E-01	.69286E-01
	3.7%	10.5%	8.9%
DEPENDENCIES	.49302	.92197	.90835

CONDITION NUMBER   43.7

CORRELATION COEFFICIENTS
```
     A 1   1.0000
     A 2    .43443    1.0000
     A 3    .21689     .92376    1.0000
```

MODE = 0, DEGREES OF FREEDOM = 14
FINAL LAMBDA =   .0000000100000000

X	Y	YFIT	RESIDUAL	Z-RESIDUAL
1.0000	.53700	.55150	-.14502E-01	-.94561
2.0000	.47300	.44308	.29925E-01	1.9513
3.0000	.42500	.40996	.15044E-01	.98092
4.0000	.40500	.39115	.13847E-01	.90291
5.0000	.36400	.37559	-.11586E-01	-.75549
6.0000	.35700	.36114	-.41384E-02	-.26985
7.0000	.34300	.34735	-.43496E-02	-.28361
9.0000	.30300	.32138	-.18376E-01	-1.1982
11.000	.28300	.29735	-.14349E-01	-.93564
12.000	.27300	.28602	-.13018E-01	-.84885
14.000	.25400	.26464	-.10635E-01	-.69346
16.000	.24000	.24485	-.48506E-02	-.31629
18.000	.23100	.22655	.44547E-02	.29047
21.000	.21500	.20162	.13381E-01	.87252
23.000	.18200	.18654	-.45399E-02	-.29603
29.000	.16100	.14774	.13258E-01	.86450
39.000	.11900	.10019	.18806E-01	1.2263

[a] FUNCTN subprogram CA3 together with MODFIT was used, with NTERMS = 3. This produced a model consisting of a reservoir and one peripheral compartment. Parameter interaction was eliminated at the expense of a clearly inferior description of the data (see Fig. 5.8)

initial concentration of PMSG in the blood plasma as a parameter for optimization. The progress of the fit is shown in Table 5.9; the fitted curve was identical to that of the double exponential process depicted in Fig. 5.1. In particular, the values found for the concentration of PMSG at time zero (A1) and the rate constant of disposal (A2) agree with those obtained using the algorithm of subprogram RESERVR as the mathematical model (Table 3.1).

The present analysis also provides estimates of the rate constants of the exchange process (A3 and A4), (0.435 ± 0.108) h^{-1} and (0.124 ± 0.030) h^{-1}, respectively. The single compartment undoubtedly represents the lumping of several compartments which cannot be resolved because of the imprecision of the measurements. Thus it would not be profitable to apply subprogram CA3 with NTERMS equal to more than 4.

Compartmental Analysis

Table 5.9. The model shown in Fig. 5.7 fitted to data on the disappearance of an intravenous injection of PMSG from the blood plasma of a sheep[a]

RES VARIANCE	A 1	A 2	A 3	A 4
8.1113	25.000	.20000E-01	.20000	.20000
.82254	25.037	.32446E-01	.28496	.93541E-01
.39077	24.835	.28137E-01	.31037	.91442E-01
.34780	25.266	.29107E-01	.44618	.12470
.34624	25.221	.28944E-01	.43290	.12309
.34623	25.229	.28954E-01	.43642	.12401
.34623	25.227	.28950E-01	.43540	.12374
STD DEVS	.46507	.96067E-03	.10842	.30347E-01
	1.8%	3.3%	24.9%	24.5%
DEPENDENCIES	.80702	.45833	.89173	.93638

CONDITION NUMBER   616.0

CORRELATION COEFFICIENTS
```
     A 1  1.0000
     A 2   .57350   1.0000
     A 3   .46987    .38023   1.0000
     A 4   .74264    .45584    .88699   1.0000
```

MODE = 0, DEGREES OF FREEDOM = 19
FINAL LAMBDA =   .0000000100000000

X	Y	YFIT	RESIDUAL	Z-RESIDUAL
0.	25.000	25.227	-.22686	-.38555
.41700	24.000	23.792	.20775	.35307
.53300	23.000	23.438	-.43812	-.74458
1.3300	23.000	21.471	1.5294	2.5991
1.8300	20.000	20.548	-.54791	-.93116
2.6700	19.000	19.355	-.35545	-.60408
3.5000	18.000	18.505	-.50491	-.85808
5.8300	17.000	16.977	.22719E-01	.38610E-01
7.6700	16.000	16.161	-.16080	-.27328
13.500	15.000	14.182	.81798	1.3901
21.670	12.000	11.828	.17199	.29229
30.000	10.000	9.8237	.17635	.29970
37.500	8.0000	8.3104	-.31037	-.52747
47.250	6.0000	6.6863	-.68632	-1.1664
53.750	5.0000	5.7832	-.78316	-1.3310
61.700	5.0000	4.8416	.15836	.26914
69.500	4.0000	4.0671	-.67078E-01	-.11400
77.500	4.0000	3.4012	.59885	1.0177
85.500	3.0000	2.8443	.15574	.26468
94.000	2.5000	2.3519	.14809	.25169
102.00	2.0000	1.9653	.34712E-01	.58993E-01
110.00	2.5000	1.6414	.85859	1.4592
117.00	1.0000	1.4022	-.40217	-.68349

[a] FUNCTN subprogram CA3 together with MODFIT was used, with NTERMS = 4. The experimental data were those described in Sect. 5.1.1. These results should be compared with those in Table 3.1, obtained with a more empirical model.

5.2.5 Extension of the Generalized Mammillary System

It is a straightforward matter to extend the approach of Sect. 5.2.4 to include those cases in which the concentration of a substance in one or more of the peripheral compartments is also measured. The calculated concentration in each compartment as defined by the model is available in subroutine CA3 for comparison with experimental data. The modifications required are minimal (Sect. 11.11).

Such an approach may not, however, be very efficient. As an example consider the luteal zinc exchange. The aim of the analysis was to describe the exchange of zinc between blood plasma and the corpus luteum. If one were to use the general mammillary model to do this it would be necessary to include exchange between plasma and at least one additional compartment. We know that zinc exchanges with other tissues and this fact must be incorporated into the model. Unfortunately, each extra compartment entails the fitting of two more parameters which do not improve our understanding of the luteal exchange. Therefore the best approach is the one used in Sect. 5.2.2 in which the plasma behaviour was used as a forcing function. In that way the need was avoided to incorporate into the model other, hypothetical exchange processes, for which no information was available.

In general, then, when the blood plasma forms a reservoir and we are interested in the exchange of material between it and another tissue, the two-stage analysis of Sect. 5.2.2 or 5.2.3 is definitely preferable. Nevertheless, it suffers from the disadvantage that there is no way in which to transfer the uncertainties arising from experimental variation in the plasma measurement to the analysis of the peripheral compartments.

6 Ligand–Protein Interaction and Competitive Displacement Assays

This chapter is in two main parts. The first deals with the modelling of associations between small molecules (typically steroids) and large ones such as the transport proteins of the blood plasma. Our chief concern is to use theoretical models to elucidate the mechanism of the interaction. The second section describes models that are particularly suitable for analysing the results of competitive protein-binding assays, radio-immunoassays and assays based on receptor interactions. Empirical models are useful there because interpolation only is required; a smooth curve well-fitted to standards suffices. The techniques of fitting mathematical models to experimental data, as described in Chap. 3 and illustrated in Chap. 5, are again emphasized here.

6.1 Interactions Between Ligands and Macromolecules

Reversible associations between hormones and large-molecular weight proteins are ubiquitous (Westphal, 1971; Wagner, 1978). Steroid hormones circulate in the bloodstream bound to transport proteins and interact specifically with target cells by binding to particular receptor proteins. The nature of the interaction is investigated by analysing the results of experiments done under well-defined conditions; plausible models are compared with one another and their parameters are estimated.

There are two kinds of theoretical models of the association process. The first assumes a macromolecule having a constant number of binding sites, each capable of simultaneous reversible interaction with a ligand, and characterized by an *association* or *equilibrium constant*. These sites are described as being *non-interactive* or *independent;* the association of a ligand with one site does not change the characteristics of another. Binding sites having equal association constants form a single class. Alternatively, there may be more than one class of sites, each with a different association constant.

The second, more general model, assumes only that the macromolecule binds some fixed number of ligands in a sequence of reactions in which the binding of the first influences the association characteristics of the next, successively. It may even be possible for sites to be created or to disappear as a result of the binding of the ligand. Interactions of this kind are referred to as being *allosteric* or *co-operative*.

Either of these models can be used to analyse not only hormone interactions but also the binding between enzymes and substrates, antigens and antibodies, or oxygen and haemoglobin. Many of the ideas presented here, which are the outcome of research in many disciplines over several decades, are treated in mathematical detail by Fletcher and Ashbrook (1973), and Rodbard and Feldman (1975).

We are concerned with the analysis of results rather than the techniques for the experimental measurement of interactions. The most widely used experimental method is equilibrium dialysis but modern developments promise great improvements in speed and convenience (see, for example, Feldman, 1978).

6.1.1 The Binding of Ligands to Non-Interacting, Independent Sites

Consider a simple model of the reversible association between a hormone P and a single kind of binding site Q on a protein. This may be symbolized by the relationship

$$P+Q \underset{k'}{\overset{k}{\rightleftharpoons}} PQ \tag{6.1}$$

where k and k' represent the association and dissociation rate constants, respectively, of the hormone-protein complex. The measure of the strength of the interaction is given by the *equilibrium* or *association constant* K which is equal to the ratio of the rate constants k/k'. That is,

$$K = k/k' = [PQ]/[P][Q] \tag{6.2}$$

where the square brackets mean "concentration of", normally given in units of [mol/litre]. $[P]$, $[Q]$ and $[PQ]$ are the *equilibrium concentrations* of free hormone, unoccupied binding sites, and sites occupied by ligand, respectively. It is useful to define symbols for the total concentrations of hormone and binding sites at equilibrium

$$T = [P] + [PQ],$$
$$q = [Q] + [PQ]. \tag{6.3}$$

Also convenient is a symbol for the ratio of the concentrations of bound to free hormone, defined as

$$R = B/F = [PQ]/[P] \tag{6.4}$$

where B is the bound, and F the concentration of free hormone at equilibrium.

We can now write

$$R_{B/F} = B/F = K[Q] = K(q-B) \tag{6.5}$$

which is similar to the model underlying the well-known graphical method of determining the characteristics of a single class of binding sites formulated by Scatchard (1949). According to Eq. (6.5) a graph of B/F against B will be a straight line with a slope of K and an intercept on the B axis of q.

It is convenient to express $R_{B/F}$ in terms of free ligand

$$R_{B/F} = B/F = Kq/(1+KF). \tag{6.6}$$

An alternative relationship, more useful experimentally, is an equation in terms of total ligand, T. Thus, using the identities

$$F = T - B \tag{6.7}$$

and

$$B/T = (B/F)/(1+B/F)$$
$$= [B/(T-B)] / [1+B/(T-B)], \qquad (6.8)$$

we define $R_{B/T}$ as being

$$R_{B/T} = B/T = \frac{\dfrac{Kq}{[1+K(T-B)]}}{1 + \dfrac{Kq}{[1+K(T-B)]}}. \qquad (6.9)$$

This model is expressed in terms of the parameters K and q, the dependent variable which is the concentration of bound ligand, and the independent variable which is the total concentration of ligand or *dose*. With this relationship it is possible to describe the interaction between a ligand and a macromolecule in terms of the total amount of ligand added to the system.

So far we have modelled a single class of binding site only. This is an idealization rarely met in prectice; the most obvious failing of the model of Eq. (6.9) is that it does not allow for *non-specific* or *low-affinity* binding, an association which by definition is weak in comparison with that at the *specific* or *high-affinity* site. For example, most steroids associate non-specifically with albumin and this would be observed experimentally if measurements were carried out using a protein preparation contaminated with albumin.

The model may be modified to incorporate non-specific binding by assuming that within the experimental frame the concentration of ligand will never be high enough to approach saturation of the weak, non-specific binding sites. All that is required is the addition of a constant term c to Eq. (6.6), yielding

$$R_{B/F} = Kq/(1+KF) + c. \qquad (6.10)$$

Often this is not enough. One may need to model a system consisting of two classes of independent binding sites, perhaps because there are two binding proteins present, each with a specific site for the ligand. The model of Eq. (6.10) is then not appropriate because c is no longer a constant, but like the first term, is a function of ligand concentration. We must instead use a model describing two specific sites, which in terms of Eq. (6.6) is

$$R_{B/F} = K_1 q_1/(1+K_1 F) + K_2 q_2/(1+K_2 F) \qquad (6.11)$$

where the K's and q's have different values for the two sites.

Lastly, it may be necessary to include a constant term to accommodate the presence of non-specific binding which, in terms now of $R_{B/T}$ rather than $R_{B/F}$, is

$$R_{B/T} = B/T = \frac{\dfrac{K_1 q_1}{[1+K_1(T-B)]} + \dfrac{K_2 q_2}{[1+K_2(T-B)]} + c}{1 + \dfrac{K_1 q_1}{[1+K_1(T-B)]} + \dfrac{K_2 q_2}{[1+K_2(T-B)]} + c}. \qquad (6.12)$$

This is analogous to Eq. (6.9) and is expressed in exactly the same terms. The independent variable is T (total concentration of ligand) and the dependent one is

B/T (the ratio of bound to total ligand). The number of parameters has increased to five: there is an association constant and concentration for each of two classes of sites, and a parameter representing non-specific or low-affinity binding. When the model defined mathematically by Eq. (6.12) is expanded and rearranged by some complicated algebra, it can be expressed as a cubic equation in B/T with the standard form

$$\alpha_0 (B/T)^3 + \alpha_1 (B/T)^2 + \alpha_2 (B/T) + \alpha_3 = 0. \tag{6.13}$$

Solving this equation necessitates finding the cube roots, which is easily accomplished by computer. A FUNCTN subprogram known as MASSACT, which embodies Eq.(6.12) will be found in Sect. 11.12, together with details of its use. It is equivalent to the special-purpose program of Raynaud (1973).

We have chosen to express the model in terms of the y variable B/T because it is easy to predict that if there is an approximately constant percentage error in the experimental measurements, the variance in this ratio, in contrast to B/F or F/B, will be constant. However, because of the consequences of Fieller's theorem (see Sect. 10.12) this variance may not in practice be found to be constant.

6.1.1.1 The Binding Properties of Human Pregnancy Plasma

In order to illustrate the application of the model defined by Eq. (6.12) we describe an experiment in which the testosterone-binding properties of blood plasma from pregnant women were measured by equilibrium dialysis. Pregnancy plasma contains a protein known as sex hormone binding globulin or SBG (Mercier et al., 1966) as well as a corticosteroid binding globulin (CBG) (Daughaday, 1956) and, of course, albumin. All three proteins bind testosterone but with very different affinities.

Two ml of pooled third trimester human pregnancy blood plasma was diluted to 40 ml with buffer (100 mM-KCl, 2 mM-EDTA, 10 mM-Tris, 0.02%-NaN$_3$; pH 7.4) and stripped of steroids by treatment with an equal volume of a suspension of 140 mg activated animal charcoal. The charcoal had been washed first with 100 ml buffer containing 14 mg dextran to reduce protein adsorption, and resuspended in 40 ml buffer.

The plasma-charcoal suspension was mixed gently overnight at 5° C, centrifuged briefly and the supernatant passed through a membrane filter (Millipore®) to give a steroid-free solution of plasma at a 40 × final dilution.

Aliquots (100 µl; 1.08 pmol) of [1, 2, 6, 7-^{3}H]testosterone in ethanol were transferred to screw-topped tubes. Unlabelled testosterone in ethanol was also added so that in the final incubation volume of 7-ml buffer (see below) the total concentration of the steroid (labelled plus unlabelled) was 0.154–7,086 nmol/litre. The ethanol was evaporated in a stream of air and 5 ml buffer was added to each tube. The tubes were capped, warmed to 37° C and thoroughly shaken.

Two-ml aliquots of the diluted plasma solution were pipetted into bags formed from approximately 0.7 cm diameter dialysis tubing by knotting (twice) one end of 20 cm lengths. The bags were closed with knots and placed in the tubes. The capped tubes were then mixed gently and continuously for 24 h at 5° C.

At the end of this time 0.5 ml aliquots were sampled from the solutions both inside the bags (by puncturing them with the needle of a microsyringe) and outside, added

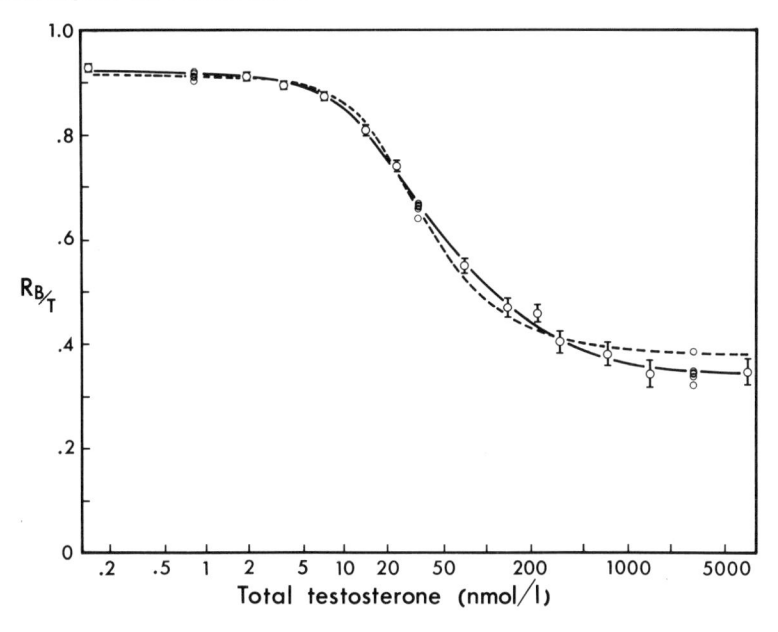

Fig. 6.1. The binding of testosterone by human pregnancy blood plasma. The *points* represent the results of an equilibrium dialysis experiment carried out as described in the text; the error bars equal one sample standard deviation of the mean, interpolated from five replicates at each of three doses (see text). At these three points error bars are omitted and the replicates (as well as their means) are indicated. The *solid line* shows the result of fitting to the data an analytical model representing two classes of independent specific sites plus a class of non-specific or low affinity sites [Eq. (6.12), and subprogram MASSACT with NTERMS = 5]. The *broken line* represents a model consisting of single class of independent specific sites plus a class of non-specific sites [Eq. (6.10), and MASSACT with NTERMS = 3]. The progress of the fits are shown in Tables 6.1 and 6.2, respectively

to a toluene scintillation solution containing a solubilizer and counted to a total of 10,000 counts in a liquid scintillation spectrometer.

It must be emphasized that this experimental procedure makes a number of assumptions that should be tested experimentally. For instance, the purities of both the tracer and unlabelled hormone must be established, and physicochemical requirements such as proof of attainment of equilibrium, absence of any partition or solubility effects, and the stability of the binding protein during the experiment, must be satisfied.

The results were interpreted as follows. The count rate of the sample from outside each bag was equated with the concentration of free testosterone. The count rate of the sample from within each bag included both free and bound testosterone. Therefore, because the free concentrations inside and outside the bags were equal, the differences between the two counts represented the concentration of bound testosterone. The ratio (count inside − count otside)/(count inside) was equal to B/T.

The results were analysed using MODFIT together with subprogram MASSACT. The experimental data in the form of a graph of B/T against *total* ligand (or dose) are shown in Fig. 6.1. The dose has been plotted on a log scale to increase legibility. The progress and results of the fit are shown in Table 6.1. One

Table 6.1. A model representing two classes of high-affinity independent binding sites plus a class of low-affinity sites (Eq. 6.12)[a]

R CHI SQUARE	A 1	A 2	A 3	A 4	A 5
2.7131	1.2000	11.000	.20000E-01	33.000	.50000
1.0934	.80744	11.678	.23272E-01	28.780	.50701
.61726	.87766	11.677	.24638E-01	28.152	.50863
.61529	.88430	11.648	.25248E-01	27.785	.50940
.61524	.88626	11.620	.25609E-01	27.603	.50979
.61522	.88772	11.599	.25849E-01	27.491	.51002
.61522	.88872	11.585	.26011E-01	27.417	.51018
STD DEVS	.16419	2.1048	.21638E-01	12.436	.38931E-01
	18.5%	18.2%	83.2%	45.4%	7.6%
DEPENDENCIES	.95960	.98579	.98753	.97657	.77723

CONDITION NUMBER   4432.9

CORRELATION COEFFICIENTS
```
     A 1   1.0000
     A 2  -.96152    1.0000
     A 3   .72137   -.81425    1.0000
     A 4  -.35684    .44158   -.85806    1.0000
     A 5   .22465   -.27071    .56517   -.76310    1.0000
```

MODE = 1, DEGREES OF FREEDOM = 11
FINAL LAMBDA =   .0000000100000000

X	Y	YFIT	RESIDUAL	Z-RESIDUAL	SIGMAY
.15400	.92600	.91939	.66109E-02	1.0493	.63000E-02
.86300	.91600	.91592	.76216E-04	.11375E-01	.67000E-02
2.0400	.91000	.90964	.36337E-03	.51911E-01	.70000E-02
3.7000	.89200	.89956	-.75595E-02	-1.0079	.75000E-02
7.2400	.87000	.87297	-.29656E-02	-.37070	.80000E-02
14.200	.80600	.80644	-.44171E-03	-.44171E-01	.10000E-01
23.800	.73900	.72422	.14781E-01	1.2317	.12000E-01
33.200	.65600	.66899	-.12991E-01	-.86609	.15000E-01
71.000	.54800	.55718	-.91762E-02	-.48296	.19000E-01
142.00	.46700	.47538	-.83767E-02	-.38076	.22000E-01
236.00	.45600	.42989	.26106E-01	1.1867	.22000E-01
331.00	.40300	.40674	-.37391E-02	-.14956	.25000E-01
709.00	.37800	.37219	.58103E-02	.22347	.26000E-01
1418.0	.34000	.35552	-.15516E-01	-.55415	.28000E-01
2835.0	.34000	.34680	-.68044E-02	-.24302	.28000E-01
7086.0	.34500	.34145	.35500E-02	.12678	.28000E-01

[a] Fitted to data from equilibrium dialysis of testosterone with human pregnancy plasma. FUNCTN subprogram MASSACT together with MODFIT was used, with NTERMS=5. The fitted model is shown in Fig. 6.1. Note the low standard deviation and dependency of the estimate of parameter A5 in comparison with the other parameters. This is because its value is a function of the horizontal asymptote of the curve at high dose. There was ample information in the data for estimating this value and it was not influenced by the other parameters. The large uncertainties in the other parameters (the %CVs are much greater than the uncertainty in the replicated data points) and the high dependencies indicate significant interaction. The large condition number means that there were too many parameters for the range of the experimental observations. The model nevertheless provides a good description of the data. Reduced chi-square was actually less than 1 and there was no systematic divergence between model and data (as shown by a runs-test).

determination was done at each of 16 concentrations of testosterone. Variance was estimated by replicating (five times) measurements at three widely spaced concentrations. The standard deviations of the replicates were found to be approximately inversely proportional to $R_{B/T}$ and the interpolated value of the expected standard deviation at each point was used to weight the fit (see Table 6.1).

The continuous curve shows the best-fitting model which was obtained with NTERMS set to 5. This represents binding by two specific processes and one non-specific one. The association constants of the two classes of specific sites, equal to parameters A1 and A3 in Table 6.1, were (0.89 ± 0.16) litre/nmol and (0.026 ± 0.022) litre/nmol, respectively. The concentrations of the sites are given by parameters A2 and A4. After multiplying by 40 (the dilution of the plasma) the estimates of the blood concentrations of the two classes of sites were (463 ± 84) nmol/litre and $(1,080 \pm 497)$ nmol/litre, respectively. Non-specific binding, expressed in terms of the model as the product of an association constant and a concentration of sites (a dimensionless value) was estimated by parameter A5. It was not possible within the confines of the experimental frame to gain information about the association constant or concentration of this class of sites.

Note that the precision with which A3 and A4 were determined was relatively low. Information about these parameters was sparse in the experiments. The data were insufficient to support five parameters as can be seen from the high condition number, and only A5 was relatively uncorrelated with other parameters.

The next simplest model, obtained with NTERMS set to 4, is of two specific sites only. This was clearly untenable because the values of $R_{B/T}$ did not approach zero at high doses.

When NTERMS is 3, a model consisting of one specific and one non-specific, unsaturable site is obtained. The result of fitting this model to the data is shown by the broken curve in Fig. 6.1. It is clear from Table 6.2 that there were systematic discrepancies between the fitted and experimental results and a runs-test (Sect. 10.6) confirmed this. What is more, reduced chi-square was too large; the divergence between model and data was greater than could be accounted for by the experimental variance. (The fact that the value of reduced chi-square in Table 6.1 was less than 1 meant that the data points just happened to lie well within the usual range of experimental variance.)

Reducing the number of parameters improved markedly the values of the condition number and dependencies. Regrettably, however, this model was inadequate. As to the identity of the binding sites, it is probable, by comparison with previously published results (Baulieu and Raynaud, 1970), that the first group was on SBG, the second on CBG and the non-specific association was with albumin. The separate contributions of the two kinds of binding site to the interaction between testosterone and pregnancy plasma are not clear from Fig. 6.1. The two association constants are not sufficiently distinct to allow the two binding processes to be distinguished by eye. In order to illustrate the effect of reducing the concentration of SBG from its high level in pregnancy, a series of simulations was done in which the concentration of SBG binding sites (parameter A2 in the five-parameter model) was progressively reduced. SIMUL and subprogram MASSACT, with NTERMS set to 5, were used. Instructions for using SIMUL to generate values of the dependent variable of a model, given a set of parameters and a range of the independent variable, will be found in Sect. 11.2.

The results are shown in Fig. 6.2. Each value of parameter A2 is given next to the appropriate curve. The effect of changing the concentration of the binding sites is made very clear by this means. The influence of the other parameters on the model could be investigated similarly. The example given in Sect. 4.2.7.1, in which the method of sequential experimental design is used to select conditions for

Table 6.2. A model representing one class of high affinity independent binding sites plus a class of low-affinity sites [Eq. (6.10)][a]

R CHI SQUARE	A 1	A 2	A 3
2.2387	.60000	18.000	.60000
1.6720	.58793	17.156	.59776
1.6696	.59527	17.054	.59937
1.6695	.59575	17.044	.59958
1.6695	.59580	17.043	.59960
STD DEVS	.43489E-01	.76968	.25937E-01
	7.3%	4.5%	4.3%
DEPENDENCIES	.77933	.81398	.38888

CONDITION NUMBER   38.3

CORRELATION COEFFICIENTS
```
    A 1   1.0000
    A 2  -.85838   1.0000
    A 3   .36788  -.52068   1.0000
```

MODE = 1, DEGREES OF FREEDOM = 13
FINAL LAMBDA =   .0000010000000000

X	Y	YFIT	RESIDUAL	Z-RESIDUAL	SIGMAY
.15400	.92600	.91434	.11655E-01	1.8500	.63000E-02
.86300	.91600	.91160	.43984E-02	.65647	.67000E-02
2.0400	.91000	.90671	.32851E-02	.46929	.70000E-02
3.7000	.89200	.89905	-.70453E-02	-.93937	.75000E-02
7.2400	.87000	.87914	-.91429E-02	-1.1429	.80000E-02
14.200	.80600	.82386	-.17860E-01	-1.7860	.10000E-01
23.800	.73900	.72985	.91531E-02	.76276	.12000E-01
33.200	.65600	.65477	.12259E-02	.81728E-01	.15000E-01
71.000	.54800	.51789	.30105E-01	1.5845	.19000E-01
142.00	.46700	.44830	.18698E-01	.84989	.22000E-01
236.00	.45600	.41944	.36556E-01	1.6616	.22000E-01
331.00	.40300	.40676	-.37600E-02	-.15040	.25000E-01
709.00	.37800	.38981	-.11813E-01	-.45435	.26000E-01
1418.0	.34000	.38234	-.42343E-01	-1.5122	.28000E-01
2835.0	.34000	.37860	-.38598E-01	-1.3785	.28000E-01
7086.0	.34500	.37635	-.31347E-01	-1.1195	.28000E-01

[a] Fitted to data from equilibrium dialysis of testosterone with human pregnancy plasma. FUNCTN subprogram MASSACT together with MODFIT was used, with NTERMS – 3. The fitted model is shown in Fig. 6.1. Note the low uncertainties and dependencies in the parameter estimates. The condition number is also low showing that there were not too many parameters for the data to support. But the model is inadequate to describe the observations as the value of reduced chi-square was too large and a runs-test showed that the signs of the residuals were not randomly distributed.

determining the properties and concentration of SBG in a sample of plasma in which CBG predominates, should be studied also.

In order to determine parameter estimates that are physically meaningful, and to calculate accurate uncertainties in those estimates, it is essential that random sampling errors are the only form of error in the experimental data. A feasible and demonstrably appropriate model must be chosen, and there must be no systematic error introduced by the experimental technique. Unknown systematic errors caused, for example, by inaccurate pipetting, will introduce bias into the parameter estimates. A common source of systematic error in experiments involving the use of radioactive tracers is the presence of radioactive contaminants. These should be eliminated by purifing the tracer before use. The presence of contaminants in the

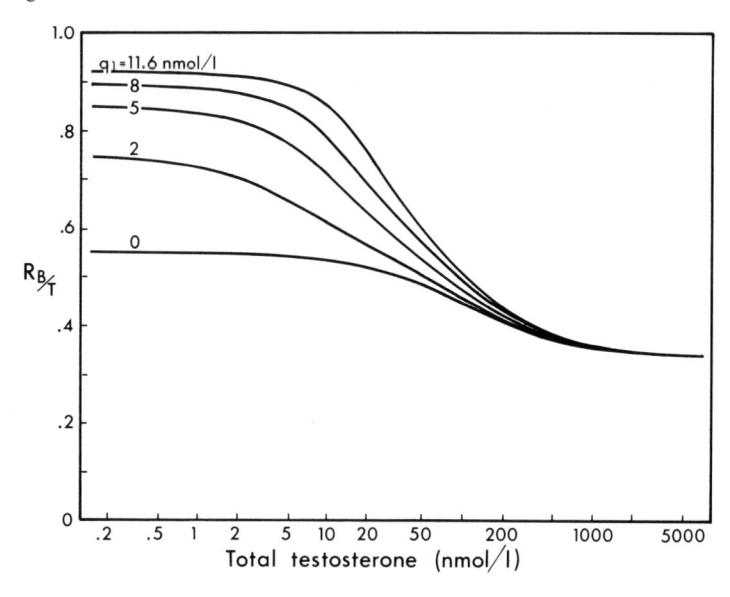

Interactions Between Ligands and Macromolecules

Fig. 6.2. Simulations of the binding of testosterone to human pregnancy plasma containing varying amounts of sex-hormone binding globulin (SBG). SIMUL and subprogram MASSACT, together with the best-fitting estimates of the parameters obtained from an equilibrium dialysis experiment (as shown in Table 6.1) were used to generate values of the response variable B/T, which were then connected by a *smooth curve*. Also shown are *curves* obtained by repeating the simulation while progressively reducing the value of the parameter representing the concentration of SBG binding sites in plasma $[A2 \equiv q_1$ in Eq. (6.12)] from the best-fitting value to zero. The figure next to each curve shows the current value of this parameter

tracer used in an equilibrium dialysis experiment will be revealed if different results are obtained when the experiment is done at two concentrations of binding protein (Builder and Segal, 1978).

6.1.1.2 Binding Expressed as a Molar Ratio

The model considered in the preceding sections can be generalized further, for instance by allowing association between a ligand and any number of classes of binding sites. Even more comprehensive is the model put forward by Feldman et al. (1972), of a system in which any number of different ligands bind to any number of non-interactive, independent sites, each class being characterized by a unique association constant. This model may be useful for predicting the equilibrium concentrations of a mixture of known concentrations of ligands and binding proteins. However, the reverse process, of fitting the model to data, would not be feasible because the number of parameters is so great that serious interaction will occur between them.

In the models already discussed the number of binding sites was expressed as a concentration (mol/litre). If the molecular concentration of the binding protein in the experiment is known, the concentration of sites may be redefined in terms of the number per molecule, a dimensionless ratio. For a pure protein this ratio must be an integer. Because the method of least squares cannot optimize to integer values, the following procedure is used (Fletcher and Spector, 1968). The best non-integer value is estimated in the usual way by introducing a parameter. This is then rounded to the nearest integer and fixed, and the fit repeated with one less parameter to be optimized. The remaining parameters adjust to allow for the integer value. The next larger and smaller integers should be tried as well. Choice of the most appropriate of the resulting models would be facilitated by applying the method of serial experimental design described in Chap. 4.

6.1.2 Sequential Binding and Co-operativity

As the number of binding sites on a macromolecule increases so does the likelihood that the sites interact, i.e. are no longer independent of one another (Fletcher et al., 1970). For this reason a sequential or co-operative model in which association occurs serially or "stepwise", provides a more realistic description of the binding of a single ligand to a number of different classes of sites on a single protein than does the independent site model described above. Indication of the need for such a model may come from an inability to find a plausible description of the data in terms of models with integer numbers of sites, especially if the number of sites is already known. Of course it must be remembered that other possible explanations for apparent non-integer numbers of sites exist: the solution of the macromolecules may contain impurities or the sites may be partially occupied by ligand other than that added by the investigator.

In order to model site interaction it is necessary to introduce sequential binding which allows the properties of the interaction at a site to depend on previous binding to other sites. The following is based on the analyses made by Fletcher and his associates, and on the summary of Fletcher and Spector (1977).

The most instructive way in which to model sequential binding is to classify together the various kinds of interactive complex, rather than the particular sites on the macromolecule where they occur. We can describe the ordered sequence of equilibria as

$$
\begin{aligned}
L + P &\rightleftharpoons L_1 P \\
L + L_1 P &\rightleftharpoons L_2 P \\
&\vdots \\
L + L_{N-1} P &\rightleftharpoons L_N P
\end{aligned}
\tag{6.14}
$$

where the nomenclature has been changed slightly to emphasize the different approach. Here L is the ligand, P is the macromolecule, and the subscript refers to the order in which the ligands interact, to a maximum of N.

This model provides a general description of interactive, co-operative or allosteric phenomena at equilibrium, being valid when binding induces changes in the characteristics, and even in the number, of sites.

Each association gives rise to a characteristic equilibrium of the form

$$K_N = [L_N P]/\{[L_{N-1}P][L]\} \tag{6.15}$$

and an expression can be derived for observed total binding in terms of these equilibrium constants [see Eqs. (10) and (12) of Fletcher and Spector, 1977].

By expressing a sequential, polynomial model in terms of the real roots of the polynomials, these authors develop an expression with the form of Eq. (6.12). In other words, the independent site model described by Eq. (6.12) is mathematically identical to the sequential one discussed here. This means that one cannot demonstrate that binding has occurred to independent sites with site-specific affinity constants, merely by fitting successfully models such as Eq. (6.12) to data. Pursuing their argument they show that, if the requirement that the roots of their factored sequential model be all real is waived, a very general relationship is obtained which incorporates the independent site model as a special case. It has a small number of parameters because, in contrast to the purely sequential scheme, it does not require a parameter for each binding step. If, when the general model is fitted to data, the estimated parameters take on values such that complex roots are formed, the possibility of co-operative binding is suggested. This evidence is far from conclusive and can be confirmed only by other kinds of experiment, such as kinetic studies.

The general model is represented by the equation

$$v = \sum_{j=1}^{p} F(2F - R_j^a) / (F^2 - R_j^a F + R_j^m) + \sum_{i=1}^{m} N_i F/(F - R_i) \tag{6.16}$$

where v is the molar ratio of bound ligand to macromolecule at a given concentration of *free* ligand, F. The real parameters $R_j^a/2$ and R_j^m represent the real parts and moduli of complex conjugate roots R_j and $\bar{R}_j$. The model allows for up to p of these pairs of parameters. The second term represents other, real, roots to a maximum of m. The total number of binding sites N is equal to $2p + \sum_{i=1}^{m} N_i$.

6.1.2.1 Use of the General Binding Model

The model of Eq. (6.16) is embodied in a FUNCTN subprogram GENBIND, a listing and details of the use of which will be found in Sect. 11.13. This subprogram together with MODFIT was used to fit the general model to values similar to those used for illustration by Fletcher and Spector (1977). (These data, on the binding of salicylate to human serum albumin, were estimated from the results shown in Fig. 1 of the article by Zaroslinski et al., 1974.)

It must be noted that the independent variable used by Fletcher and Spector for their general model, the concentration of free ligand at equilibrium, is inappropriate, because it is a response variable of the system, is not fixed by the investigator, and includes experimental uncertainty. The usual assumption of the method of least squares is, therefore, invalidated and the uncertainties in the parameters will be underestimated. For this example, however, we shall assume that the independent variable is without uncertainty.

The results of fitting a model consisting of one of the first terms of Eq. (6.16) and one of the second, are shown in Table 6.3. The parameter estimates may be compared with those in the last line of Table 3 in the report by Fletcher and Spector (1977). The values estimated for parameters A1 and A2 represent a pair of complex roots, which can be taken as evidence of site interaction. The authors point out, on the basis of Monte Carlo experiments and from theory, that this could be an artefact of fitting a model with too few parameters. When they generated data using a stepwise model with six independent sites and then fitted the four-parameter general

Table 6.3. The general binding model [Eq. (6.16)] fitted to data on the interaction between salicylate and human serum albumin[a]

```
RES VARIANCE        A 1           A 2           A 3
-------------------------------
GENBIND -   P      SITES
            1        2
-------------------------------
   .24299E-02 -5.6000       476.00      -2.2000
   .22041E-02 -7.5892       499.96      -2.1729
   .22037E-02 -7.6802       501.35      -2.1722
   .22037E-02 -7.6800       501.37      -2.1722
   .22037E-02 -7.6800       501.37      -2.1722

STD DEVS          3.0981         39.876        .11070
                 -40.3%           8.0%         -5.1%

DEPENDENCIES    .46364         .33609         .56323

CONDITION NUMBER     507.5

CORRELATION COEFFICIENTS
    A 1   1.0000
    A 2    .96653E-01   1.0000
    A 3    .59015        .43964       1.0000

MODE =  0, DEGREES OF FREEDOM =   13
FINAL LAMBDA =    .0000010000000000

      X            Y          YFIT        RESIDUAL     Z-RESIDUAL
  .17300E-01  .21100E-01  .16069E-01   .50311E-02    .10717
  .54200E-01  .52700E-01  .49530E-01   .31699E-02    .67527E-01
  .20900      .21100      .17891       .32092E-01    .68364
  .28200      .23200      .23443      -.24279E-02   -.51721E-01
  .30500      .29500      .25127       .43734E-01    .93163
  .75000      .50600      .52688      -.20876E-01   -.44471
  .80800      .58000      .55703       .22972E-01    .48936
 1.2800       .72800      .76712      -.39118E-01   -.83331
 1.5400       .92800      .86184       .66159E-01   1.4094
 2.3100      1.0200      1.0849       -.64925E-01   -1.3831
 4.1800      1.4500      1.4378        .12221E-01    .26034
 4.6900      1.4900      1.5099       -.19947E-01   -.42492
10.000       2.1100      2.0513        .58750E-01   1.2515
12.200       2.1800      2.2238       -.43836E-01   -.93381
37.100       3.3600      3.2940        .66016E-01   1.4063
38.600       3.2600      3.3256       -.65568E-01   -1.3968
```

[a] FUNCTN subprogram GENBIND together with MODFIT was used, with NTERMS = 3, $p = 1$, $m = 1$ and $N = 2$. Notice the low dependencies of this well-conditioned model. Data are from Zaroslinski et al., 1974, with kind permission.

model, they forced the parameter values to adjust in such a way as to suggest cooperative binding when none existed. One must, therefore, have prior knowledge of the number of sites that are actually present, before applying the general model.

Parameter A3 is a third root. The way in which the compound term in Eq. (6.16) is interpreted and the method for calculating the stochiometric binding constants from the roots, are explained by Fletcher and Spector (1977).

It turns out to be very difficult to choose between all these different models when confronted with experimental data. Both the independent and sequential ones often give very similar fits. But the most important conclusion is that just because the independent site model of Eq. (6.12) provides a good description of a set of data, and an estimate of an affinity constant, the latter cannot be unequivocally interpreted as being associated with any particular binding site. It is impossible to distinguish by means of equilibrium dialysis between the behaviour of independent binding sites and those that interact in a negatively co-operative way.

These are common difficulties in parameter estimation. Selection of a unique model may be possible only if the experimental data are very precise and lie within as wide an experimental frame as variation in the independent variables can provide. This area is ripe for systematic experimentation to differentiate between models using the sequential design approach of Chap. 4.

6.2 Competitive Protein-Binding Assays

The most important analytical technique to be applied to research and clinical investigation in endocrinology is undoubtedly that of the competitive protein-binding assay, also known as saturation analysis, which includes radio-immunoassay and radio-immunometric methods. This importance is due to an extraordinary sensitivity resulting from the use of radioactively labelled tracers, which allows concentrations to be determined, even of polypeptide hormones, of 10^{-10} M or less.

The subject grew from a combination of new immunological methods and well-established analytical procedures (Berson et al., 1956) to develop in many different directions, so that now there are assays based not only on immunogenic substances reacting with their antibodies, but also on the interactions between ligands and transport proteins, and hormones and receptors. All share the feature of being essentially radioisotope dilution methods, i.e. a small amount of a pure, radioactively labelled substance is added to a biological fluid containing an unknown amount of unlabelled substance to be analysed. To make quantitation easy, identical aliquots of tracer are added to standards containing known concentrations of the substance. Samples of equal mass of the substance are then isolated from each mixture by an appropriate specific procedure and their contents of label are determined: because of dilution the greater the amount of substance in the total material assayed, the less tracer will be found in the isolated sample. Comparison with the results from the known standards allows estimation of the unknown amounts in the biological material examined. The difficult part is to devise an appropriate procedure for isolating the sample of substance after label has been added. This is the role of the specific antibody, binding protein or receptor.

It is not our itention to discuss the basic principles or experimental procedures of competitive protein-binding assays. So important is this subject to endocrinology that the reader is probably already expert or at least familiar with the technique.

We are concerned here with the methods for analysing the results of assays so as to best interpret their meaning. We will emphasize only those aspects concerned with the design and analysis of these assays, important in endocrinology, that are based on principles of mathematical modelling.

Two main paths of development are clear in the many published mathematical analyses of competitive protein-binding assays. One is theoretical modelling with the aim of optimizing conditions of assay, while the other is the empirical approach with a concern for the problems of fitting models to data. We shall summarize both the theoretical and empirical models and illustrate their differences.

The aim of practical assays is not to distinguish models or to estimate parameters but to interpolate between standards so as to determine the concentrations of unknowns. Empirical modelling has therefore an important role.

On another level, theoretical modelling with the estimation of physically meaningful parameters, is valuable when one is attempting to optimize an assay for maximum sensitivity and precision (Sect. 6.2.5). The conditions under which assays are carried out, such as the failure often to attain equilibrium or separate completely the free and bound fractions, preclude accurate parameter estimation. It is preferable when seeking to characterize the physical parameters of an assay to use a more reliable experimental approach, such as equilibrium dialysis, for establishing their values.

6.2.1 Theoretical Models

A systematic, theoretical approach to modelling competitive protein binding assays was chosen by Ekins et al. (1968). They derived expressions analogous to Eqs (6.9) and (6.12) (but in terms of the ratio R_{F_B} instead of R_{B_T}) and drew theoretical curves for systems consisting of one or two kinds of binding site. Simulations of this sort are readily generated using the program SIMUL, together with a suitable subprogram and values of K and q appropriate to the system being investigated.

One can also do this in reverse and, using MODFIT and MASSACT, for example, fit the model of Eq. (6.12) (as was done in Sect. 6.1.1.1) to the results of a competitive protein-binding assay. Rodbard and Tacey (1978) have advocated this approach and noted its advantages and limitations. Choice of the value of NTERMS to use depends on the data. A single binding site is modelled with NTERMS set to 2; when NTERMS is 3, non-specific binding is taken into account as well. If this is insufficient to obtain a good fit one might try using NTERMS equal to 4 to model a system of two independent sites, or set NTERMS to 5 if non-specific binding occurs as well. An example of the use of MASSACT to model a radio-immunoassay is given below (see Sect. 6.2.1.2).

However, in contrast to its use in analysing dialysis experiments, there are pitfalls in applying a theoretical model such as that incorporated into subroutine MASSACT to data obtained by radio-immunoassay. Care must be used in interpreting the parameter estimates because there are many systematic errors such as tracer impurity (see the end of Sect. 6.1.1.1), adsorption of labelled material to the tubes or other misclassification phenomena, which will lead to a possibly erroneous conclusion that more than one kind of binding site exists. In other words, one may be using a theoretical model in an unwittingly empirical way. This does not matter provided all that is desired is an accurate interpolation model, but the parameter estimates obtained will have diminished physical significance.

An apt illustration comes from the experiments of Naus et al. (1977) who used a transformation of the model given in Eq. (6.17) below, to analyse six different kinds of radio-immunoassay. Although couched in terms of parameters with physical significance, it was clear that the estimates yielding the best fit of the model to the data failed to correspond to physically meaningful values.

6.2.1.1 Effects of Labelled Ligand and Cross-Reactants

It may happen that the presence of a label on the ligand alters the association constant. This is most likely when the tracer is labelled with a bulky iodine atom as is common in assays for peptide hormones. Ekins et al. (1968; 1970) have specifically analysed this situation. With the assumptions that there are unequal association constants for labelled and unlabelled ligands, that there is a single kind of binding site, and that equilibrium has been attained, they derived the equation

$$R_{F/B}^2 + R_{F/B}\left(1 + \frac{p^*}{A_3} - \frac{1}{A_2 A_3}\right) - \frac{R_{F/B}\left(\frac{x}{A_3}\right)(R_{F/B} + 1)}{\left(\frac{A_1}{A_2}\right)R_{F/B} + 1} - \frac{1}{A_2 A_3} = 0 \qquad (6.17)$$

where $A_1 = K$ and $A_2 = K^*$, the association constants of unlabelled and labelled ligand, respectively, $A_3 = q$, the concentration of binding sites, p^* is the total concentration of labelled ligand, and x is the concentration of unlabelled ligand or dose.

Ekins and his associates make a further very important point about interpreting experimental data. It concerns the possibility of a third ligand, an "unknown" or cross-reacting hormone not identical with the standard and with a different association constant K_u. If an assay is carried out over a restricted range of values of $R_{F/B}$ then, although the position with respect to the dose axis of the response curve of an unknown at several dilutions depends on the value of K_u, this curve can be superimposed on that of the standards (with equilibrium constant K) simply by displacing it along the dose axis. This is not the case if $R_{F/B}$ ranges from very low to very high values. Therefore the commonly used criterion for the identity of two hormones that their standard curves be superimposable or, if plotted on a logarithmic scale, be parallel, may be ineffective. Ekins presents a number of experimental results to verify this theoretical prediction, showing that determinations of very high precision are required to identify cross-reactants at values of $R_{F/B}$ greater than 1. The recent report by Rodbard (1977) emphasizes this point, while Laurence and Wilkinson (1974) show how to optimize the conditions of assay so as to differentiate most clearly between different ligands.

6.2.1.2 Analysis of a Radio-Immunoassay for Testosterone

The results of a testosterone radio-immunoassay will be used to compare the application of both theoretical and empirical models. The assay procedure used was developed by M. M. Ralph and R. F. Seamark (Janson et al, 1978). The antibody was raised against testosterone-3-(O-carboxymethyl) oxime-BSA in a sheep. The tracer was [1, 2, 6, 7-^{3}H] testosterone. After addition of antibody and tracer (10,000 cpm/tube) to standards or samples, the assay tubes (containing a total volume of 0.2 ml of 0.1 M-phosphate buffer, pH 7.0) were incubated for 5 min at 37° C, and then for 30 min in ice-water. The final dilution of antibody was 1 : 20,000. One mg of gamma-globulin was added to aid precipitation, followed by polyethylene glycol 6000 (to a final concentration of 20.5% wt:vol.), and the tubes were centrifuged. The precipitates were counted in a liquid scintillation spectrometer. Previous experiments had shown that equilibration was rapidly attained, well before the addition of the polyethylene glycol.

The standard curve is shown in Fig. 6.3. Duplicate determinations of $R_{F/B}$ were made at eight concentrations of testosterone. Dose was expressed in terms of nmol/litre incubation mixture.

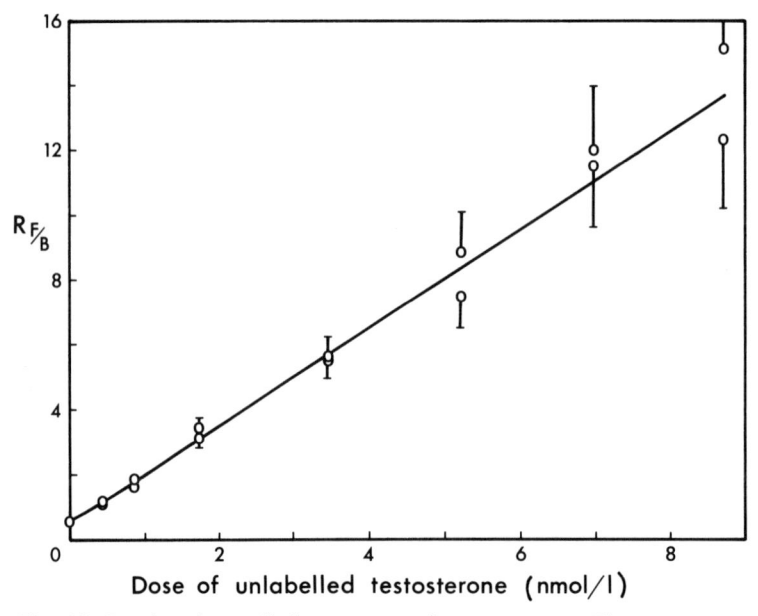

Fig. 6.3. Results of a radio-immunoassay for testosterone. The *points* represent experimental determinations obtained as described in the text and transformed into terms of the response variable $R_{F/B}$. The *line* shows the result of fitting the analytical model of Eq. (6.17) to the data, using MODFIT together with subprogram RIA. The *error bars* represent sample standard deviations in the means estimated by pooling the results of 20 previous assays. Notice the greatly increased standard deviations at high values of the response variable, corresponding to low counts bound before transformation. The progress of the fit is shown in Table 6.4

The first example of the analysis of these data uses the model of Eq. (6.17) incorporating non-identical behaviour of tracer and unlabelled ligand. It is embodied in FUNCTN subprogram RIA, a listing of which is given in Sect. 11.14. The mass of labelled hormone (0.080 pmol; 0.40 nmol/litre) was entered into subprogram RIA as a constant. The count rate of the free (unbound) hormone was calculated by subtracting the count rate of the bound fraction from the total counts added. Note that the bound count must then be corrected by subtracting the non-specifically bound counts determined experimentally, because in this model no allowance is made for non-specific binding. Values used for weighting were the standard deviations calculated from the results of the experimental data from twenty previous assays (Sect. 6.2.3).

The results of the fit are shown in Table 6.4. It will be seen that the dependencies were very high indicating interaction, while the condition number was low reflecting the small number of parameters. Reduced chi-square was less than 1 because the data in this particular experiment were more precise than was usual.

Assuming that the parameter estimates have physical significance the values of K and K^* were found to be (5.9 ± 1.0) litre/nmol and (8.7 ± 3.1) litre/nmol, respectively. There was no evidence, therefore, that the association constants of the unlabelled and labelled hormones differed. This was not unexpected considering that the tracer was ^{3}H-labelled. If iodine labelling had been used, the association constants might well have been unequal. The concentration of binding sites was estimated to be (0.45 ± 0.07) nmol/litre.

Table 6.4. The model of Eq. (6.17) fitted to data from a radio-immunoassay for testosterone[a]

```
R CHI SQUARE         A 1          A 2          A 3
-----------------------------------
RIA - TRACER CONCENTRATION:
         .40000      UNITS
-----------------------------------
  3.5825             6.0000       9.0000       .40000
   .45091            5.8879       8.7563       .44170
   .41321            5.8564       8.5766       .45092
   .41316            5.8575       8.5765       .45115
   .41316            5.8575       8.5765       .45115

STD DEVS             .99265       3.0225       .65633E-01
                     16.9%        35.2%        14.5%

DEPENDENCIES   .94393             .99364       .98903

CONDITION NUMBER         431.0

CORRELATION COEFFICIENTS
        A 1    1.0000
        A 2     .93679            1.0000
        A 3    -.88813            -.98796      1.0000

MODE =  1, DEGREES OF FREEDOM =   14
FINAL LAMBDA =      .0000010000000000

        X           Y            YFIT       RESIDUAL     Z-RESIDUAL   SIGMAY
  0.            .58606         .58606     -.60055E-04   -.15014E-02   .40000E-01
  0.            .57900         .58606     -.70601E-02   -.18103       .39000E-01
  0.            .59400         .58606      .79399E-02    .19366       .41000E-01
   .43500      1.1200         1.1438     -.23827E-01   -.29058        .82000E-01
   .43500      1.1900         1.1438      .46173E-01    .52469        .88000E-01
   .87000      1.8700         1.7773      .92742E-01    .62243        .14900
   .87000      1.6200         1.7773     -.15726      -1.2581         .12500
  1.7400       3.1500         3.0846      .65389E-01    .22863        .28600
  1.7400       3.4600         3.0846      .37539       1.1586         .32400
  3.4800       5.6600         5.7193     -.59340E-01   -.92719E-01    .64000
  3.4800       5.5600         5.7193     -.15934      -.25535         .62400
  5.2200       7.4900         8.3555     -.86550      -.89596         .96600
  5.2200       8.5000         8.3555      .49450       .39560        1.2500
  6.9600      12.000         10.991      1.0089        .49697        2.0300
  6.9600      11.500         10.991       .50886       .26782        1.9000
  8.7000      15.100         13.626      1.4736        .49617        2.9700
  8.7000      12.300         13.626     -1.3264       -.62564        2.1200
```

[a] FUNCTN subprogram RIA together with MODFIT was used; the fitted model is shown in Fig. (6.3). The concentration of labelled testosterone in the final incubation volume (0.40 nmol/litre) was supplied to the subprogramm on the file UNIT 2. Notice the particularly large uncertainty in the estimate of parameter A2, the association constant of labelled ligand, and its negative correlation with A3, which estimates the concentration of binding sites. The large dependencies indicate significant parameter interaction which reduces the reliability of the uncertainties. The condition number shows that this model is not over-parameterized.

Because this analysis showed that there was no difference in the association constants the refinement of Eq. (6.17) was unnecessary. Let us, therefore, compare the results with those of fitting the model of Eq. (6.12) (subprogram MASSACT) to the data. The response variable is now $R_{B/T}$ and the weights were calculated in the same way as for counts bound (see Sect. 6.2.3). A model consisting of one specific binding site plus non-specific association was necessary and sufficient to describe the data. The experimental points and the line representing the fitted model are shown in Fig. 6.4. The parameters will be found in Table 6.5 together with other

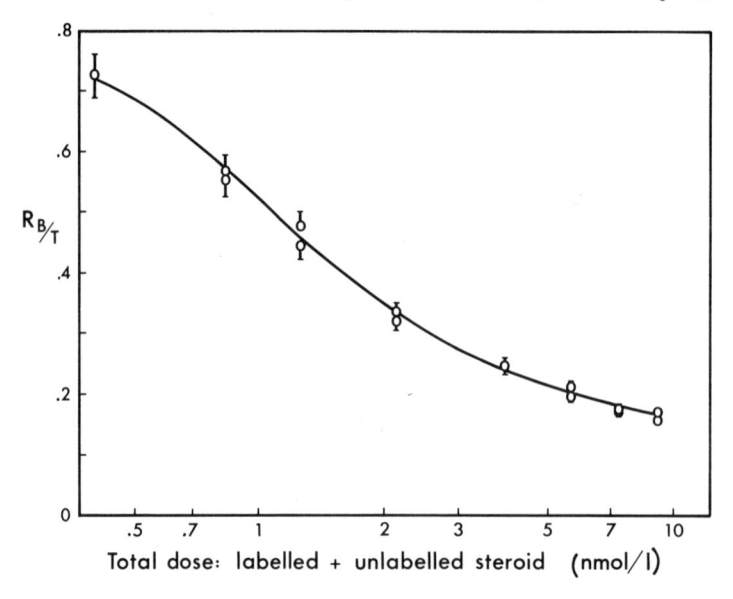

Fig. 6.4. Results of a radio-immunoassay for testosterone. The *points* are the same as those in Fig. 6.3 but are expressed here in terms of the response variable $R_{B/T}$. The *line* shows the result of fitting to the data the analytical model of Eq. (6.10) (using MODFIT together with subprogram MASSACT, and NTERMS=3). Notice the greater homogeneity in the variance in comparision with Fig. 6.3, as reflected by the sample standard deviations in the means. The progress of the fit is shown in Table 6.5

details. Notice in particular that, in comparison with the previous model, the dependencies were smaller in size and consequently the uncertainties in the parameter values were diminished.

The association constant K was estimated to be (7.7 ± 1.7) litre/nmol and the concentration of binding sites q to be $(0.59 \pm .04)$ nmol/litre. Parameter A3, the estimate of non-specific binding, represents the association of hormone with protein other than the antibody and also with the insides of the assay tubes, as well as incomplete separation resulting in unbound hormone contaminating the bound fraction. The estimates of K and q were not significantly different from those obtained using the model of Eq. (6.17) (*t*-test).

In summary, theoretical models of competitive protein-binding assays are essential for estimating physically meaningful parameters that are necessary when optimizing assays for sensitivity and precision. It is preferable, however, to estimate these parameters from the results of experiments carried out by means of a reliable technique such as equilibrium dialysis rather than the more rapid and convenient methods used for assay purposes.

6.2.2 Empirical Models

The aim of an empirical model of a competitive protein-binding assay is to define a smooth curve through results obtained from standards, so as to allow the determination of unknowns. The practical advantages of empirical models of competitive protein-binding assays were recognized even before the difficulties of making meaningful estimates of the parameters in theoretical models were fully

Table 6.5. A model representing a single class of high-affinity independent binding sites plus a class of low-affinity sites [Eq. (6.10)][a]

R CHI SQUARE	A 1	A 2	A 3
25.022	5.0000	1.0000	.10000
1.1786	5.0909	.60973	.12139
.50717	7.0968	.58845	.12296
.45250	7.6617	.59124	.12278
.45241	7.7031	.59090	.12286
.45241	7.7049	.59086	.12286

STD DEVS	1.6569	.38689E-01	.89069E-02
	21.5%	6.5%	7.2%

DEPENDENCIES .76731   .87976   .75506

CONDITION NUMBER   361.6

CORRELATION COEFFICIENTS
```
     A 1   1.0000
     A 2  -.85063    1.0000
     A 3   .66096   -.84203    1.0000
```

MODE = 1, DEGREES OF FREEDOM = 14
FINAL LAMBDA = .0000001000000000

X	Y	YFIT	RESIDUAL	Z-RESIDUAL	SIGMAY
.40000	.72700	.71944	.75576E-02	.19994	.37800E-01
.40000	.73000	.71944	.10558E-01	.27856	.37900E-01
.40000	.72400	.71944	.45576E-02	.12121	.37600E-01
.83300	.56800	.57241	-.44139E-02	-.14962	.29500E-01
.83300	.55300	.57241	-.19414E-01	-.67409	.28800E-01
1.2700	.44500	.45802	-.13025E-01	-.56384	.23100E-01
1.2700	.47900	.45802	.20975E-01	.84238	.24900E-01
2.1400	.33800	.33477	.32328E-02	.18368	.17600E-01
2.1400	.32100	.33477	-.13767E-01	-.82438	.16700E-01
3.8700	.24700	.23965	.73530E-02	.57445	.12800E-01
3.8700	.24900	.23965	.93530E-02	.72504	.12900E-01
5.6100	.21400	.20058	.13420E-01	1.1876	.11300E-01
5.6100	.19800	.20058	-.25798E-02	-.25047	.10300E-01
7.3400	.17400	.17960	-.55976E-02	-.61852	.90500E-02
7.3400	.17700	.17960	-.25976E-02	-.28234	.92000E-02
9.0800	.15900	.16640	-.73951E-02	-.89420	.82700E-02
9.0800	.17200	.16640	.56049E-02	.62695	.89400E-02

[a] Fitted to data from a radio-immunoassay for testosterone. FUNCTN subprogram MASSACT together with MODFIT was used; the fitted model is shown in Fig. 6.4. Notice the lower, acceptable dependencies in comparison with those in Table 6.4, and the improved uncertainties.

appreciated. It was realized that a host of experimental uncertainties such as the purity of the antibody, imperfect separation of free and bound fractions, and incomplete equilibration, could defeat attempts to determine values of physical parameters accurately; one might as well seek for no more, in a routine assay, than an accurate and precise method of comparing unknowns with standards.

A further stimulus to the development of empirical models was the finding that the simple theoretical ones described above are incapable of providing a good fit to the results of every assay, even if no attempt is made to interpret the parameter estimates as physical constants. Adding more parameters may improve the fit, but parameter estimation then becomes very sensitive to poor initial guesses, and parameter interaction increases to a point where convergence of the fitting procedure may be prevented. Elaborations of the model of Eq. (6.17) were particularly unsatisfactory in these respects, possibly because of the inhomogeneity of variance caused by transformation of the values of the dependent variable $R_{B/T}$ into terms of $R_{F/B}$.

The more flexible of the empirical models described below, even though over-parameterized, provide good fits to most assays while remaining sufficiently robust.

6.2.2.1 Logit-Log and Non-Linear Regression Models

A simple empirical model yielding a linear or approximately linear dose-response curve advocated by Rodbard et al. (1969) turned out to be very successful and popular. This was the logit-log plot, a transformation long used in the analysis of bio-assays (Colquhoun, 1971) which made linear the sigmoidal plot of B/B_0 against log (dose), where $B=$ the concentration of bound ligand, $B_0 = B$ at zero dose, and dose is the total concentration of ligand in the reaction mixture.

The most important reason for introducing a linearizing transformation was to allow weighted linear least squares fitting with its straightforward error analysis. Unfortunately, there were shortcomings in the logit-log transformation. Much depended upon an accurate and precise estimate of B_0, which was in fact a point on the standard curve. It was also necessary to estimate accurately and precisely the value of non-specific association so as to subtract this from all observations. This is not always easy to do accurately: either one determines the counts bound in the absence of antibody or receptor, or one effectively displaces all labelled ligand from specific binding sites by the addition of a large excess of unlabelled ligand. Neither approach may achieve the desired end.

Difficulties of this sort, particularly in dealing with the results of radio-immunometric assays (Rodbard and Hutt, 1974) or in vitro bio-assays (Rodbard, 1974), combined with the availability of increasing computing power, led to the development of non-linear empirical models. One of the more generally useful of these, suggested by Healey (1972), is couched in terms of four parameters, as follows

$$y = A_1 + A_2 [Z/(1+Z)] \qquad (6.18)$$

where $Z = \exp[A_3 - A_4 \ln(x)]$, y is the response variable which may be counts bound B or the ratio B/T, A_1 represents non-specific binding or the response at infinite dose, A_2 is the response at zero dose, A_3 is the natural logarithm of the dose at a point at which the response is midway between that at infinite dose (A_1) and zero dose (A_2), A_4 is a slope factor also known either as the Hill or the Sips coefficient (approximately equal to 1 for most assays), and x is the dose.

Similarity in form between Eq. (6.18) and the theoretical model of a single binding site given by Eq. (6.6) is clearer from Rodbard's version of the above which is

$$y = (A_2 - A_1)/[1 + (x/A_3)^{A_4}] + A_1 \qquad (6.19)$$

where the symbols have the same meanings, (except for A_2 and A_3 which are defined slightly differently). Rodbard et al. (1978, Appendix A) show how the model of Eq. (6.19) can be fitted using linear regression methods. This is accomplished by applying the logit-log transformation to linearize the function and carrying out alternately linear optimization on parameters A_3 and A_4 (using this linearized form), and on A_1 and A_2 with Eq. (6.19) itself.

In the models of Eqs. (6.18) or (6.19), the zero and infinite dose-responses appear as parameters. Information for their estimation comes from all the experimental data rather than just a few points, which is much more satisfactory than the earlier logit-log model. The response variable y can be B, F, B/T or various other quantities, which means that the same model can also be used for analysing bio-assays or radio-immunometric assays.

Healey's model [Eq. (6.18)] has been incorporated into a FUNCTN subprogram named RIAH, a listing of which will be found in Sect. 11.15. This, together with MODFIT, can be used to fit most radio-immunoassays, protein-binding assays, receptor assays, radio-immunometric assays or bio-assays. It is routinely used in our laboratory in an expanded form in which MODFIT reads raw data as either bound or free counts, punched on paper tape by a liquid scintillation or gamma-spectrometer. Using a Data General Nova 2 minicomputer, the standard curve is drawn on a plotting device and the doses contained in the unknown samples are interpolated and printed automatically. We use this system to analyse the results of assays for a variety of steroid hormones, prostaglandins, melatonin, LH, FSH, GnRH and cAMP.

Subprogram RIAH has been applied to the results of the assay for testosterone shown in Sect. 6.2.1.2. In the present case the response variable was counts bound. Weighting was applied as described in the first part of Sect. 6.2.3 below. The fitted curve is shown in Fig. 6.5 and the progress of the fit in Table 6.6. In this particular assay the experimentally determined value of non-specific binding was 1,065 cpm, which agrees with the estimate (A1) of $(1,134 \pm 249)$ cpm from this model. Note that the value of parameter A4 is approximately 1. Only if an assay is unusual does this power term change. It is often possible to set it constant to 1 and so reduce the

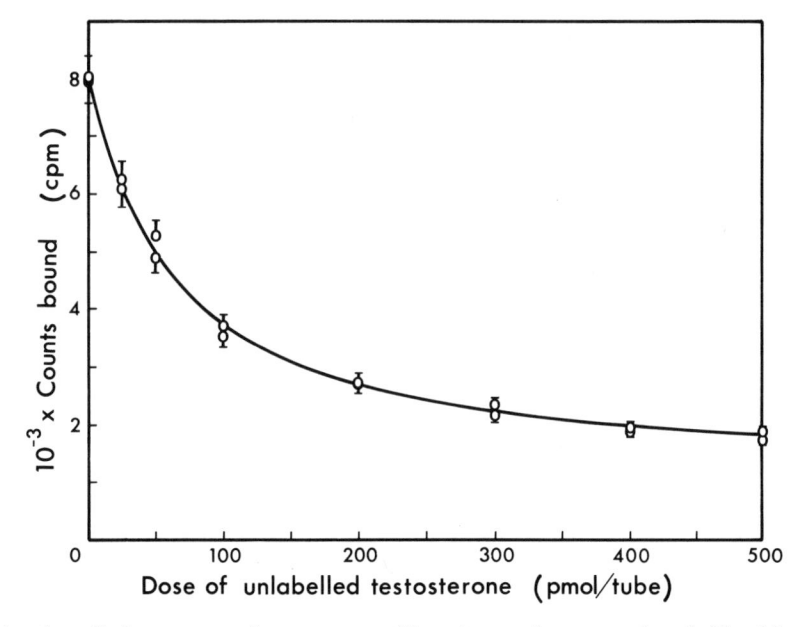

Fig. 6.5. Results of a radio-immunoassay for testosterone. The *points* are the same as those in Figs. 6.3 and 6.4 but are expressed here in terms of the bound counts. The *line* shows the result of fitting to the data the empirical model of Eq. (6.18) (using MODFIT together with subprogram RIAH). The uncertainties are equivalent to those in Fig. 6.4. The progress of the fit is shown in Table 6.6

Table 6.6. The empirical model of Eq. (6.18) fitted to data from a radio-immunoassay for testosterone[a]

R CHI SQUARE	A 1	A 2	A 3	A 4
64.005	1000.0	7000.0	5.0000	1.0000
4.5981	1357.3	6540.7	4.0151	.97648
.44659	1136.9	6888.0	4.4334	1.0711
.44658	1134.5	6890.0	4.4288	1.0699
.44658	1134.4	6890.1	4.4287	1.0698
STD DEVS	248.93	378.71	.51406	.12686
	21.9%	5.5%	11.6%	11.9%
DEPENDENCIES	.98338	.90285	.99573	.99745

CONDITION NUMBER   61951.8

CORRELATION COEFFICIENTS
```
     A 1   1.0000
     A 2   -.78776    1.0000
     A 3    .83422    -.85461   1.0000
     A 4    .92185    -.83239    .97798   1.0000
```

MODE = 1, DEGREES OF FREEDOM = 13
FINAL LAMBDA =   .0000010000000000

X	Y	YFIT	RESIDUAL	Z-RESIDUAL	SIGMAY
0.	8011.0	8024.5	-13.521	-.32424E-01	417.00
0.	8044.0	8024.5	19.479	.46601E-01	418.00
0.	7977.0	8024.5	-47.521	-.11451	415.00
25.000	6255.0	6151.1	103.91	.31974	325.00
25.000	6088.0	6151.1	-63.085	-.19901	317.00
50.000	4900.0	4996.7	-96.739	-.37937	255.00
50.000	5274.0	4996.7	277.26	1.0119	274.00
100.00	3719.0	3738.8	-19.764	-.10240	193.00
100.00	3535.0	3738.8	-203.76	-1.1074	184.00
200.00	2718.0	2681.2	36.799	.26099	141.00
200.00	2745.0	2681.2	63.799	.44615	143.00
300.00	2362.0	2222.8	139.19	1.1316	123.00
300.00	2183.0	2222.8	-39.810	-.34921	114.00
400.00	1912.0	1969.4	-57.418	-.57998	99.000
400.00	1946.0	1969.4	-23.418	-.23186	101.00
500.00	1748.0	1809.5	-61.462	-.67541	91.000
500.00	1893.0	1809.5	83.538	.85243	98.000

[a] FUNCTN subprogram RIAH together with MODFIT was used; the fitted model is shown in Fig. 6.5. Notice the high dependencies and condition number. These do not matter in this empirical model because the uncertainties are reasonable and the parameter estimates are irrelevant. The important feature is that this model is capable of analysing the results of most assays and allowing ready interpolation.

number of parameters optimized to three. It will be seen that even though the dependencies and condition number are high, the parameter uncertainties are very reasonable, reflecting the reliability of this model.

6.2.2.2 Simulation of the Testosterone Radio-Immunoassay

It is somewhat surprising, in view of the dependency values, that the parameter uncertainties obtained above were not greater. To gain more information on this point a Monte Carlo simulation was done. The aims were (1) to simulate a series of radio-immunoassay experiments having uncertainties in the response variable equal to those observed in the laboratory experiments, (2) to analyse them by means of the model of Eq. (6.18) and (3) to determine from the results whether the calculated uncertainties in the parameter estimates shown in Table 6.6 agreed with the uncertainties obtained by replication. This approach assumed to some extent the very fact at issue, namely that the model of Eq. (6.18) was suitable for generating radio-immunoassay results as if they had been determined in the laboratory. Nevertheless, there is no evidence in Table 6.6 to suggest that Eq. (6.18) was inadequate as a model of the testosterone radio-immunoassay. What is more, the results of the simulation were found to compare favourably with genuine data from replicate laboratory assays.

The simulation was done using SIMUL and subprogram RIAH. Instructions for using SIMUL will be found in Sect. 11.2 and a detailed example of its use in Sect. 3.7.1.1. The input data were identical to those used by MODFIT when fitting the model of RIAH as shown in Table 6.6, except that the initial parameter guesses were replaced by the optimized estimates. A total of 50 sets of assay results was generated by SIMUL and to each value of the response variable the program added a normally distributed random error from a population with a mean of zero and a standard deviation equal to that observed for the particular dose. The model was then fitted to each set of data.

The results of the simulation are shown in Table 6.7. The parameter estimates obtained on fitting RIAH to the 50 sets of data are not shown, in order to save space (KEY in SIMUL was set to zero). Notice the standard deviations in the parameter estimates. Comparison of these uncertainties with the means of the uncertainties as calculated in the 50 simulations (as well as those from the single experiment in Table 6.6), shows that the calculated values were similar to those found by replication.

We were able also to compare the results of the simulation with parameter estimates from the fitting of Eq. (6.18) to data from 20 genuine laboratory assays. The means and standard deviations of the parameter estimates from the latter are shown in Table 6.8. By comparison with Table 6.7 it is clear that the simulation was accurate, and that the uncertainties as calculated in any one fit were reliable. Therefore, from the results of both simulation and the analysis of laboratory experiments, we can assert that even though the dependencies and condition number obtained in the course of fitting the empirical model of Eq. (6.18) to the data from the testosterone radio-immunoassay were very high, the uncertainties in the parameter estimates were accurate.

It can sometimes happen that the four-parameter model of Eq. (6.18) or (6.19) does not fit experimental data well owing to anomalies in the shape of the response curve. Rodbard et al. (1978, Appendix A) have suggested a number of extensions involving the addition of extra parameters. The most general of these is a model of the form

$$y = (A_2 - A_1)/\{1 + \exp[f(x)]\} + A_1 \qquad (6.20)$$

where $f(x)$ is some suitable continuous, monotonic function such as a polynomial, exponential or spline (see below). Interaction is increased by the addition of extra parameters but because one is interested only in accurate interpolation, this does not matter, unless the fitting process becomes unstable and fails to converge. However, in our experience it has not been necessary to go beyond the four-parameter model of Eq. (6.19).

Table 6.7. Monte Carlo simulation of the testosterone radio-immunoassay, for determining the accuracy of calculated uncertainties in the parameter estimates[a]

```
NUMBER OF SIMULATION RUNS =   50
DEGREES OF FREEDOM         =   13
MODE = 1

PARAMETERS          A 1           A 2           A 3           A 4
                  1134.4        6890.1        4.4287        1.0698

              X            YFIT         SIGMAY
            0.            8024.5        417.00
            0.            8024.5        418.00
            0.            8024.5        415.00
           25.000         6151.3        325.00
           25.000         6151.3        317.00
           50.000         4997.0        255.00
           50.000         4997.0        274.00
          100.00          3739.1        193.00
          100.00          3739.1        184.00
          200.00          2681.5        141.00
          200.00          2681.5        143.00
          300.00          2223.0        123.00
          300.00          2223.0        114.00
          400.00          1969.6         99.000
          400.00          1969.6        101.00
          500.00          1809.6         91.000
          500.00          1809.6         98.000

MEAN VALUES OF PARAMETER ESTIMATES
                  1142.3        6837.0        4.5711        1.1009
STD DEVS          34.839        54.705        .77549E-01    .19372E-01

MEAN BIAS         -7.8981       53.073        -.14236       -.31138E-01

STANDARD DEVIATIONS OF PARAMETER ESTIMATES
                  246.35        386.82        .54836        .13698

MEAN VALUES OF CALCULATED STANDARD DEVIATIONS
                  251.61        383.45        .52949        .13003
STD DEVS          10.424        8.1978        .76539E-02    .12441E-02

DEPENDENCIES      .98459        .91080        .99597        .99759

CONDITION NUMBER     62649.5

CORRELATION COEFFICIENTS
        A 1    1.0000
        A 2    -.79963        1.0000
        A 3    .83431         -.86288       1.0000
        A 4    .92234         -.84368       .97796        1.0000

MEAN R CHI SQUARE     1.0750
STD DEV               .57970E-01
MEAN ROOT MEAN SQR    1.0189
```

[a] FUNCTN subprogram RIAH together with SIMUL was used. Fifty assays were simulated and the results are interpreted as follows (see also Table 3.2 and Sect. 3.7.1.1). The mean values of the 50 sets of parameter estimates are printed under the data, together with the standard deviations in the means as measures of precision. The latter are used in assessing the significance of the values of bias, which follow. Bias is the amount by which each parameter estimate differs from the value used to generate the data. It can be seen that the mean parameter estimates were within twice the calculated standard deviations of the true values. The sample standard deviations of each of the four sets of 50 parameter estimates obtained by replication are then printed. These should be compared with the means of the standard deviations calculated from each fit appearing in the following line. Again, the uncertainty in each mean is shown as a measure of precision.

Table 6.8. Standard deviations of the parameter estimates from 20 replicated testosterone radio-immunoassays, compared with the means of the standard deviations in each parameter calculated by MODFIT[a]

	A1	A2	A3	A4
Standard deviations of the replicates	244	460	0.44	0.12
Means of the standard deviations calculated by MODFIT	247	385	0.68	0.16

[a] FUNCTN subprogram RIAH together with MODFIT was used to fit the model of Eq. (6.18) to the results of laboratory assays for testosterone. The standard deviations of the four parameters were then calculated from the 20 replicates. Also shown are the means of the 20 sets of standard deviations produced by MODFIT from an analysis of the experimental uncertainty. Comparison of these results with the values obtained by Monte Carlo simulation (Table 6.7) shows that all are in good agreement. In particular, it is clear that the uncertainties estimated by MODFIT were accurate, whether or not the data were obtained from laboratory experiments or generated by simulation. This shows that the non-linearity of the model was not sufficiently great to invalidate the linearization method used by MODFIT to calculate the parameter uncertainties.

6.2.2.3 Spline Functions

Spline functions can provide excellent empirical models and the methods described in Sect. 2.3.1.1 have been used to interpolate in competitive protein-binding assays. Selection of knot-points is a problem; too few knots yield poor results if the data do not lie on a simple, smooth curve, while too many knots may allow the function to fluctuate widely between them and prevent accurate interpolation.

Splines can be fitted to transformed or untransformed data but problems do occur with some co-ordinate systems (Rodbard et al., 1978, Appendix C). Mosley and Bevan (1977) describe a method for the analysis of human placental lactogen assays in which a quadratic spline was fitted to the standard curve expressed in terms of B against ln (dose). So far as we are aware no other empirical interpolation method has much to commend it.

6.2.3 Weighting

Regardless of whether the model is theoretical or empirical, it is essential to weight the fit because the variance in the response variable is different at different points on the standard curve. These differences have been predicted theoretically (Rodbard and Lewald, 1970) and confirmed by experiment. Rodbard and Hutt (1974) suggested that the relationship between the variance and the dependent variable (whether it be B, F, $R_{B/T}$ or $R_{F/T}$), can be described adequately either by a straight line with non-zero slope or, in the case of radio-immunometric assays, by a quadratic. As usual (Chap. 3) a weight is expressed as the reciprocal of the variance.

In our experience, when analysing assays by means of the empirical model of Eq. (6.18) where the response variable is counts bound (B), it is convenient to work in terms of the percentage coefficient of variation (%CV), rather than variance. This is because the value of B may change considerably from one assay to another and use of the %CV effectively eliminates the effect of this change. It is impracticable to estimate the variance in the response at each dise level in every assay: instead, the results are pooled from as many assays as possible. We have found that the relationship between the %CV of B and dose is effectively constant over the dose ranges of a number of assays run in our laboratory. For example, the following relationship was found for 20 testosterone assays,

$$\%CV = (0.0025 \pm 0.0023)x + (5.20 \pm 0.58) \tag{6.21}$$

where x is the dose in pg ranging from 0 to 500 and the uncertainty is expressed as the standard deviation. (The linear regression was done using FUNCTN subprogram POLYNOM together with MODFIT, and with NTERMS set to 2). The coefficient of x is not significantly different from zero and so the %CV was assumed to have a constant value of 5.2% for this assay. Actual variances were calculated from this percentage value, and the appropriate standard deviation was entered with each data point (Tables 6.5 and 6.6).

One must, of course, determine weightings in the co-ordinate system used for the fitting. A different result is obtained if the procedure above is repeated on the response variable $R_{F/B}$. It is then unnecessary to express uncertainties as %CV because the variable $R_{F/B}$, being already a ratio, does not require normalization. The %CV was retained, however, to allow comparison with the previous analysis. Values of $R_{F/B}$ were calculated after subtracting the experimentally determined non-specific binding; no allowance was made for non-specific binding in the model of Eq. (6.17), which is a considerable practical limitation. A regression of %CV in $R_{F/B}$ against $R_{F/B}$ itself was used rather than against dose, because the uncertainty in $R_{F/B}$ depends strongly on the value of this ratio. This yielded

$$\%CV = (0.89 \pm 0.09)x + (6.3 \pm 1.1) \tag{6.22}$$

in the same terms as Eq. (6.21). The slope was significant, and was included in the calculation of weights (Table 6.4). It can be seen how much larger the uncertainty was in $R_{F/B}$ than in bound counts alone, and how it increased with dose. This was caused by the subtraction of the non-specific binding, a figure of similar magnitude [Eq. (10.6)]. These examples clearly demonstrate the need for weighting when fitting transformed mathematical models to data (see Sect. 2.8.1). Notice the difference in variation of the weights (standard deviations) in Tables 6.4 and 6.5 caused simply by transforming the co-ordinates of the data, particularly the changing (inhomogenous) variance in the response variable $R_{F/B}$.

6.2.4 Sensitivity and Precision

The most useful definition of assay sensitivity is the *minimum detectable concentration* or *minimum detectable dose* of hormone (Rodbard, 1978). This is calculated by determining the dose level corresponding to a response that differs significantly from the response obtained from a sample containing no hormone. It is appropriate to use a one-tailed t-test (Sect. 10.9) for this purpose.

The calculation is illustrated with the results of the testosterone assay analysed in Sect. 6.2.2.1. The aim is to estimate the bound count which is significantly lower (for instance, at the $p=0.05$ level) than that of the zero dose, and then to interpolate to find the corresponding dose of hormone.

Consider a certain dose giving in the assay a response of 7,000 cpm bound. From Table 6.6 the mean response for the three zero points was 8,011 cpm bound. The %

CV of any count was found by replication to be 5.2% (see Sect. 6.2.3); this will be used to estimate the standard deviation in the difference of the two counts. Thus

$$t = (8{,}011 - 7{,}000)/[(8{,}011 \times 0.052)^2 + (7{,}000 \times 0.052)^2]^{1/2}$$
$$= 1{,}011/554$$
$$= 1.83.$$

We find from tables that one-tailed t for 13 degrees of freedom and for $p=0.05$ is about 1.8. Therefore a response of 7,000 cpm bound in this assay can, at the 5 percent level of probability, just be distinguished from the response at zero dose. By interpolation a response of 7,000 cpm bound is equivalent to a dose of about 10 pmol. We conclude that 10 pmol testosterone/assay tube is the minimum detectable dose for this assay procedure.

The precision in an interpolated dose at any point on the standard curve may be calculated using the mean standard deviations in the responses obtained for purposes of weighting by pooling the results of many assays. We shall estimate the 95 percent confidence interval for a dose causing a response of 5,000 cpm. From the constant %CV of 5.2 percent the standard deviation in the count is found to be 260 cpm. We calculate the 95 percent confidence interval in the response (Sect. 10.12), using a value of t (d.f. = 13, two-tailed) equal to 2.16 to be $5{,}000 \pm (2.16 \times 260)$ cpm bound, or from 4,438 to 5,562 cpm bound. This is equivalent, by interpolation on the standard curve (Fig. 6.5), to an approximate confidence interval in the dose of 40 to 70 pmol/tube.

The precision of the particular assay illustrated was somewhat higher than the average (notice the low value of reduced chi-square in Table 6.6), but the confidence limits were calculated assuming the usual level of precision for this type of assay. In our experience, it is not worth attempting a more sophisticated calculation of uncertainty in each interpolated dose. If a reliable measure of precision is desired it is best not to calculate it as above but to replicate measurements on the sample in several assays and from these values determine the mean and uncertainty.

6.2.5 Optimization of Assays

To achieve the highest possible sensitivity and precision in an assay it is necessary to minimize the variance arising from each step in the experimental procedure. The aim is to make experimental variance negligible in comparison with the uncertainty due to biological variability.

Not only must all pipetting and other manipulations be maximally precise but also the assay conditions must be optimized. It is essential to check all the factors involved in an assay to ensure that the response is at a maximum. The duration of incubation, the temperature, the pH value and the concentrations of tracer and binding protein, all influence the response, and may interact. The methods referred to in Sect. 3.4.5 on optimizing the response of a system can be applied to advantage. Carefully designed factorial or EVOP-simplex experiments usually produce satisfactory results, showing the effects of varying parameters and variables and facilitating the selection of the best conditions. The EVOP-simplex approach is, of course, an empirical one. The assay conditions are varied until the difference between the responses at the two ends of the dose range is maximized. Care must, however, be taken to ensure that such a choice of conditions does not lead to greatly reduced precision or the advantage will be lost.

The methods of Chap. 4 are also useful. Application of the design criterion for parameter estimation will indicate how to distribute the points on a standard curve in such a way as to give the highest precision in the parameters, which in turn will lead to increased overall precision of response. This method is limited, in its present form, to giving information on optimizing the choice of the value of a single independent variable.

A theoretical approach to optimization which depends on a knowledge of the physical parameters of the assay was tried out by Ekins et al. (1968; 1970). They first developed expressions assuming that all experimental uncertainty was due to errors in the measurement of radioactivity. Then, having made a number of additional assumptions concerning the effects of other sources of variance, several useful conclusions were drawn. For example, it was shown that use of tracer with a very high specific activity does not automatically give greater sensitivity, but that an upper limit is approached which depends on the association constant of the binding sites and the pipetting errors. However, accurate predictions from theoretical considerations are extremely difficult to make unless accurate information about the distribution of experimental errors is available.

Rodbard and his colleagues have emphasized the need to characterize fully the nature of the association between ligand and protein when attempting to optimize an assay. As well as estimating the values of association constants, it is helpful to know the rate constants of association and dissociation (Rodbard, 1973; Ketelslegers et al., 1975; Rodbard, 1977, Appendix D), the effect of delayed addition of binding protein (Rodbard et al., 1971), the thermodynamics of binding and the influence of incubation temperature (Keane et al., 1976), and the effect of the technique used to separate the free ligand from that bound to the protein (Rodbard and Catt, 1972).

Accurate estimates of association constants, concentrations of binding sites and other parameters may not be easily obtained from analysis of competitive protein-binding assays carried out to determine unknowns. It is preferable to obtain data for estimating the parameters of theoretical models from measurements made under carefully controlled conditions, such as those used in equilibrium dialysis experiments. Yanagishita and Rodbard (1978) have summarized the present position regarding assay optimization and report that predictions of optimum conditions made by simulation using a combination of computer programs, were in reasonable agreement with the results of subsequent experimentation. Optimization by these methods is a complex procedure, probably still beyond the capacity of most laboratories. Such methods may come into general use in the future but meanwhile investigators will undoubtedly rely on the fact that in most binding assays there is much latitude in the conditions suitable for producing near-optimal results.

7 Mathematical Modelling of Biological Rhythms

Biological organisms live in a multi-rhythmic environment. Light, heat, nutrients and other stimuli are supplied from the surroundings with a variety of frequencies and amplitudes. There are also internal rhythms including, for example, the supply of blood containing gases, nutrients and hormones, as well as rhythms in nervous impulses, and autonomic and other muscular contractions. Hormones are important transmitters of information within the body on both the state of the external environment (through the central nervous system) and of states of other internal organs; they are therefore intimately involved with these rhythms.

According to the well-known principle of homeostasis, biological systems contain mechanisms for adjusting their internal environments within a limited range of effector values; these confining limits, outside which survival may be endangered, are often considerably narrower than the range of values encountered in the environment. The model of negative feedback (Sect. 2.5) is evoked as a major mechanism for maintaining homeostasis. It is interesting that this model, which is designed to produce constancy of variables in the internal environment, also permits (mathematically) the expectation of stable rhythms under some circumstances. Non-linear negative feedback systems which display time delays combined with high gain as expected in biological organisms, can have solutions to their equations described not by stable steady states, but by stable oscillations, known as limit cycles, the characteristics of which are described in Sect. 2.6.2. Any values taken by the variables of the system change with time towards those describing the limit cycle, thereby ensuring stability of the rhythm (Fig. 2.13). Stability is a characteristic also of biological rhythms.

There are mathematical models other than negative feedback which predict stable limit cycle behaviour, and these also may be appropriate for describing biological rhythms (Sect. 2.6.4). The mathematical concept of stable rhythms produced by limit cycles has inspired some intriguing biological experiments confirming its predictions and has explained data difficult to interpret in other ways. Interpretations using this model, as well as the important potential of such internal rhythms to provide mechanisms for control of biological function are major concerns of this chapter.

7.1 Biological Rhythms: Experimental Evidence

The evidence for persistent internal rhythms in biological organisms is described in a vast literature, augmented by attempts at explanation (see Palmer, 1976, and Sollberger, 1965). For example, Palmer lists some 80 enzymes, hormones and metabolites in organs and tissues of higher animals and plants which, at that time, had been demonstrated to have a circadian fluctuation in concentration or activity.

It is thus hardly surprising that the behaviour of organisms also varies with a daily rhythm. In humans, for instance, apart from the obvious cycles of activity, rhythms have been found in responses shown to drugs and allergens, ability at psychomotor tests, tolerance to pain, time perception, metabolism of alcohol and many other characteristics.

It used to be thought that rhythms which are entrained to geophysical cycles may be controlled from a master clock in the central nervous system, perhaps by hormones from the pineal gland, the secretions of which are known to be influenced by cycles of light and dark. However, it is now evident that individual organs, cells and also certain cell-free biochemical mixtures can sustain their own independent rhythms even when isolated from the intact animal. Single heart cells can maintain a circadian rhythm of contraction: isolated adrenal glands from the golden hamster when cultured in a defined medium have been shown to consume oxygen and secrete corticosteroids in a 24 h rhythm (Palmer, 1976). Chance and his colleagues (Chance et al., 1967) have shown that oscillations in the concentration of NADH in the glycolytic pathway can occur not only in yeast cell cultures, but also in cell-free extracts. These latter rhythms have been modelled in terms of the rate constants and non-linearities of the interactions between enzymes and substrates.

Do the rhythms of whole organisms or isolated cells depend upon external stimuli or are they inherent, being merely synchronized by environmental cues? The effects of removing circadian signals from animals and humans have been extensively studied. Some rhythms have thus been shown to become desynchronized (no consistent relationship between rhythms) while others take up a new phase relationship to each other (Aschoff and Wever, 1976). However, those rhythms tested generally persist, and appear to be inherent in the absence of at least obvious entraining cues.

In contrast, Yates (1974) holds the view that periodicites observed in the performance of isolated components of the adrenal system in vitro are not caused by intrinsic oscillators. In his opinion, such data demonstrate merely that the components have non-linear memory properties and that if they have been driven in an oscillatory fashion, their parameters will continue to vary periodically. The mathematical models of the functioning of the adrenal system so far devised do not use as a basis the concept of an inherent oscillator.

Hitherto, the emphasis has been on circadian rhythms but

> only a tone-deaf biologist would insist on hearing merely the circadian pitch in the symphony of processes that characterize life.

In spite of the previous paragraph, this quotation is from enthusiastic advocates (Yates et al., 1972) of the view that the ultimate explanation of the design principles of life must be based on the oscillator in its many frequencies and forms, and that periodicities, cycles or repeated motions are the only known stable behaviours of non-linear systems.

Biological rhythms are not confined to simple frequencies designed with ease of investigation in mind. Many are multiple and interact with other systems in the organism. Simple examples concerning the menstrual cycle are the release of LH from the pituitary in women, which shows a monthly peak associated with ovulation, but also exhibits small oscillations with a frequency of about 90 min.

Similarly, body temperature has a 24-h period as well as a monthly variation correlated with the menstrual cycle (Sect. 7.5.1.1).

7.2 The Contribution of Mathematics

What has mathematical modelling to contribute to the elucidation of biological rhythms?

(1) Mathematics proposes models of relationships which produce rhythmic outcomes. (2) It suggests ways in which external influences can affect rhythms. (3) Equations can be written to describe these processes, allowing comparison of model with data. (4) Modelling suggests critical experiments for testing ideas about rhythms. (5) Mathematics gives guidance in collecting and analysing experimental data to ensure that the rhythmic characteristics determined are meaningful.

A few aspects of all these functions that have caught our interest are briefly outlined here.

Mathematics cannot discover the purposes served by biological rhythms, their components, causal connections, structures, precise parameters of space and time, and which inter-relationships occur between rhythms; that is the role of inspired experimentation. However, combined searches by both experimentalists and mathematical modellers for physical and mathematical descriptions of biological rhythms can give mutual guidance by suggesting possible approaches to explore. Benefits from such combined activities are demonstrated clearly in the following brief descriptions.

Several of our examples have been selected not because the concepts and methods are applied to endocrinological systems, but rather that they illustrate some significant aspect in the understanding of all rhythms.

7.2.1 Description of Rhythms

The most characteristic property of rhythms, oscillators or cycles is that a sequence of events or measured values is found to recur regularly with the passing of time. A rhythm is characterized by its *frequency* – the number of times the sequence of events recurs in a given interval of time (for example, cycles/h). The inverse of frequency measures the interval between each repeated event and is known as the *period*. If a quantity is varying rhythmically, then half the difference between its maximum and minimum values is termed the *amplitude*. *Phase* describes some arbitrarily chosen fraction of a cycle, such as that traversed since the most recent occurrence of a conspicuous event. A biological clock is a cyclic system providing a rhythm which controls the regular timing of an event external to it. A rhythmic change in a quantity may be plotted as a function of time, or represented independently of time as a closed loop produced by a rotating arrow (Fig. 7.1). A circle can also be used to represent a rhythmic series of events. Each rotation of 360° represents one complete cycle of defined values or events. Sect. 7.5 describes methods of characterizing the frequencies, amplitudes and relative phases of rhythmic measurements from biological systems.

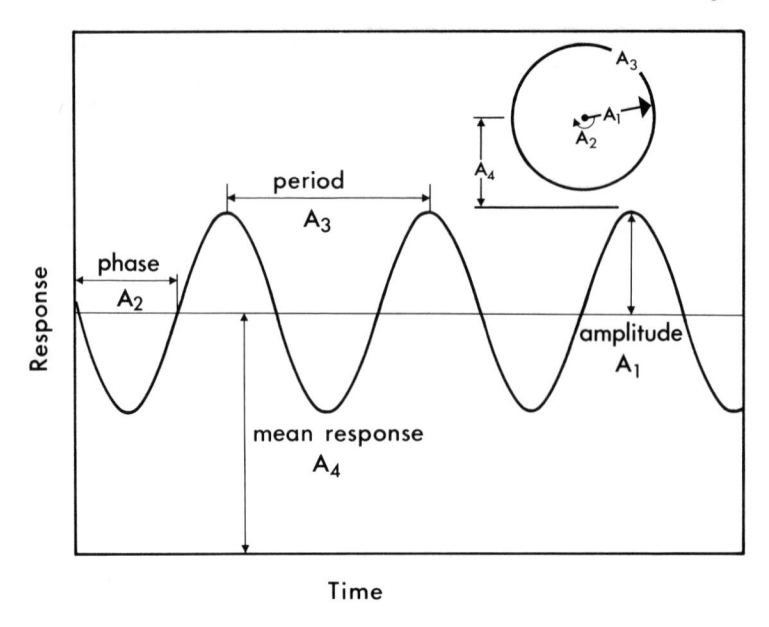

Fig. 7.1. Representations of rhythmic changes in a variable. The variations with time are here shown as a *sine wave*. The parameters A_1 to A_4 are explained further in the description of Eq. (7.3). The phase relationship is not a fixed characteristic of the rhythm but is defined by the user for a particular purpose. Here it measures the displacement from a reference curve in which sin (0) occurs at zero time

7.2.2 Mathematical Models of Response to Stimuli

Three types of mathematical models may be proposed to account for the responses of biological systems to stimuli. Living processes appear to be described by all three models.

1) The effect of a stimulus may be rapidly reduced by a mechanism in the biological system so that a nearly constant internal steady state is maintained at which the organism is adapted to function optimally, as in homeostasis. Such a return may be monotonic or exhibit damped oscillations which decline with time, and therefore cannot constitute a sustained rhythm. These systems are modelled using differential equations where possible, or in terms of negative feedback loops. Linear mathematical methods have been most highly developed (Sect. 2.5.2).

2) A set of stimuli controls the initiation or maintenance of a response. If the stimuli are removed, the rhythm or response ceases; the organism is required to follow the rhythm presented to it. Such a passive biological system would rely upon outside forces to initiate and sustain its behaviour. While such environmental interdependence provides for adaptation, total dependence is unlikely to sustain the life form except in very consistent environments. If a shadow is cast at the wrong moment the system may be doomed.

3) An internal rhythm in the organism (such as a stable limit cycle) persists in isolation. A charcteristic of a limit cycle, for example, is that it maintains a stable rhythm even in the absence of stimuli, or if stimuli are non-rhythmic. Such a persistent internal cycle may respond to rhythmic external or internal inputs by *entraining* (matching) its frequency to that of the stimulus. Response may not occur

to all disturbances but only at appropriate sensitive phases. In a reasonably hospitable environment, such a system could select those couplings and interactions with its environment required for both adaptation and persistence. The entrained internal rhythms might also act as stimuli or controllers of other internal events, thus synchronizing the functioning of the whole organism. It has been proposed that a network of interacting limit cycle oscillators provides a basis for control and organization of life processes (see, for example, Iberall, 1972). The descriptions in Sect. 7.3 will help to clarify the nature of limit cycle behaviour and possible responses to stimuli.

An event observed to occur cyclically may thus be modelled as being triggered by a rhythmic stimulus which is independent of it (second model above), or as an inherent part of a limit cycle (third model). The timing of mitosis, for example, has been modelled in both ways. In a model of the second kind, described in Sect. 7.3.2.3, a clock external to mitosis acts as a trigger at regular intervals. This interpretation appears to explain more experimental results than do other models. In a model of the third kind, mitosis is one event in a cyclic sequence of discrete states, each stimulating the next to produce the rhythm (reviewed by Mitchison, 1971). Other models in which mitosis is a necessary part of the limit cycle, propose the accumulation of a "mitogen" which at a critical level initiates mitosis, is itself consumed in this process, and then must accumulate again before mitosis can recur.

Evidence for spontaneous stable internal rhythms implied by the third kind of model is being actively sought. For example, Rapp and Berridge (1977) have suggested that in cells Ca^{2+} and cAMP are linked in a negative feedback loop capable of producing such behaviour. Concentrations of these components are proposed to fluctuate with a frequency of between 0.1 s and 5 min. Such oscillations would rhythmically alter membrane potentials, thus affecting many biochemical reactions within cells, and influencing frequency and amplitude effects of hormone stimulation. The authors invoke such a mechanism as a possible basis for explaining diverse biological rhythms including oscillations of potential in cardiac pacemaker cells, neurones and insulin secreting beta-cells, cAMP pulses in *Dictyostelium* and rhythmical and cytoplasmic streaming in *Physarum*. They suggest also that the rhythmic release of pituitary hormones and adrenocorticoids might be explained by this mechanism.

Like many such potentially important models for explaining rhythms, the necessary supporting experimental data were incomplete at the time of publication. Elucidation of the linkages between cAMP synthesis and Ca^{2+} concentration was still required, as were simultaneous measurements of cAMP and Ca^{2+} oscillations in the same tissue in order to test the sustained limit cycle nature of their relationships. The availability of non-obtrusive techniques for measuring dynamic changes in concentrations of substances in individual cells appears crucial to elucidating such problems on the molecular level.

7.3 Response of Rhythms to Stimuli – Rhythm Coupling

While there has been much speculation on the mechanisms bringing about couplings between rhythms and stimuli, few structural mechanisms have been proposed to explain the nature of inherent biological cycles themselves. Membranes are clearly implicated in the maintenance, if not the control of biorhythms. Treatment of cells with substances affecting the structure of membranes (as do valinomycin, ethanol, lithium or lipids), or altering important membrane-bound enzymes (such as by caffeine), is one of the remarkably few consistent ways found for changing the timing of biological clocks, other than by stimuli naturally entraining the rhythms. A membrane model of a circadian controlling clock based on feedback oscillators has been proposed by Njus et al. (1974). Several other feedback models for circadian controlling rhythms at the level of gene transcription are described by Edmunds (1976). Any physical model of circadian rhythms must allow for entrainment by 24-h geophysical phenomena.

Suggestions for physiological and biochemical mechanisms which might bring about the coupling of rhythms and events include all of the known cellular components related to kinetic parameters and variables in living systems. Alterations in the concentrations of hormones, enzymes, metabolites, inhibitors or activators, the rates of synthesis of enzymes, the transport properties of membranes, the numbers of hormone receptors, the kinetic constants of enzymes or the properties of a rate controlling enzyme in a series of reactions, are but a few of the possible ways in which biological rhythms may be disturbed, or have their behaviours altered by external or internal stimuli, rhythmic or non-rhythmic.

The aim of modelling the mechanisms of many of these ubiquitous rhythms theoretically in terms of components appears currently to be unattainable. Much directed experimentation is needed to identify the components responsible, their individual kinetics, and their interactions, before concise differential equations with identifiable independent variables and parameters can be written (i.e. if differential equations are appropriate).

However, "black box" methods of investigating the interactions of rhythms have yielded some very interesting interpretations of particular mechanisms. It has been rewarding to measure the responses of a system to stimuli of various kinds and intensities applied at different times during a cycle, and then to look for similarities or discontinuities in these responses. Simplified descriptions follow of some insights into unexpected experimental observations obtained by these means.

7.3.1 Phases Sensitive to Stimulation

We consider here models devised to explain experimental investigations of the links between biological rhythms and environmental stimuli.

An annual rhythm is evident in the behaviour of many animals and insects. Some means of measuring the absolute duration of either light or dark, or the ratio between them, would appear to provide obvious mechanisms for relating these annual responses to geophysical phenomena.

An effect related to patterns of light and dark controls the release of hormones in insects which bring about or prevent diapause, a period of dormancy between stages of active growth and development. Saunders (1976) has described some unexpected experimental results concerning the interplay of light–dark rhythms on the diapause of a fly. The larvae of the flesh fly *Sarcophaga argyrostoma* were observed to develop without diapause in lighting periods of more than 14 h per 24 h. As expected, diapause was induced with 12 h light : 12 h dark. However, many larvae continued to develop without diapause with 12 h light and *longer* periods of darkness of about 24 and 48 h. Interpretation of this phenomenon in terms of the simple, direct mechanisms proposed in the previous paragraph is inadequate; instead, the existence of a sensitive phase in an internal controlling circadian oscillator, which responds to incident light by preventing diapause, provides an explanation of the results, as follows. Dusk is assumed to entrain the circadian oscillator, and the sensitive phase would occur 10 h later. Under natural lighting stimulus, nights longer than 10 h produce diapause. During experimentally prolonged dark periods the circadian oscillator continues to cycle, and if this sensitive phase happens to coincide with the lighted interval during one of several following circadian cycles, diapause may still be inhibited.

The sizes of golden hamster testes show a similarly unexpected and very marked response to artificial lighting rhythms (Elliott et al., 1972). At least 12,5 h light per 24 h period are required to maintain testicular function and weight in this hibernating animal. While 6 h light alternating with either 18 or 42 h darkness caused the expected regression of the testes to about one fifth their active weight, periods of only 6 h light combined with 30 or 54 h darkness were sufficient to maintain testicular weight, even over 89 days (35 cycles of 6 h light : 54 h dark). Figure 7.2 shows one possible model with an entrained circadian oscillator containing a light sensitive phase, as marked. Coincidence of the internal rhythm entrained by dusk with external light rhythms is postulated to be required for promoting hormonal action on the hamster gonads. This observed sensitivity to light is probably mediated by the inhibitory action of dark-induced secretions of the pineal gland because pinealectomy abolishes the gonadal regression during continued darkness. The regrowth part of the cycle appears to be controlled by yet another longer-term internal clock, independent of light. After 20–25 weeks of constant darkness, the testes will spontaneously regenerate without light. This latter mechanism is presumably designed to allow breeding to occur immediately after the animals emerge from hibernation (Reiter, 1974).

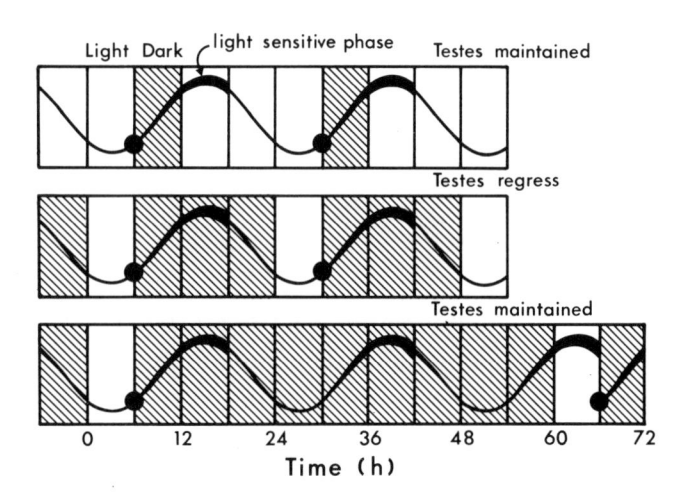

Fig. 7.2. Possible model for the response of hamster testes to artificial lighting rhythms. The *sine waves* represent a circadian rhythm in the hamster entrained by dusk (●). Coincidence of a sensitive phase of this rhythm with light results in maintenance of the weights of the testes even during unnaturally extended intervals of darkness

Adaptive interaction of a persistent internal oscillator at a particular phase with external stimuli (Sect. 7.2.2, model 3) therefore appears necessary to explain both the annual onset of diapause and the annual regression of testis weight. A model in which these events are induced by direct stimulation (model 2) from a particular length of day or night, or their ratio, will not suffice.

Similar models are possible in which two or more internal cycles must be synchronized separately by different cues in the environment to ensure coincidence of a sensitive phase in each at an appropriate time of year. Diapause control in the wasp *Nasonia vitripennis*, a parasite of the flesh fly (Saunders, 1976) appears to be described by such a model. If the female wasp is exposed to more than 15.2 h light in 24 h, the eggs will give rise to larvae which are prevented from entering diapause. With shorter days diapause does occur. However, very short days can, unexpectedly, also prevent diapause. The interaction of daylight and internal oscillators affecting the control of diapause is not by means of a photo-sensitive period as in the fly because, in constant darkness, suitably timed changes in temperature can also bring about or prevent diapause. Temperature or light must act merely as entrainers of internal rhythms. The model proposed (Fig. 7.3) has two internal oscillators, one entrained by dawn and the other by dusk. At suitable day lengths, sensitive phases of the oscillators coincide to bring about development without diapause. One can imagine schemes in which concentrations of two or more substances must reach certain levels simultaneously in order that another controlling enzyme or hormone be produced. The lower part of Fig. 7.3 shows that in this model the coincidence of oscillators preventing diapause may be produced not only by long days but also by very short ones, as is observed experimentally. The finding of a "short-day" effect such as this provides good experimental evidence for the proposed model.

Wallen and Yochim (1974) have suggested a model similar to that in Fig. 7.3 for producing cycles longer than circadian by the interplay of circadian rhythms with similar, but not identical, periods. They propose, on the basis of regrettably inadequate data, that the activity of the enzyme hydroxyindole-*O*-methyltransferase (HIOMT) involved in the production of melatonin in the rat

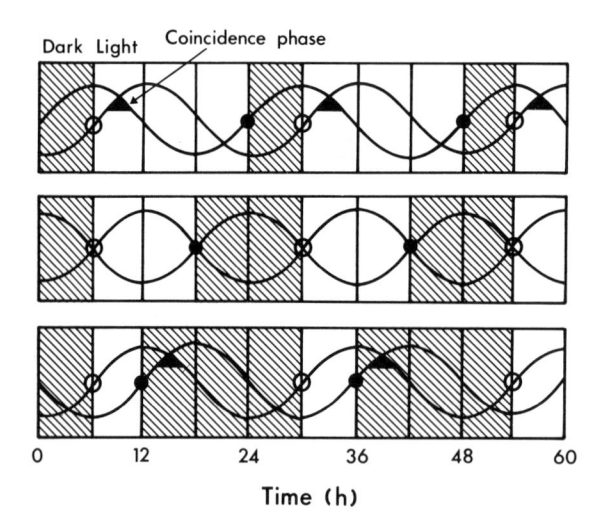

Fig. 7.3. Model of the induction of diapause in the larvae of the wasp *Nasonita vitripennis*. The *sine waves* represent two circadian rhythms in the female wasp, one entrained by dawn (○) and the other by dusk (●). When the rhythms coincide at a sensitive phase, diapause is inhibited in the larvae from her eggs. Both long and very short days produce this result. Redrawn from Saunders, 1976, The Biological Clock of Insects. Copyright by Scientific American, Inc. All rights reserved. With kind permission of W. H. Freeman and Co. for Scientific American, Inc.

pineal gland, is regulated by the interaction of a 24-h rhythm with an approximately 20-h one. This is suggested to form a repeating pattern of enzyme activity in the gland over four or five days, which the authors have attempted to correlate with the phases and length of the rat oestrous cycle. Figure 7.4 shows their experimental data together with curves calculated from their model. Where the two rhythms postulated by the model coincide, there is a maximum amplitude of summed activity, but when the rhythms are 180° out of phase two days later, a reduced peak of activity of longer duration should occur. By such a mechanism either the high peak or longer duration of enzyme activity produced by these combined rhythms might be the sensitive phase instrumental in triggering some process related to the oestrous cycle. If the 24-h rhythm is entrained and the other is free-running, this may account for the observed variability in the length of the cycle. Note that the first four days of the five-day cycle shown in Fig. 7.4 use the same data as the four-day cycle. (Where animals are killed for each measurement it is not possible to measure successive cycles – all are averaged for one cycle.)

This graph also shows clearly the difficulty of estimating periods and amplitudes from small numbers of discrete measurements of periodic phenomena. The analysis given relies heavily on the last point of the four-day cycle on the graph and if this were by chance too high it appears possible to draw, within the uncertainty of the other points, four regular oscillations of approximately equal period and amplitude. Further data collected around the maximum and minimum peaks, together with

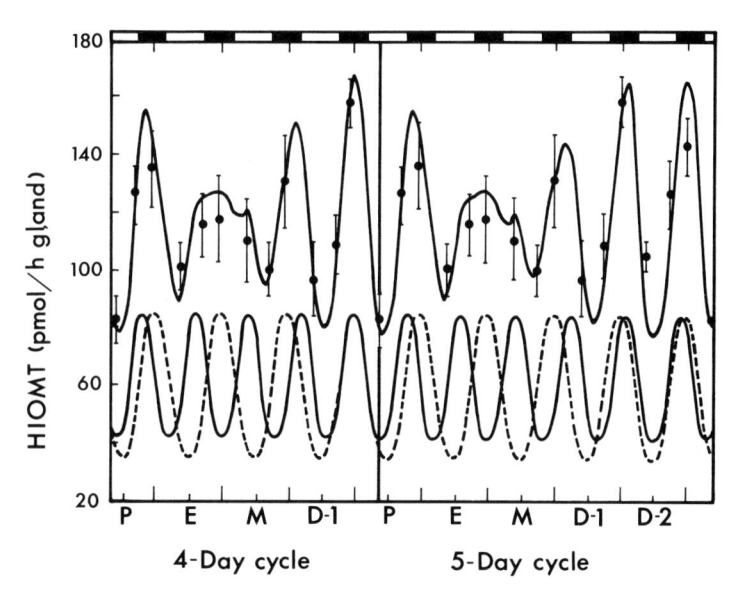

Fig. 7.4. Suggested model for producing four and five-day rhythms from two circadian rhythms in HIOMT activity during the rat oestrous cycle. The *lower curves* represent hypothetical component rhythms of 24 h and 19.2 or 20 h. The sum of these is shown above, with measurements of the enzyme activity (● ± sample standard deviation of the mean), during the different stages of the oestrous cycle (*P* = pro-oestrus; *E* = oestrus; *M* = metoestrus; *D* = dioestrus). Light and dark periods are shown at the top of the graph. Redrawn from Wallen and Yochim, 1974, with kind permission

other methods of analysis, would have shown whether the published interpretation was feasible.

Let us consider the kinds of experimental information needed to test the physiological implications of four or five-day rhythms in the activity of HIOMT. For example, is this enzyme involved in any sort of "control" of the timing of the rat oestrous cycle, or is the cycle controlling the concentration of enzyme? The enzyme activity was assayed after homogenization which would have disrupted any structural control of its kinetic behaviour that might have operated in vivo. This enzyme is the last in a series which converts tryptophan to melatonin. Only if this enzyme is rate limiting will it affect the rate of production of melatonin. Much larger increases occur during periods of darkness in the activity of another enzyme, N-acetyl transferase, which precedes HIOMT in the sequence of reactions producing melatonin (Klein and Weller, 1970). However, it is possible that the increase in activity of the latter enyzme may make that of the HIOMT relatively less, and therefore rate limiting. In this case melatonin should show the same kinds of four or five-day variable oscillations. Whether such variations in melatonin secretion would be received by some target tissue influencing the oestrous cycle depends also on the kinetics of transport and clearance rates, so that simple measurements of peripheral blood concentrations of melatonin, for example, may not be relevant to its action in tissues reached by other means of transport. Furthermore, the nature of any target tissue or tissues of melatonin in rats is still in doubt because pinealectomy does not seem to affect in any way the reproductive performance of rats in laboratory experiments.

Considerably more experimental work and basic knowledge of the relationships of enzyme concentrations in the pineal gland to reproductive function are required to test the hypothesis that the proposed rhythm has any influence on the oestrous cycle of the rat. Mathematical models may suggest new possibilities to seek but, as ever, sound experimental evidence is needed to give such models credence.

The pineal gland itself does not appear to respond directly to the influence of light. A model using an intermediate controlling clock with sensitive phases is needed to explain the production of melatonin by this gland. Darkness during night time causes synthesis and release of melatonin by a well-studied mechanism, including the large increase in the synthesis of N-acetyl transferase mentioned earlier (Klein, 1978). However, contrary to the implications of a model in which the pineal responds to light directly (the second kind of response to stimuli listed in Sect. 7.2.2), darkness during daylight hours does not cause production of melatonin. There appears to be a circadian oscillator located in the suprachiasmic nucleus which is capable of activating the mechanism leading to melatonin production during only part of the daily cycle. Light at any stage of the cycle prevents the production of melatonin. A cyclical model such as that proposed by Pavlidis (1971) appears to be appropriate. During daylight the system traverses a non-productive phase of the cycle, at the end of which it stops. Darkness must occur before the cycle can continue to other phases. Stimulus by light during the dark phase immediately resets the cycle to the daylight one. In continued darkness the cycle can oscillate through both phases unimpeded, producing melatonin in a circadian rhythm.

The models outlined in this section are metaphoric – the important physiological and biochemical aspects of both the internal, inherent rhythms and their sensitive phases have not been described in detail. In addition to the sensitive phases, all models depend on the entrainment of an inherent oscillator, that is, matching of an internal rhythm to the period of an external one. A possible way in which this can be modelled is described in Sect. 7.3.3.

7.3.2 Disturbances in Models Involving Limit Cycles

If inherent biological rhythms can be modelled as limit cycles, what kinds of responses would be predicted to disturbances from stimuli? Some relevant properties of limit cycles are discussed here, a model of phase changes in biological rhythms is presented and interpreted in terms of limit cycles, and several experimental tests of the predictions of a limit cycle model are described.

Some kinds of non-linear interactions within systems which may produce limit cycles are described in Sect. 2.6.4. The rhythmic changes in the levels of components can be plotted as a function of time (Fig. 2.13), or in phase space forming a closed loop (Fig. 2.14).

The important characteristic of limit cycles is their stability; if the values of the variables y and/or z are perturbed instantaneously away from the limit cycle, the equations driving the trajectory of the perturbed point ensure that it winds back towards the cycle (Fig. 2.14), where it continues to oscillate. An exception occurs if the perturbation drives the point (y, z) outside the area of attraction of the limit cycle, whereupon it moves to some other stable region of the topology. Another exception occurs if the system is perturbed exactly to S (Fig. 2.14), the unstable steady state. The slightest disturbance from S will, however, cause y and z to spiral out to the limit cycle. If the parameters of the cycle are altered or the disturbance is maintained, the characteristic frequency of the cycle and the repeating values of the variables may change (Fig. 7.9) or the cycle may be eliminated altogether (dotted line in Fig. 2.14).

Winfree (1970) describes a useful concept related to limit cycles called an isochron. The initial value of any point (y, z) not on the limit cycle cannot be assigned a phase of the cycle, but the determination of latent phase is helpful. The latent phase of (y, z) is the same as the phase of the corresponding point on the cycle towards which the trajectory of (y, z) will move with time. If a dot is put on the trajectory of (y, z) at time intervals equal to the period of completing one traverse of the cycle, then the path of these dots will be seen to move towards a particular point on the cycle. The line joining the dots is an *isochron*. All points on an isochron have latent phase equal to the phase of the point on the limit cycle at which the isochron intersects it. Isochrons of a limit cycle are illustrated in Fig. 7.8. Isochrons all meet at S; points very close to each other near S may eventually take up phases very different from one another on the limit cycle.

All these interesting and perhaps unexpected behaviours of components y and z are consequences of the nature of the interaction between them, and may be deduced by the theoretical or quantitative application of mathematics.

7.3.2.1 Pulse Stimuli Causing Phase Changes

One of the characteristics of biological cycles entrained to periodic external events is the appearance of apparent discontinuities in the phase of their responses when pulse stimuli are applied at successive intervals of time. A simplified model of this behaviour is as follows. Figure 7.5 represents a cycle which may be interpreted as a

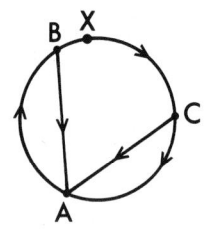

Fig. 7.5. A cycle represented as a circle. At X an observable event is initiated. A pulsed stimulation by an entraining signal at any stage of the cycle resets it to phase A. Stimulation at B causes a delay in the expected occurrence of X whereas at C the cycle and X are advanced in time

rhythmic repetition of events, the concentration of a substance or the like. When this rhythm is free-running, phase X recurs each time one traverse of the cycle is completed. At X an observable event is initiated for which this cycle acts as a clock. Suppose that an instantaneous entraining stimulus such as the switching off of a light immediately resets the cycle to A. If the cycle is at B when the light is switched off, the arc A to B must be traversed again, and the observable event X will be delayed. If, however, the cycle is at C when the light is switched off, the cycle will be advanced when reset to point A, and X will occur sooner than expected. There will be a short time interval near point X encompassing responses of both maximal advance and maximal delay in X in response to the light being switched off, thus producing an apparent discontinuity.

This kind of discontinuous response to pulsed stimuli applied at successive intervals of time has been demonstrated to occur in many light-entrained biological systems, as follows. After being entrained to normal 24 h daylight patterns, the system is kept continuously in the dark with an entraining pulse of light applied to different samples of it at various times over 24 h. Plots of apparent phase shifts in X as a function of the time of applying pulsed light have the general characteristics of Fig. 7.6. Events which have been studied in this way, include such various circadian behaviours as the hatching of the pupae of fruit fly, the onset of activity periods of flying squirrels and of hamsters, the luminescence in dinoflagellates, and the movements of leaves in beans and petals of houseplants (Pittendrigh, 1965).

7.3.2.2 Limit Cycle Interpretation of Phase Changes

If Fig. 7.5 is considered to be a limit cycle in phase space (Sect. 2.6.2) showing the rhythmic relationships between two variables y and z, this models predicts several other interesting and unexpected properties for which good experimental support has been found.

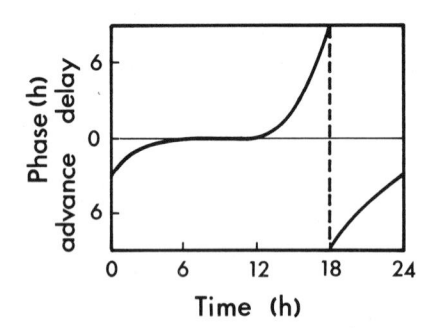

Fig. 7.6. A generalized phase response curve for biological systems having light-entrained circadian rhythms. Resulting phase advance or delay of an appropriately observed circadian event is plotted against the time of day (initial phase) at which a sample of the system was stimulated with a pulse of light

It is unlikely, for example, that a stimulus will alter the values of y and z so that they fall exactly on the cycle at A. In Fig. 7.7, if for simplicity z only were reduced by stimuli applied at P, X, and Q, then the trajectories of its resulting states would wind out again to the limit cycle to reach the same phases as their isochrons on the cycle at P', X, and Q'. Thus each new phase would be either advanced or delayed with respect to the old, with a gradual change rather than the abrupt one shown for the special case of Fig. 7.5.

It might also be expected that different intensities of stimuli would cause different degrees of displacement from the limit cycle, thus altering the shapes of the curves of phase displacement versus phase of stimulus application (time) shown in Fig. 7.6 (Pavlidis, 1973, Chap. 3). Winfree (1977) constructs a three-dimensional diagram from such experiments with axes corresponding to the phase of the cycle at which the stimulus is applied, the intensity of the stimulus, and the resulting phase of activity. These values, which have been measured for a number of biological rhythms, form a surface which resembles a screw rotating about the equivalent of the singular point in a limit cycle. The phase discontinuity in Fig. 7.6 can be explained in terms of this structure.

From his experimental results on the change in the time of eclosion (emergence of pupae) of the fly *Drosophila* with phase and intensity of applied light signals, Winfree constructed a physical model of such a screw. He was able to calculate the conditions (intensity of stimulus and phase of application) required to displace the system to the singularity, and to test the biological significance of this theoretical point by measuring the new phase produced. It was anticipated that either no circadian rhythmicity in eclosion would be observed, or alternatively one of unpredictable phase. Experimentally, it was shown that this state corresponded to the arhythmic condition occurring in pupae reared from the egg stage in total darkness; the first light signal moves dark-reared pupae away from this state by "turning on" the clock producing the usual circadian cycle of eclosion. Similar calculations applied to the oscillating fluorescence of NADH in a yeast cell suspension predicted the conditions necessary to force the system to its singular point, where the oscillations were seen experimentally to disappear.

Winfree (1977) points out that such phenomena may not be observed with all biological rhythms as this model ignores effects from transients. The stimulus must be of short duration, as sustained signals may alter the form of the limit cycle making comparison of phases meaningless. The dynamics of the system must be such that it rebounds quickly to the limit cycle – a very long trajectory may result from disturbance, or it may not return to the same cycle. A stimulus sufficiently intense for the system to reach the singularity may not be physically attainable.

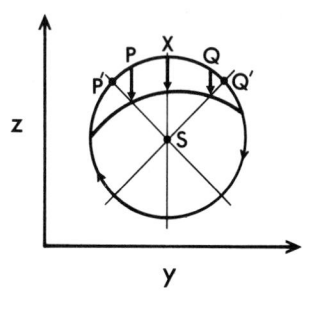

Fig. 7.7. A limit cycle model of phase resetting. The *circle* represents a stable limit cycle in the concentrations of y and z. Isochrons of the phase space are marked from the singularity of the cycle, S. If a pulsed stimulus resets P, X and Q as marked by the *arrows*, P', X and Q' denote the resulting phases of the cycle. Stimuli applied near X produce a gradual change in the resulting phase from delay to advance

7.3.2.3 Application of a Limit Cycle Model

A model based on a limit cycle oscillator which has been extensively investigated is that applied to the timing of mitosis in the slime mould *Physarum polycephalum* (reviewed by Kauffman, 1977). This model successfully predicts complicated responses in the timing of a rhythmic event (mitosis) to various stimuli. Earlier models do not readily account for these responses without ad hoc embellishments. Although the physical details of this metaphoric model are not directly relevant to endocrinology, the principles involved in the timing of an event by an internal clock have wide-ranging implications.

The model of Kauffman and his colleagues is based on an internal limit cycle clock which is proposed to trigger the experimentally observed event (mitosis) at a threshold concentration of one of its components (z in Fig. 7.8). The clock need not be dependent on any of the processes leading to the event. Such a model has been shown to be consistent with the observed complex effects of heat shock on the advancement or delay of mitosis in *Physarum polycephalum*, and also in timing of mitosis in fused pieces of plasmodia (Sect. 7.3.4). Interpreted generally, their method of studying this dynamic system was to perturb it by applying stimuli over a range of intensities at different phases of the cycle, and to map the locations of stationary states, thresholds, limit cycles and so on, as shown by the responses. Such a "black box" approach yields results given a metaphoric interpretation and is not used to propose any particular physical mechanism.

The effects of heat shock on the timing of mitosis were found to depend both on the stage of the cycle at which the shock was applied and its duration, as follows. Heat shocks immediately after mitosis produced a phase advance, while short shocks just before mitosis caused delay. Longer shocks given near one particular phase brought about discontinuities in the response, transitions occurring from short delays to ones of up to two complete periods, with mitosis, where it occurred, being almost in phase with unshocked controls. When the durations of the heat

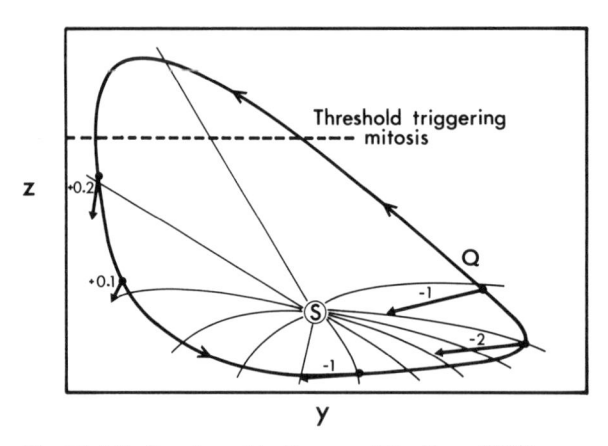

Fig. 7.8. A limit cycle used by Tyson and Kauffman (1975) as a metaphoric model for a clock in which mitosis is triggered by a threshold in the concentration of z. The equations of the limit cycle are similar to Eqs. (2.19) and (2.20), namely $dy/dt = A - By - yz^2$ and $dz/dt = By + yz^2 - z$, where $A = 0.5$ and $B = 0.05$. Isochrons are drawn from the singularity at equal time intervals. The dark *arrows* indicate 20% reductions in y and z due to heat shocks at different phases of the cycle. The significance of the region around Q is described in the text. Redrawn with kind permission

shocks were further increased near this phase another discontinuity occurred, the delay diminishing from two or three cycles to one of only a fraction of a cycle.

The effects of heat shock are interpreted in terms of reductions in the concentrations of the two relevant unidentified variables (y and z), these being displaced from their phase of the limit cycle by amounts proportional to their concentrations, and to the duration of the shock. Figure 7.8 shows a "metaphoric" limit cycle used to interpret the experimental observations. Isochrons are marked, as are displacements of y and z by heat shocks towards zero. The time of crossing the threshold is advanced or delayed depending on the direction of the disturbance relative to the isochrons. It is easy to see that shocks applied immediately after crossing the threshold would advance the cycle, so that the threshold trigger would be reached sooner than usual in the next cycle. Displacements later in the cycle would delay it.

There is a short region near Q on the cycle from which heat shocks may cause displacement to a point close to the singularity. As will be clear from the similar limit cycle shown in Fig. 2.14, the trajectory of a point near the singularity may make several revolutions before reaching the limit cycle, or, in Fig. 7.8, crossing the threshold and triggering mitosis. Thus, heat shock applied at the correct phase should delay mitosis for several cycles. However, if the shock is even longer and (y, z) passes from the region of Q to a point well beyond S, then the cycle might merely be delayed several hours but still undergo mitosis. Such variable behaviour in the responses to different intensities of shock would not be expected at other phases of the cycle. The behaviour of this limit cycle model was able to account very successfully for the complex experimental obsevations described above. An extension of the model is described in Sect. 7.3.4.

7.3.3 Entrainment of Oscillators by Rhythmic Forcing Functions

In the preceding models the stimuli applied to the limit cycle oscillators have been of very brief duration; when no longer perturbed, the interactions between the components control the return of the system to the same limit cycle. The model described here concerns the effect of imposing a sustained external rhythm on an internal one, which has no reciprocal effect. Such a forcing function will alter the phase of the internal rhythm continuously, and can have the interesting property of causing its frequency to decrease or increase, until it matches that of the imposed rhythm. The closer the values of the natural and imposed frequencies, and the larger the amplitude of the forcing function, the more likely is this entrainment to occur. A rhythm known as a relaxation oscillator is particularly easily entrained by a wide range of forcing frequencies. These rhythms show a relatively slow increase of variables compared to an abrupt decreasing phase. The oscillator equations producing the results shown in Fig. 2.13 are of this sort.

Figure 7.9 is an illustration of the phenomenon. It shows the result of applying a sine wave input forcing function to the variable z in the equations producing the traces of Fig. 2.13. In this case

$$dy/dt = A - (B+1)y + y^2 z, \tag{7.1}$$
$$dz/dt = By - y^2 z + E \sin(2\pi t/P) \tag{7.2}$$

where E and P denote the amplitude and period of the forcing function, respectively. Addition of this term is equivalent to adding z to the system at the rate of

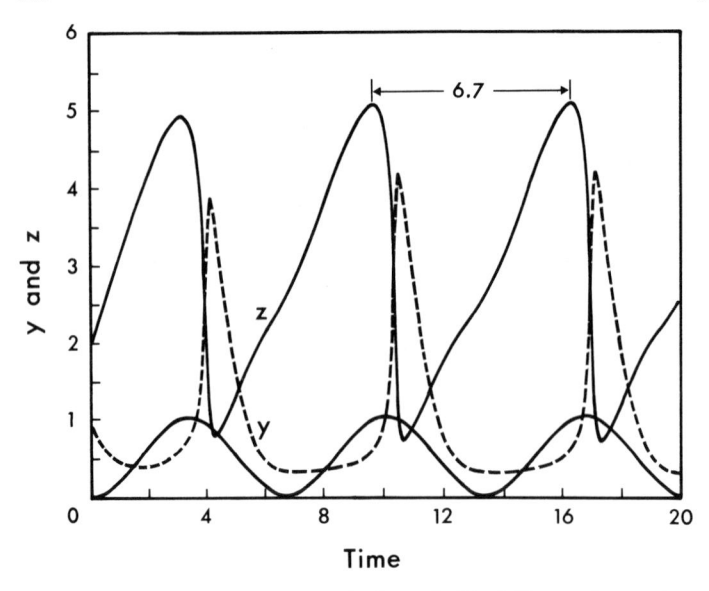

Fig. 7.9. Entrainment of the limit cycle shown in Fig. 2.13 to an imposed continuous forcing function (*lowest curve*). Initial values of $y=1$ and $z=2$ were on the original cycle. A new cycle was rapidly approached (*upper curves*) having the same period as the forcing function (6.7 time units). Values of y and z were calculated by computer using program SIMUL run with option (1) (Sect. 11.2) together with FUNCTN subprogram LIMIT (Sect. 11.17), modified by the addition of a sinusoidal forcing function term [Eq. (7.2)]

$E \sin(2\pi t/P)$. When $E=0.5$ and $P=6.7$ the system rapidly attains a new stable cycle in which the frequency has been reduced from 7.1 units in the unforced system (Fig. 2.13) to 6.7 units, equal to that of the entraining rhythm (Fig. 7.9). The use of a cosine forcing function with the same parameter values produces an identical limit cycle after a longer transition period; the form of the final result is not dependent on the relative phases of the initial limit cycle and the forcing function. Entrainment may also occur to pulsed, periodic stimuli. Pavlidis (1973, Chap. 4) discusses the mathematics of entrainment in detail.

Models of this sort provide possible descriptions of mechanisms producing observed synchronization of biological function. An imposed rhythm may be used to entrain inherent biological oscillations. Synchronized timing of behaviour occurs internally between cells and organs, and also allows adaptation to environmental rhythms such as circadian oscillators. Another possible biological mechanism involving entrainment is suggested by the experiments of Basar (1976); the measured effect of various frequencies of acoustical stimulation on the evoked potential patterns recorded from the cat auditory cortex, showed a strong resemblance to the behaviour of similar entrainment models. Nerves in the cat brain appeared to be entrained to the frequency of the noise stimulus.

7.3.4 Interactive Coupling of Limit Cycles

Section 7.3.3 describes the behaviour of a model of one cycle driven by another to demonstrate one-way coupling of rhythms. Interactive coupling can also occur and is more complex.

Winfree (1974b) discusses a simple model of the mixing of two systems described by the same limit cycle but having different phases. In this case the averaged values of the concentrations of y and z will be inside the limit cycle, and it is necessary to determine the resulting phase of the mixture. Let us consider an idealized, symmetrical limit cycle (Fig. 7.10) having straight isochrons SM and SN joining the symmetrically placed, unstable singularity to the limit cycle. It can be seen that if equal amounts of material exhibiting phases A and B are mixed to give (y, z) at J, the resulting phase (M) of the mixture will be quite different from that obtained if phases C and A are mixed at J' to produce phase N. This is true even though B and C may be very close together in time. There is a range of concentrations of y and z near the singularity from which all phases of the limit cycle are accessible. Winfree has predicted the results of mixing two phases in different proportions, to yield beautiful patterns of phase changes in three dimensions. These behaviours include the locus of singularities where no phase (i.e. cessation of the rhythm), or indeterminate phase, may result. Less symmetric cycles and singularities, and curved isochrons would yield different, more complex results. Winfree has shown that relaxation oscillators (as in Fig. 2.14) produce patterns of resultant phases different from the circular one in Fig. 7.10. The pattern of resulting phases of mitosis arising from the fusing of plasmodia of slime mould at different phases was able to be related by Kauffman and Wille (1975) to patterns predicted in a similar fashion for a moderate relaxation oscillator.

We shall illustrate some possibilities of coupled rhythms using the analysis of Tyson and Kauffman (1975) on the effect of coupling two systems displaying behaviour modelled by limit cycles of the kind shown in Fig. 7.8. Their metaphoric model was applied to the observed timing of mitosis of *Physarum polycephalum* after interaction of parts of the organism at different stages of the cycle. When pieces were cut from two plasmodia at different phases of the mitotic cycle and fused side-by-side, veins soon formed and pumped cytoplasmic material between the pieces. The model simplifies this arrangement to two well-stirred compartments separated by a membrane through which the two unidentified limit cycle variables can diffuse. Combining Fick's law describing diffusion of y and z with the equations of the limit cycle oscillations of these variables, mathematical expressions similar to Eqs. (2.19) and (2.20) are obtained describing the rate of change of y and z in each compartment. The eventual steady state in each compartment after the transients have disappeared is obtained by equating these rates of change to zero and solving for y and z. With similar diffusion coefficients for both variables, the solutions show that similar stable limit cycles develop for both compartments. With different diffusion

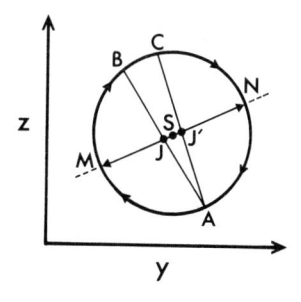

Fig. 7.10. A model of interactive coupling of two systems having identical idealized limit cycles with straight isochrons intersecting at the singularity S. The systems are mixed in equal quantities at different phases A and B or A and C to yield the resulting phases M and N, respectively

coefficients for y and z, the stable limit cycle of each uncoupled oscillator becomes unstable on fusion. Inhomogenous solutions to the equations result, where each compartment may have different unstable steady states and different stable limit cycles — a bifurcation of the sum of the initial cycles. These solutions (yielding the trajectories of the final limit cycles) were shown by Tyson and Kauffman to depend on the parameters of the limit cycle equations, the rates of diffusion of y and z, and the initial phases of the two compartments at which diffusion begins.

Figure 7.11 gives an example which shows an effect with potentially general significance: on mixing samples of material having widely separated initial phases P and Q, two limit cycles result, both of which are unable to reach the threshold value of z necessary to trigger the biological event. In this particular case, contact inhibition of growth should therefore ensue. It is proposed that by gradually altering the ratio of the diffusion coefficients of y and z, the cells might suddenly change from ones which synchronize rhythms on fusion to ones which induce stable contact inhibition of the controlling rhythms.

Transient effects on the timing of mitosis observed experimentally, such as discontinuities in delays of one of the fused parts or the formation of abnormal states, are also explicable in terms of this limit cycle model containing a triggering threshold (Kauffman and Wille, 1975).

This model of the interaction of two limit cycle oscillators is a further example of a possible control mechanism for biological behaviour resulting from the dynamic properties of the system rather than the production of a new component such as a specific substance.

Interaction among a large number of identical oscillators produces systems such as those described in Sect. 2.6.3 having spatial as well as temporal dependence of response to stimuli. Pavlidis (1973) discusses possible approaches to the very complex behaviours of which interacting oscillators are capable.

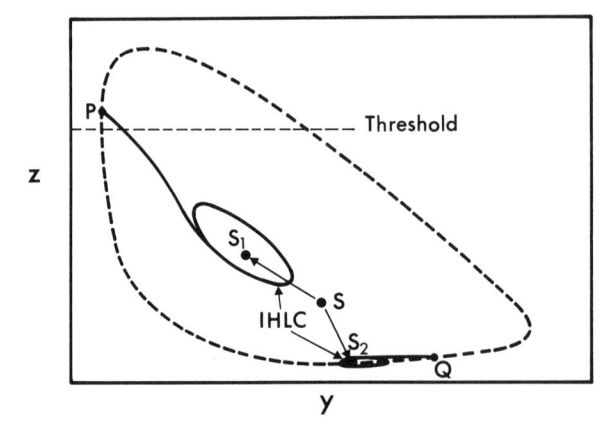

Fig. 7.11. Results of interactive coupling between two systems having the homogenous limit cycle of Fig. 7.8 (*dotted line*) with singularity s before being linked via a semi-permeable membrane. Variables y and z have diffusion coefficients $D_y = 0.5$, $D_z = 0$ across the membrane. When started at phases P and Q the trajectories of the systems move to inhomogeneous limit cycles (IHLC) each having a singularity S_1 and S_2. Redrawn from Tyson and Kauffman, 1975, with kind permission

7.4 Rhythms, Endocrinology and Biological Control

It is clear that rhythms are an important concept in understanding biological control. Organization is based not simply on structural components but also on the dynamics of their interaction. The correct interplay of time-varying, rhythmic components or concentrations controls the initiation of many events. The metaphoric models described above (Sect. 7.3) indicate some of the possible varieties of outcomes and potential for control arising from the interactions of rhythms. The actions of external rhythms on internal ones provide means of adaptation to environment, while interplay of internal rhythms is unavoidable because one rhythm in the supply or removal rates of metabolites, activators, inhibitors or products will affect other cell processes; multiple internal rhythms are necessarily linked.

The concept of a single persistent cycle oscillator as a means of controlling timing is, therefore, probably too restrictive. A more adequate picture might be obtained from visualizing a network of biochemical conversions embedded in an overall oscillating pattern, which accepts stimulation from those external events providing adaptive functioning. The outcome of this oscillating network may be tuned by several parameters, different ones dominating where some goal-seeking behaviour is required. Hastings (1972) goes so far as to propose a biochemical hologram for biological timing mechanisms.

How does the concept of endocrine control fit into such complexity? The idea of interplay of neurosecretions and hormones with internal rhythms allows a great many possible mechanisms for describing control of function. Endocrine control might be but one influence that provides information on environmental and internal states; hormones may be used not to drive but to modify internal rhythms by changing, for example, rates of membrane transport, synthesis of enzymes or mitosis. While acceptance of such complexity, however organized, may not be conducive to enthusiastic experimentation, lack of awareness of the possibilities of rhythm interplay leads to confused and contradictory interpretations of experimental results. It is very important for the experimenter to be always aware that internal rhythms of synthesis, sensitivity, clearance, transport rates, concentrations, receptor sensitivity and so on may, and probably do, exist. Measurements on individuals may be essential to detect these rhythms, as data from groups will obscure all but the most striking features.

Evidence is accumulating that production of each hormone is not confined to a single organ in the body (see, for example, Pasteels, 1977), that production in different places may result from different stimuli, and that cell receptors for these hormones may not be absolutely specific but may respond to several endocrine secretions. Such observations support the concept of a network control of body processes with major emphasis placed on the state of the cells or organs themselves determining to which environmental cues they will respond, and how.

Another dimension has been added to the use of rhythmic models in biological control by a suggestion of Bogumil (1974). He proposes an important function for the rhythmic, pulsatile nature of hormone release. Rhythmic secretions of pulses of hormones are potentially capable of exchanging larger amounts of information more quickly between organs than signals involving small continuous changes in absolute levels over longer periods.

Bogumil gives examples of the way in which time-varying signals may be encoded in a series of pulses. Not only is the dimension of level able to be used to convey information, but so also are the time intervals between pulses, and the pulse widths. The pituitary may release a pulse of hormone. At the target organ both short term response in secretion of steroids to this pulse, as well as long term morphological changes from accumulation of pituitary signals would produce a corresponding response signal returning to the brain. If the information in the returning signal of, for example, ovarian secretions describing the state of this organ, could be analysed by the hypothalamic-pituitary complex, there is potential for very sensitive monitoring of disturbance in ovarian function, and rapid correction through further release of gonadotrophin in the next pulse. The aim of the feedback loop is, of course, to achieve suitable development or maintenance of some state during, say, the reproductive cycle.

Endocrine communication and control is conducted over a communication channel composed of the circulatory system and other tissues, including those involved in the degradation of hormones. The maximum rate at which distinguishable signals can be received depends on the plasma clearance rates of the hormones involved. The use of the same channel for many other purposes may tend to reduce its effectiveness, and this is particularly true for a non-pulsed continuous signal involving small changes. For example, cross-linking of systems may occur; sex hormones produced by both the adrenal glands and the gonads will be interpreted indiscriminately by the hypothalamic-pituitary system. (This may, of course, have a function.) The common circulatory communication path may make hormone signals and their reception susceptible to other rhythms in blood such as flow rate, clearance of hormones and production of active substances from other systems. Noise and distortion would therefore affect each signal. Interpretation of the sequential feedback pulses must be designed to depend mainly on the condition of the target organ and not on the properties of the channel. Those aspects of a hormone signal controlling response are determined by the complex properties of hormone receptors, presently the subject of intense study.

The energy involved in the response of a biological system is usually considerably greater than that apparent in an encoded signal, such as the low energy stimulation of the optic nerve or a pulse of hormone. Responses therefore require coupling to endogenous power sources and are dependent upon them. The nature and effects of such receptor-mediated coupling within target cells are of interest in endocrine systems. As stated by Yates et al. (1972) an ant cannot control a horse without some very special arrangements for energy conversion.

Other requirements of control systems must be met if their function is to be achieved. The mathematical concepts of controllability and observability (see, for example, Kalman, 1962) are important. The relationships necessary for these attributes have been investigated algebraically for linear systems in communication and control theory. Controllability implies the ability of a component of the system to be controlled by suitable inputs. Observability means the ability to determine the relevant condition of a component by observing outputs. In terms of a feedback control model of the ovulatory system, the condition of the ovary must be controllable by the rhythmic signals of the pituitary, while the pituitary must be capable of detecting the condition of the ovary from endocrine signals. Bogumil (1974) applies these concepts to a hypothetical system showing, amongst other things, the possible importance of intra- as well as inter-organ interactions to system control. He suggests that the concept of negative feedback is inadequate for describing endocrine regulation and needs to be extended by tests for controllability and observability. Quantitative measurements demonstrating the conditions under which these apply are needed. The requirements of these latter concepts may explain the time delays characterizing endocrine relationships, because long "codes" (proposed to be transmitted as pulsed rhythms) may be necessary to span the controllable/observable space in endocrine systems.

While metaphoric postulates of the functions of rhythms in controlling endocrine and other systems are interesting, it can be difficult to evaluate the significance of these ideas in particular instances. Examples of attempts to construct theoretical models based on real physical components to describe an endocrine cycle, and the comparison of the models' behaviour with experiments, are given in Chap. 8.

7.5 Empirical Characterization of Rhythms from Data

Having detected a rhythm in a biological system, it is necessary to determine its characteristics. Biological rhythms are seldom very accurate; they differ from the physical or mathematical idea of a precisely defined period or oscillation. Care must therefore be taken in interpreting the results of applying analytical methods developed originally for describing physical systems to biological ones. For instance, many biorhythmic variations occur about a *central mean*, otherwise known as a *resting value*, *baseline* or non-cyclic *trend*. The concept of amplitude (Sect. 7.2.1), which is clearly defined in precise physical and mathematical terms, may be elusive when applied to biological data with a variable baseline.

The most obvious property of a rhythmic process is its period. The period may be very variable in a biological system and the extraction of repeating periods from biological responses, often buried deeply in "noise", is an important aspect of mathematical modelling in biorhythm research. The methods briefly described below are capable of dealing with data which, to the eye, are highly ambiguous.

Parametric statistical tests, such as the t-test and analysis of variance, have been much used in the past to prove the existence of a rhythm. They are not well-suited to this purpose, being designed to compare the means and dispersions of groups, and they demand assumptions inappropriate to rhythms. It is now accepted that biological rhythms occur, and modern methods of analysis are needed to unravel subtle complexities obscured by random fluctuation. In rhythm analysis it is particularly difficult to combine data from individuals into meaningful averages; individual rhythms may be thus obscured by differences in phases, means, amplitudes or frequencies.

Two basic techniques have been applied to the analysis of time-series or ordered sequences. The first is the *auto-correlation function* which aims to describe the evolution of a process through time; this is known as analysis in the time domain. The second is the *spectral density function*, a technique for analysing complex rhythmical variations as the sum of cyclic components with differents periods, and referred to as analysis in the frequency domain. In spite of the confusing nomenclature in the literature, most techniques are concerned with elaborations of these two ideas only.

Sollberger (1965, Chaps. 19 and 20) and Halberg (1969) discuss the intuitive basis of early biological rhythm analysis. More advanced descriptions of suitable mathematical methods will be found in books such as those by Jenkins and Watts (1968), or Chatfield (1975).

7.5.1 The Sine Wave Model

Ordinary statistical analysis is concerned with values distributed about a mean without regard to their order in time. In contrast, when analysing a time series it is this order, or relationship between the values in time, that is important. The basic model of the former analysis is the normal distribution; of the latter it is the sine curve, a repetitive oscillation evolving in time.

A *stationary* or *random time-series* arises if one plots a sequence of random values along a time axis: they will oscillate about a mean value in an irregular manner. Within limits, any period should be as likely to occur as any other although an impression of rhythmicity may be given. Truly random oscillations are improbable in real data and some sort of cyclic tendency is to be found in most variables.

There is great danger in searching intuitively for rhythms in a response. For example, Sollberger (1965, p. 205) describes how even in a random time series peaks will tend to occur at particular average intervals, these being dependent upon the criteria used to judge the presence of a peak. Clearly there is a need for a quantitative approach, if only a suitable non-parametric test for detecting a trend, such as the runs-test (Sect. 10.6).

The simplest kind of rhythmical variation is illustrated by the sine wave. This well-known curve (Fig. 7.1), traced out in time by the vertical component of a point on the circumference of a wheel revolving at a constant speed, has intersting properties. The frequency of the oscillation can be expressed in two ways: it is either the angular distance (measured in radians) swept out in unit time and known as the angular frequency ω, or it is the number of cycles covered in unit time, f, which is equal to $\omega/(2\pi)$. The period (or wavelength) is then the reciprocal of the frequency.

A mathematical model based on the sine wave and suitable for describing many experimental, rhymical time-series is

$$y = A_1 \sin\left[6.2832 \; (A_2 + t)/A_3\right] + A_4 \tag{7.3}$$

where y is the dependent variable and t, the independent one, is time (Fig. 7.1). Parameter A_1 matches by multiplication the maximum value of the sine curve (which is equal to 1) to the amplitude of the observed rhythm. A_2 is a parameter for synchronizing the phases of the model and the data; it has the effect of displacing the calculated curve along the time axis. Parameter A_3 modifies the period or distance between peaks of the sine wave. A_2 and A_3 are expressed in units of the time variable: the constant 6.2832 (equal to 2π) provides the necessary conversion so that the angle (in square brackets) is in terms of radians. Parameters A_4 represents the displacement of the central mean from zero.

7.5.1.1 Temperature Variation During the Menstrual Cycle

The cyclical change in body temperature accompanying variation in hormone levels during the menstrual cycle in women is a typical example of a biological rhythm. A consistent monthly rhythm is apparent, but there is variation from one cycle to another in an individual. The major rhythm is readily modelled by a sine function.

Temperature records were kept for almost a year by a woman with normal menstrual cycles who was not taking oral contraceptives. Temperatures were measured orally on wakening each morning; records were omitted on a total of 94 days. The model of Eq. (7.3) was fitted to the data by means of FUNCTN subprogram SIN (Sect. 11.16) together with program MODFIT. The progress of the fit is shown in Table 7.1, and the first 90 days of experimental data together with the fitted model are depicted in Fig. 7.12.

The cyclicity is readily apparent to the eye. The sine curve provides a reasonable approximation to the data (considering its scatter) although this model is purely empirical. The response of body temperature to hormone levels is unlikely to actually follow a sine curve, and a better model could possibly be found. The parameters of the model were estimated with great precision and there was no trace

Table 7.1. Results of fitting the model of Eq.(7.3) to observations on daily body temperature variation[a]

RES VARIANCE	A 1	A 2	A 3	A 4
.24259	.20000	12.000	28.000	37.000
.32599E-01	.16379E-01	16.039	28.180	36.563
.30813E-01	.22613E-01	17.786	27.888	36.562
.24816E-01	.82994E-01	15.200	26.990	36.560
.22734E-01	.14257	11.049	27.223	36.560
.16791E-01	.15141	13.612	27.093	36.561
.15763E-01	.18857	12.638	27.065	36.561
.15733E-01	.19054	12.850	27.073	36.561
.15733E-01	.19068	12.846	27.072	36.561
.15733E-01	.19068	12.846	27.072	36.561
STD DEVS	.11243E-01	.47407	.62236E-01	.78777E-02
	5.9%	3.7%	.2%	.0%
DEPENDENCIES	.16074E-01	.72827	.72847	.17554E-01

CONDITION NUMBER   60.8

CORRELATION COEFFICIENTS
```
      A 1   1.0000
      A 2  -.28558E-01  1.0000
      A 3  -.12749E-01   .85114     1.0000
      A 4   .55423E-01   .17478E-01  .41107E-01  1.0000
```

MODE = 0, DEGREES OF FREEDOM = 251
FINAL LAMBDA =   .0000010000000000

X	Y	YFIT	RESIDUAL	Z-RESIDUAL
1.0000	36.560	36.547	.12765E-01	.10177
2.0000	36.500	36.504	-.38584E-02	-.30761E-01
3.0000	36.450	36.464	-.13543E-01	-.10797
4.0000	36.530	36.428	.10155	.80961
5.0000	36.560	36.400	.15954	1.2719
6.0000	36.450	36.381	.68920E-01	.54947
.				
.				

[a] FUNCTN subprogram SIN together with MODFIT was used. Notice the high precision of the parameter estimates, the exceptionally low dependencies of parameters A1 and A4, and the low condition number. Extremely small correlations between all parameters except A2 and A3 are features of this model when fitted to large sets of data. Careful choice of initial parameter estimates ensured a stable solution in spite of a sizable residual variance and an objective function which is known to display many local minima. The data and fitted model are shown in Fig. 7.12.

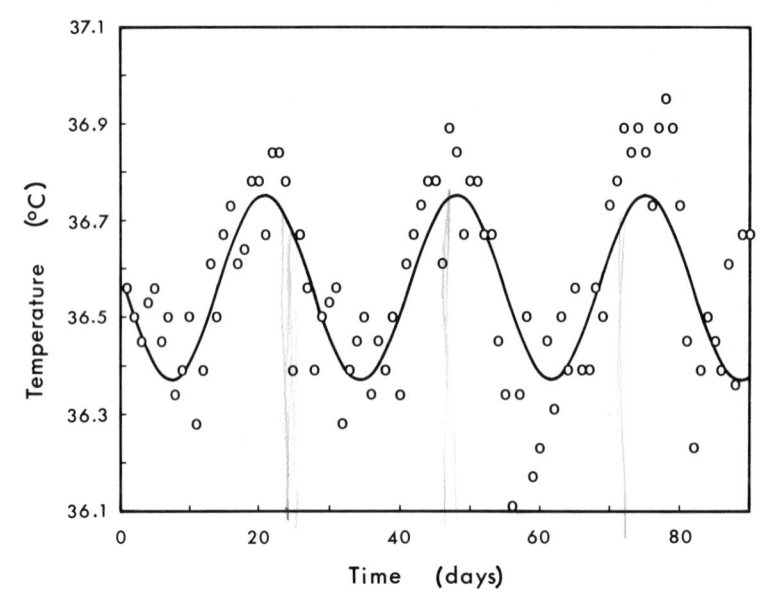

Fig. 7.12. Variation in body temperature recorded daily, as described in the text. The *smooth curve* represents the results of fitting the sine curve model described by Eq. (7.3) to 255 measurements over a period of 349 days. The progress of the fit is shown in Table 7.1

of parameter interaction. Notice in particular the very small uncertainty of 0.008° C in the estimate of parameter A_4, the mean body temperature (36.561° C) at this time of day. The estimate of parameter A_1, approximately 0.191° C, is a measure of the mean maximum amplitude of the positive and negative variation of temperature about the mean level.

Parameter A_3, the period of the rhythm, is of most interest. The estimate of (27.07 ±0.06) days is also very precisely determined, the reason for which is as follows. Imagine a very small change in the period of the sine curve model. Amplified over eleven cycles this small shift becomes much larger. Furthermore, the fact that variance about the fit is measured in the vertical direction means that a small horizontal displacement of the model produces a relatively large difference between it and the measured data.

The response surface of the objective function of this model is littered with local minima, and great care must be taken to make accurate initial estimates of the parameters. Many combinations of starting values lead to stable minima that are considerably inferior to the true one. These local minima result from parameter values corresponding the harmonics of the basic rhythm and are quite stable. Fortunately, it is obvious when the wrong minimum has been found.

7.5.2 Auto-Correlation: Analysis in the Time Domain

Another approach to the analysis of a time series is to calculate the correlation between all pairs of values of a variable, the *auto-correlation coefficient*, at each different *lag* or time interval apart. This correlation coefficient is calculated from the covariance between values of the same variable displaced in time, rather than between values of different variables, as is usual (Sect. 10.2).

A graphic representation of the variation of correlation with lag is known as a *correlogram*. A graph of this kind begins with the maximum correlation of 1 when the lag is zero (because each measurement is then correlated with itself), diminishes as the lag increases, and reaches another peak at a lag value corresponding to the period of the cyclic process. If there is more than one rhythm in the time series then a corresponding number of peaks are found in the correlogram, their positions measuring the period of each process. Correlograms of time series displaying obvious cyclicity may not provide new information because they tend to mirror closely the rhythm of the data. Peaks may also occur at harmonics of the basic frequencies, and these can confuse the interpretation. An example of a correlogram is given in Sect. 7.5.3.1.

For a truly random series, the correlation coefficient is approximately zero for all lags greater than zero. Even so, one can expect to find on average an apparently significant (at the 5% level) correlation coefficient every twenty values (compare this with the reason for not applying *t*-tests indiscriminantly, explained in Sect. 10.10).

The variance of the auto-correlation coefficient r at a particular lag is

$$V(r) \cong 1/N \tag{7.4}$$

where N is the number of observations. Approximate 95 percent confidence limits are then $\pm 2/(N)^{1/2}$; this allows an estimate to be made of the significance of a peak.

When there are many measurements within each period of the cyclic process, the correlation coefficients obtained with small lags will tend to be high. If the number of measurements is low, the correlation coefficients at small lags will again be high but will tend to alternate in sign. If there is a trend or steady change in the data, either an increase or decrease which has a period long in comparison with the time scale of the observations, the values of the correlation coefficients will never reach zero. Finally, if the raw data exhibits a clear, regular, sinusoidal pattern, the correlogram will have the same form and little information will have been gained.

A related concept is that of *auto-regression* in which the value of a response is expressed as a function of past values of itself rather than on an another variable, which is the usual way of calculating a regression. A first order auto-regressive process, also known as a *Markov process*, is expressed by

$$y_t = A_1 y_{t-1} + A_2 \tag{7.5}$$

where A_1 and A_2 are parameters. Substitution of values of y at successive intervals of t yields an infinite-order Markov process. (A stochastic process which has a series of possible successive states is called a *Markov chain* if the probability for passing into the next state is completely determined by the present state of the system.)

Details of models of this kind for analysing time series are given by Chatfield (1975, Chaps. 3 and 4). A number of the models are non-linear and the techniques presented earlier (Chap. 3) are suitable for fitting them to data.

7.5.3 Frequency Analysis of Rhythms

A particularly appropriate way of analysing rhythms is to describe them as the sum of an arbitrary number of sine waves of different frequencies, phases and amplitudes.

This is known variously as *frequency, spectral, harmonic* or *Fourier analysis*. The method represents a generalization of the single sine curve model of Eq. (7.3). A model consisting of a sum of sine waves is known as a *spectral representation*, and it can be shown that every frequency in the range of zero to infinity may contribute to an observed time series.

From the spectral representation it is possible to construct a *spectral density function* or a *spectrum*. This is a graph showing the contributions of each frequency to the observed process. It is worth noting that this spectrum is the Fourier transform of the auto-covariance function from which auto-correlations are calculated (see above). Thus analyses in the time and frequency domains are equivalent, and are related by Fourier transforms. This approach can be used to identify periodic components in the presence of noise.

Fourier analysis has been very useful for describing complex phenomena in the physical and engineering sciences, but there are many biological rhythms for which models in terms of the sum of multiple sine curves are inappropriate. It may be difficult to determine the biological significance (if any) of the harmonics required to ensure a good fit of a Fourier function to data; this model is purely empirical.

Two practical points must be emphasized. Consider the daily temperature records analysed in Sect. 7.5.1.1. These data give no information about temperature variation within each day. If this required at least two measurements must be made at intervals during that time; the higher the frequency of interest, the more often must observations be recorded. Conversely, the lowest frequency which can be identified in 365 daily temperature records corresponds to a period of one year, and to define this period precisely two, three or even more years of data are required. The lower the frequency, the longer the time over which measurements must be made.

The second point is easy to appreciate when one analyses continuous time series. The daily temperature records are an example of discrete data obtained by sampling a continuous variable – the measurements were made at specific times and, in this case, were evenly spaced. In fact, regular spacing of observations is essential for making the analyses. In general, a continuous variable must be sampled for analysis and the problem arises of how often this should be done. Very short intervals become expensive in analysis time, but as the interval increases information is lost. If the interval between samples is too long then an effect known as *aliasing* may occur. Consider Fig. 7.13. When the sampling is done at points ● a smooth curve can be drawn through these with a period longer than that of the original series. This misleading outcome arises whenever a rhythmical process is measured at intervals which happen to be similar to or more widely spread than the period of a dominant oscillation in the response.

An example of the dangers of aliasing is provided by Gallagher et al. (1973), who report measurements of ACTH and cortisol made at 5 min intervals in plasma. They showed by simulation that 20 min sampling of the data would have led to erroneous conclusions.

7.5.3.1 Auto-Correlation and Frequency Analysis of Temperature Data

For illustration, we shall apply the methods of Sects. 7.5.2 and 7.5.3 to the daily temperature data analysed previously.

Auto-correlation and frequency analyses were done using the SPSS subprogram SPECTRAL described by Aarons and Reagan (1977). The input data consisted of

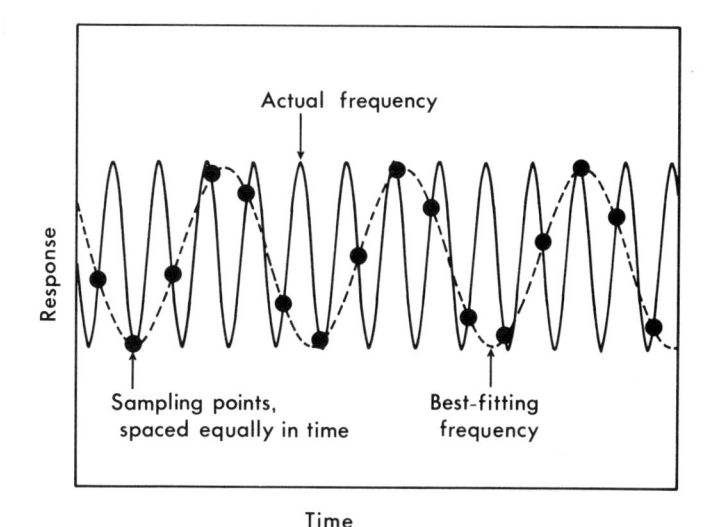

Fig. 7.13. An illustration of aliasing. If sampling is done at intervals longer than the period of a time series (e.g. at points marked ●) a false picture will be obtained of its true period

temperature measurements over 349 consecutive days; missing observations were indicated as such. Univariate analysis was selected using Tukey's smoothing function (window), and a maximum of 170 lags were used. Weighted auto-covariances, weighted auto-correlations, and spectral densities corresponding to a range of periods were calculated.

The relationship between auto-correlation and lag is shown in Fig. 7.14. The values of the correlation coefficients between pairs of measurements separated by a range of lags or time intervals varied in a sinusoidal manner which clearly mirrored the dominant cyclicity of the data. The peak in the trace at a lag of about 27 days shows that there was a mean correlation of 0.33 between all measurements separated by this interval. Needless to say, a correlation also existed between observations 54 days apart, and so on. A correlogram is not useful when applied to data with such an obvious rhythm.

The spectral density graph is shown in Fig. 7.15. It is clear that the variation of early morning temperature with the stage of the menstrual cycle could be expressed in terms of a Fourier analysis having a single major component with a frequency of about 0.037 cycles/day (corresponding to a period of 27 days). This justifies fitting the model of Eq. (7.3) to the data described in Sect. 7.5.1.1. Note that there is no significant contribution at an infinite period (or zero frequency) as would be the case if there was a trend, or constant positive or negative slope in the data. It is important that trends or dominant low frequency variations are removed prior to harmonic analysis lest they obscure other frequencies.

This example does not demonstrate the power of frequency analysis. The month-long cycle is obvious without elaborate calculation. Given a long time-series with many observations, the methods described are, however, capable of revealing periodicities that are so immersed in random noise as to be completely invisible on inspection. It is certainly possible to assert in the present case that there is no

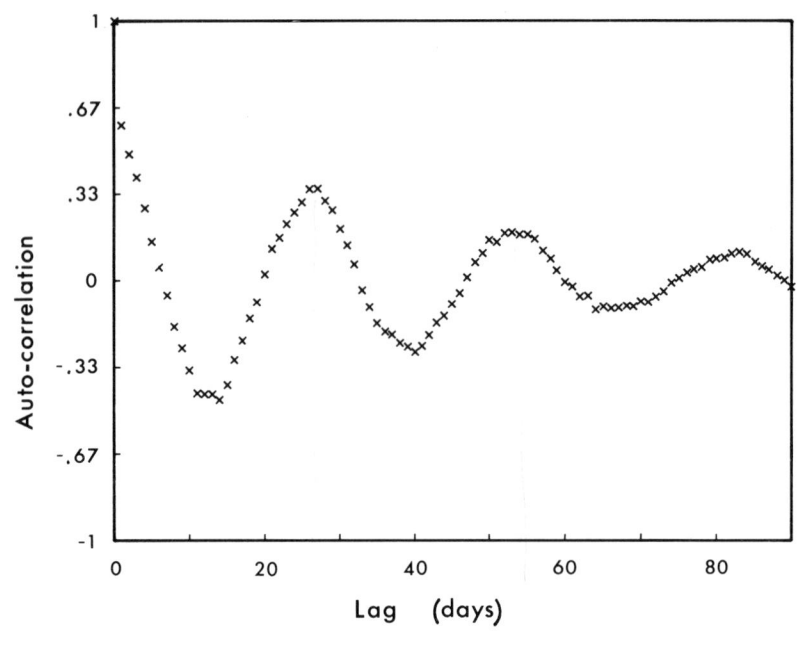

Fig. 7.14. Auto-correlation as a function of lag for the daily temperature data. A total of 170 lags were calculated but for clarity only 90 are plotted here. Notice how auto-correlation decreases from the theoretical maximum of 1 when the lag is zero (each point is correlated perfectly with itself), rises again to a maximum at a lag of about 27 days and then oscillates at lower values about multiples (harmonics) of 27 days. A correlogram of an obviously rhythmic process, such as the temperature data, is not very helpful

evidence whatever for any rhythm in the temperature data other than that of 27 days. Rhythms with periods of less than one day, however, cannot be tested for unless a shorter sampling interval is used.

7.5.4 Bivariate Processes; Cross-Correlation and Cross-Spectra

The relationship between two time-series is frequently of interest. For instance, one may wish to search for a possible correlation between two variables changing simultaneously. Another important reason for comparing the time sequences of two variables is when one is the input to a linear system, the other the output, and the aim is to determine the properties of the system. Frequency analysis for the latter purpose is discussed in Sect. 2.3.5, and it will be helpful to relate the concepts used earlier with those presented here.

A process having two variables (bivariate) is characterized by the same properties as univariate ones, but using the *cross-covariance function*. A full description is given by Chatfield (1975, Chap. 8) who points out certain dangers in interpretation.

If a time domain analysis similar to that of auto-correlation with one variable, but known in this case as *cross-correlation* is carried out, a lag will be discovered corresponding to the time required for input to pass through the (linear) system, and emerge as output. This lag is equivalent to the phase angle displacement discussed in Sect. 2.3.5.

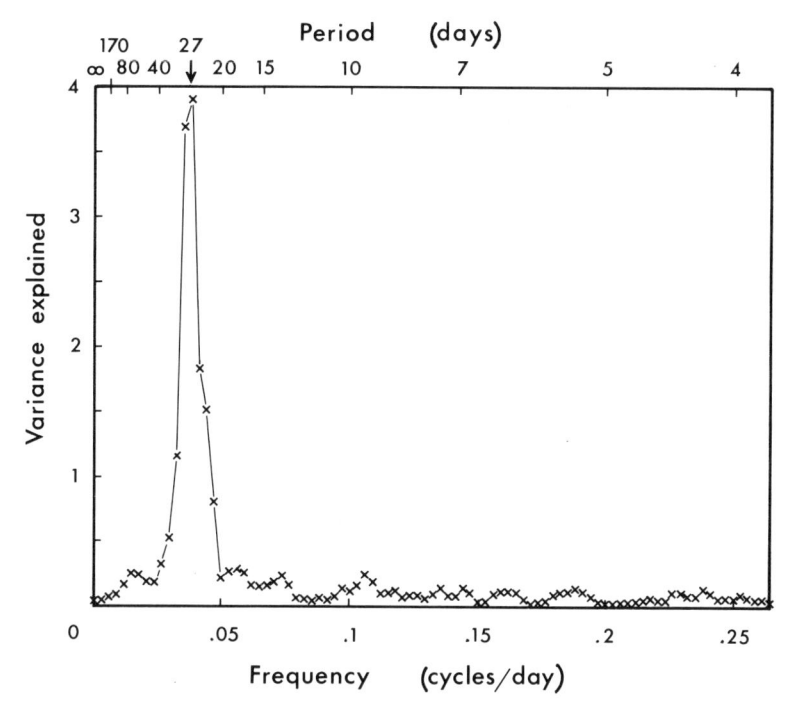

Fig. 7.15. Spectral density function of the daily temperature data. The contributions of different frequencies (also expressed as periods) to the total variance about the mean of the data is represented as a function of the frequencies. Notice how most variance is explained by a process with a period of between 26 and 28 days. Traces of other components are also visible. For clarity, periods of less than 3.8 days are not shown

The frequency domain analogue of the univariate spectral density function is the *cross spectral density function* or *cross-spectrum*. Following the same approach as for the single variable, the cross-spectrum of a bivariate process measured at unit intervals of time is the Fourier transform of the cross-covariance function. This technique is suitable for examining the relationship between two time-series over a range of frequencies. It should be noted that the Fourier transform is a special case (Chatfield, 1975, pp. 233–237) of the Laplace transform, used for analysing linear input–output systems (Sect. 2.3.2).

A useful measure of the correlation between two processes at a particular frequency is given by the *squared coherency* derived from the cross-spectrum; the closer this is to 1, the closer the relationship between the two processes. Also relevant are the *gain spectrum*, a graph of the regression coefficient of the output on the input as a function of frequency (see Bode diagrams, Sect. 2.3.5), and the transfer function in the frequency domain (Sect. 2.3.5).

It must be remembered that many biological processes cannot be even approximated by linear systems and so the practical application of these methods to the analysis of system behaviour is severely curtailed (Sect. 2.2).

Examples of the use of the methods discussed above will be found in the report of Vagnucci et al. (1974). Both auto-correlation and frequency domain analyses were used to demonstrate a 24-h periodicity in plasma levels of aldosterone, cortisol, corticosterone, growth hormone and renin activity in a small sample of normal individuals whose plasma was analysed at 30 min intervals. Cross-correlation suggested synchrony of aldosterone and renin, and cortisol and corticosterone, and showed a lag of 5 between the levels of the two pairs. It was concluded that 30 min sampling was not rapid enough to accurately define high-frequency oscillations because of the danger of aliasing.

Another example of the application of frequency analysis comes from the work of Holaday et al. (1977) on rapid fluctuations of cortisol release in monkeys. They point out that the broad, confused power spectra obtained are caused by the episodic rather than smooth rhythmic nature of the release. This is probably a common phenomenon in biology and may diminish the usefulness of spectral methods designed for the analysis of mechanical systems. Another, practical constraint on the application of these methods to endocrinological studies is the requirement for many data points. These may not be obtainable for ethical, economic or other reasons.

8 Large Systems: Modelling Ovulatory Cycles

Mathematical model building consists of (1) abstracting relevant aspects of a process, (2) expressing their relationships in formal mathematics, (3) studying the implications of this formalization on the behaviour of the model and (4) comparing this with observations or experimental results. It is hoped that the aspects abstracted are the important controlling features of the process, and that the formalizations are appropriate. However, a particular model can only be a product of (a) the experimental data available, (b) the concepts currently held and (c) the developed mathematical techniques of the time. (Endocrinologists are well aware that experimental data also depend heavily on the development of experimental techniques.) A major function performed by model building is to detect limitations for further investigation in all three of these areas.

To many endocrinologists mathematical modelling seems to be synonymous with so-called "whole system" modelling. In such investigations, mathematical methods have been used to simulate quantitatively whole system behaviour by combining data obtained from separate subsystems. However, the modelling of whole systems is but one aspect of a much more fundamental activity required for any quantitative (and many qualitative) investigations in endocrinology, or science in general.

This chapter investigates attempts made to describe an endocrine system in terms of the relationships between glands, organs and brain structures, hormone secretions, morphological and behavioural changes, and environmental influences. Most of the examples used concern a particularly complex system, the female menstrual or oestrous cycle. A critical appraisal is given of some achievements of the models described.

The descriptions here aim to illustrate general principles involved in modelling, to use words rather than mathematical symbols; to show the application of mathematical methods described in Chapts. 2 and 7, not to give particulars or details. We adhere to a uniform terminology rather than explain the proliferation of symbols existing in the literature. It is hoped that these descriptions will form a useful introduction to this kind of modelling and provide a coherent approach to a complex literature.

8.1. Modelling the Ovulatory Cycle

There was a burst of activity in modelling the ovulatory cycle in the late 1960's and early seventies. This coincided with the development both of radio-immunoassays for determining hormone levels in blood, and of an awareness of the potential in applying systems analysis to biology. Since then many experimental investigations and conceptual developments have expanded our understanding of interactions in this system, helped also by better procedures for assaying the variables. Mathematical techniques have also advanced. The challenge now is to improve on these first attempts with new models; we believe that several are in the process of being devised (R. J. Bogumil; S. S. C. Yen, personal communications, 1978).

The current models are instructive in revealing the deficiencies in our understanding of the fundamental processes involved. The basis of all the models describing the cycle is a negative feedback loop (Sect. 2.5.2) in which the interactions between components are described by empirical equations or postulated relationships; simplifications and assumptions (many extrapolated from physiological observations) are made, and such parameters estimated as are required to ensure that simulations of the model fit experimental data. While the models are derived from a wealth of careful and sensitive observations and experiments, insufficient information has been available to propose mechanisms for interactions of the feedback components based on a quantitative understanding of these events.

Hypotheses concerning the cause of events are also used. Causality in rhythms can be difficult to establish without carefully designed experiments. The observation that two events occur in the same system with the same frequency may be interpreted to mean that both events are necessary for cyclicity, that one event drives the other with no reciprocal effect, or that both are driven by some other rhythm which is independent of them.

A reasonable intention in devising these models of ovulatory cycles appears to be to test whether known or postulated relationships can adequately describe experimental observations. To formulate a model which merely simulates observations on a normal cycle is shown below to be inadequate; with a few hypotheses, assumptions, simplifications and fitted parameters, a good approximation to such data is too easy to achieve using a variety of models. Predictions must be tested, as must the effects of manipulating variables and parameters; in some cases identification of parameters with physiological or cellular components is required. Only then will these or future models have a sound theoretical basis from which reliable predictions can be made.

Four major themes can be discerned in the structures of the models discussed below.
1) Finding a mathematical form which yields cyclic variation of the components of the system.
2) Reproducing the shapes of rhythmic peaks of the variables.
3) Defining the interactions between components essential to the cyclic behaviour of the real system.
4) Reconstructing the behaviour of the whole system from a knowledge of the functioning of the subsystems. Most models involve several of these.

In spite of the inadequacies and incomplete nature of the models of large systems presented here, such modelling exercises appear to be essential to advances in knowledge, and to the use of that knowledge. This is because it is extremely difficult to predict even qualitative outcomes intuitively in all but the very simplest feedback systems. The guidance of a mathematical model is needed which incorporates the extent of the interactions between components and the timing of responses. There are many instances, particularly in humans, where suitably controlled experiments cannot be performed and simulations on strongly based quantitative models appear to be the only approach possible.

8.2 A Description of the Ovulatory Cycle

The function of the ovulatory cycle is to prepare and release eggs in limited numbers from the ovaries at regular intervals of time, and to co-ordinate the involvement of the reproductive tissues in the fertilization of the eggs, their transport to the uterus and implantation. If pregnancy ensues the cycle ceases. The organs primarily involved are thought to be the ovaries, the uterus, the anterior pituitary, the hypothalamus, the adrenals and the central nervous system. The following brief summary refers to the normal human cycle.

The ovary contains many follicles each apparently capable of discharging an egg. Some of these follicles increase in size during the first half (follicular phase) of the cycle but usually only one eventually releases its egg at midcycle. In the luteal phase that follows, a corpus luteum, formed from the follicle which has ovulated, secretes hormones affecting the other reproductive tissues, including the preparation of the uterus. If pregnancy does not intervene the corpus luteum atrophies and menstruation occurs.

Growth of the follicle, release of the egg and maintenance of the corpus luteum are affected by secretions of gonadotrophins from the anterior pituitary, namely follicle stimulating hormone (FSH), luteinizing hormone (LH) and prolactin. Secretion of these hormones is known to be influenced by gonadotrophin releasing hormone (GnRH) produced by the hypothalamus.

The ovarian structures secrete steroids including oestradiol (E_2) and progesterone (P), and also other non-steroid hormones. Oestradiol and progesterone appear to both activate and inhibit the release of FSH and LH, affect GnRH secretion, and produce growth and morphological changes in the follicles and corpora lutea themselves. The actions of follicular androgens (A), are not clearly defined. The adrenals are also responsible for the production of some oestrogen precursors and progesterone which are released into the blood plasma.

The uterus responds to the variation in plasma hormones with morphological changes, including menstruation, and apparently has little influence on the other components of the cycle, at least when pregnancy does not intervene.

The complexity of the system is indicated schematically in Fig. 8.1, in which the major component cycles, known interactions and some of the important phases are sketched. A more detailed and general description of the female reproductive system is given by Greep et al. (1976).

Measured experimental variables include the concentrations of steroids, gonadotrophins and releasing hormones, and observations of morphological changes. Understanding of the components of the ovulatory cycle and their interrelationships is based on extensive investigations. These include the effects of controlled stimulation by exogenous hormones, natural, synthetic or radioactively labelled; the effects of the removal of hormones by antigens or the extirpation of organs followed by controlled hormone replacement; the measurement of rates of synthesis, release, metabolism, interconversion, protein binding and clearance of hormones; and related morphological and chemical studies on end organ response in intact or pathological systems, organisms at different stages of their life cycles, isolated tissues and cell cultures. Useful references in this field are provided by Greep et al. (1976) and Schwartz et al. (1977).

Phases

Short pulses
Possibly longer term
  modulations
___

LH synthesis subcycle
LH release modulations
  including LH surge

FSH modulation

Short LH, FSH pulses
___

Follicular growth

Luteinization

Ovulation

Corpus luteum growth
  and degeneration

Phases

One or more
  major peaks of
  steroid hormones
___

Endometrial changes

Menstruation in
  humans
___

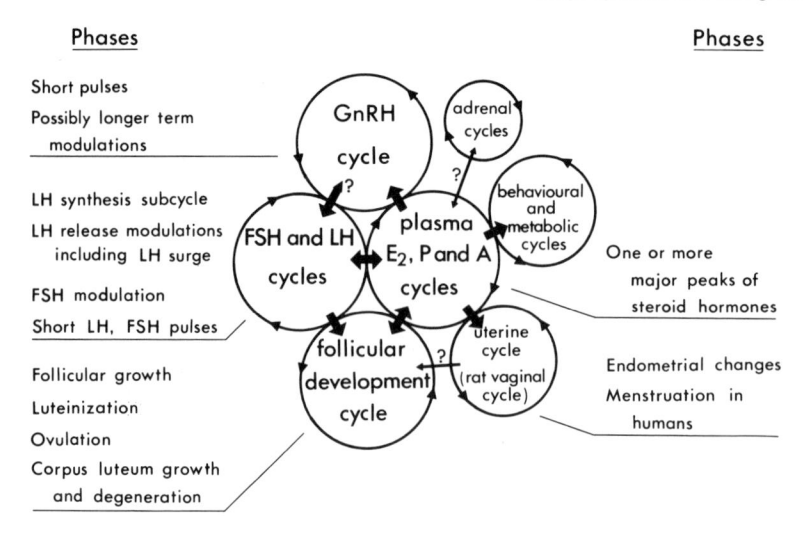

Fig. 8.1. Proposed interaction of cycles of major components involved in the ovulatory cycle and some of their phases

Different species exhibit considerable variation in both the events and lengths of their ovulatory cycles. Some animals, such as the rabbit and cat, do not show oestrous cycles at all, ovulation occurring in response to copulation. Luteal function in some species (such as the rat) does not develop as far as it does in the human. Menstruation occurs in a few species only. Environmental influences are species dependent and various; for instance, many species have seasonal breeding times, while timing in the example of the cycle of the rat is linked also to the daily lighting schedule.

In the models to be discussed the chosen experimental frame is confined usually to averaged observations on mature, healthy, cycling females uninfluenced by drugs, and who do not become pregnant. Figure 8.2 shows typical experimental data for two women individually, which illustrate the changes in the concentrations of four hormones measured daily in blood plasma during normal menstrual cycles. Other events relevant to the cycle which are not considered in these models, are the inception of rhythmicity at puberty or its resumption after pregnancy and lactation, the cessation of cycling at the menopause, and seasonal breeding. Environmental and neural interactions with the system, possible influences from other organs and body systems, such as the pineal gland or adrenals (other than the constant output of steroids), have not yet been included. Influences other than those named in each model are assumed to be negligible, constant or to vary identically during the course of each and every cycle.

8.3 Use of Differential Equations with Cyclic Solutions

In an early attempt to model the relationships between variables in the menstrual cycle, Lamport (1940) showed that two simple linear differential equations

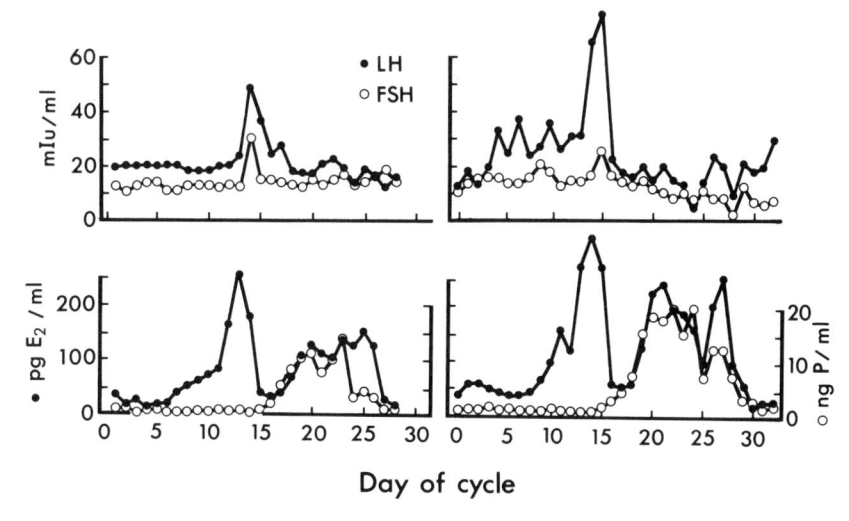

Fig. 8.2. Changes in blood plasma levels of hormones measured daily in two individual women during a menstrual cycle. Redrawn with kind permission from Mishell et al., 1971. Serum gonadotrophin and steroid patterns during the normal menstrual cycle. Am. J. Obstet. Gynecol. 111: 60–65

describing a negative feedback loop between oestradiol and gonadotrophins were insufficient to produce a stable cyclic solution for these variables. It was not possible to simulate experimental data from the menstrual cycle using these equations unless a discontinuity was introduced.

In the feedback equations that Lamport considered, FSH stimulated the production of E_2, while E_2 diminished the secretion of FSH. The rates of change of the levels of the hormones in blood are assumed to be simply the rates of release of the hormones into the blood stream, less the rates of their removal therefrom (Sect. 2.1.1.1). The actual mechanism of the release of E_2 is approximated as being proportional to the blood plasma level of FSH, while a constant maximum rate of FSH release is reduced by a term proportional to E_2. That is

$$d[E_2]/dt = \text{secretion rate } E_2 - \text{clearance rate } E_2$$
$$= f_1([\text{FSH}]) - b_1[E_2]$$
$$= a_1[\text{FSH}] - b_1[E_2] \quad (8.1)$$

and

$$d[\text{FSH}]/dt = \text{secretion rate FSH} - \text{clearance rate FSH}$$
$$= \{\text{a constant} - f_2([E_2])\} - b_2[\text{FSH}]$$
$$= c - a_2[E_2] - b_2[\text{FSH}] \quad (8.2)$$

where a_1 and a_2 are rate constants governing release, b_1 and b_2 are rate constants controlling clearance, c is a constant representing the maximum rate of FSH secretion, and the square brackets denote concentrations. Rapoport (1952) and Danziger and Elmergreen (1957) elaborate further on the failures of such equations.

There are, however, forms of non-linear differential equations that *can* produce stable periodic solutions (Sect. 2.6.4). Use has been made of these latter equations and of discontinuities (another form of non-linearity) in constructing models of periodicity in physiological systems. Sufficiently detailed physiological data on the significant feedback mechanisms in the ovulatory cycle are not available to give strongly based forms to such non-linear differential equations.

Smith (in press) has devised a model of the feedback between GnRH, LH and testosterone (T) secreted by the testes. The model of this simpler system has been devised using differential equations chosen to yield stable cyclic solutions. This model is included here as an illustration of a metaphoric one in which the mathematical form is shaped by consideration of dynamic behaviour of the system rather than the details of known physiological components. Short-term pulsatile oscillations observed in the level of LH in plasma are postulated by Smith to be dominated by this particular feedback loop. Such variations in LH concentration, with periods of 1 to 6 h, are found in both males and females; the mechanism causing these pulses is possibly similar in both sexes, oestradiol acting in the female analogously to testosterone in the male. In mature females similar, short-term pulses are found in addition to the large-scale release of LH prior to ovulation that occurs once in each menstrual or oestrous cycle.

The causal relationships between morphological structures and hormones modelled by Smith are shown in Fig. 8.3. Processes for removing hormones are not shown. The model is simplified by omitting the influence of additional feedback loops inhibiting the pituitary directly by testosterone, and inhibition of the hypothalamus by LH. Neural influences on GnRH secretion are not included. Variable numbers or responses of hormone receptors, and any effects of hormone-binding proteins in plasma are also excluded.

Smith's equations [Eqs. (8.3) to (8.5)] are based on the same principles as those of Lamport [Eqs. (8.1) and (8.2)] except that in this case the function describing the negative feedback effect of testosterone on GnRH has a different form. The equations are

$$d[\text{GnRH}]/dt = f([\text{T}]) - b_1[\text{GnRH}], \tag{8.3}$$

$$d[\text{LH}]/dt = a_1[\text{GnRH}] - b_2[\text{LH}], \tag{8.4}$$

$$d[\text{T}]/dt = a_2[\text{LH}] - b_3[\text{T}] \tag{8.5}$$

where a_1 and a_2 are positive rate constants governing release of the respective hormones, and b_1, b_2 and b_3 are rate constants for clearance. It is assumed that the parameters are constant both with time and with changing concentrations of the variables; these assumptions require experimental support because a_1 and a_2 include receptor response which might vary with both present hormone con-

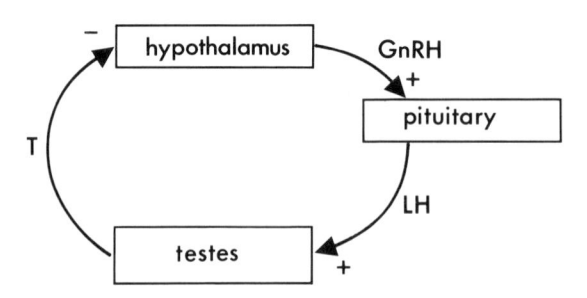

Fig. 8.3. Major components of a feedback model for the pulsatile release of LH in males. *Arrows* indicate release of hormones and their transport through the appropriate blood system. Adapted from Smith, in press

centration and previous exposure. The function $f([T])$ describing the negative feedback was chosen for mathematical reasons. It was the simplest function allowing solutions of the equations which, depending on the parameter values, showed either periodic variations in the plasma hormone concentrations or a stable steady state. That is,

$$f([T]) = \{c - h[T]\} \{1 - H([T] - c/h)\} \tag{8.6}$$

where c and h are fitted parameters, and H is a discontinuous operator being zero for $T = 0$ and 1 when $T > 0$. Details are given in the references.

The solutions of Eqs. (8.3) to (8.6) can show oscillations in plasma hormone levels similar to those displayed by limit cycles having only two variables (see Figs. 2.13 and 2.14). Such oscillations are observed in the hormone levels of mature males. Different parameter values yield a solution showing a single stable steady state value for each hormone which might explain the lack of these oscillations in pre-pubertal males.

The use of the particular mathematical form for Eq. (8.6) simulates the observed dynamics but does not have a structural basis in terms of known components and measured interactions. The equations used by Smith were suggested previously by Danziger and Elmergreen (1956) to model proposed interactions between an enzyme and hormones believed to cause periodic catatonic schizophrenia. Similar interactions must be shown for the effect of testosterone on the hypothalamus to give this particular mathematical model greater weight than other mechanisms yielding cyclic solutions. Only then will parameters determined from experimental data have direct interpretation in terms of real physical quantities. Otherwise the model remains metaphoric and, therefore, non-unique (Sect. 1.1.1).

One aspect of the behaviour of such equations which might have experimental significance in the real, physiological system is this: if the level of one of the variables (in this case T, LH or GnRH) is maintained artificially constant above certain values, then the rhythmic changes of *all* the variables of the feedback system cease and a steady state ensues. Experimental changes in other parameters may also bring about this altered behaviour. In practical terms this means that reduction or cessation of pulsatile release of hormones may be induced unintentionally by, for example, infusion of one hormone at a constant rate. The model cannot account for any modification in receptor response or stimulation of hormone removal in this situation.

This simplified model predicts incorrectly that castration should cause cessation of the pulsatile nature of GnRH and LH secretion. Smith proposes that while the feedback mechanism is the dominant cause of pulsatile release of hormones, further processes, less important in the intact animal, also contribute to the fluctuations and synchronize with them.

It is also possible that other mechanisms such as cyclic permeability in the membranes of one or more of the tissues involved may allow pulsatile release of hormone which drives pulsed secretion in the rest of the loop.

Smith's model for the male is greatly simplified and by excluding, amongst other effects, feedback of the steroid hormone directly to the pituitary. In the female this feedback plays a significant part in an apparently much more complex system. The complexities of the physiological interactions of oestradiol on the secretion of LH from the pituitary of the female have been studied experimentally by Yen and his colleagues. The summary by Yen (1977) on the qualitative interactions operating during the female menstrual cycle is shown in Fig. 8.4. LH in the pituitary is divided into two dynamic pools, a synthesis/storage pool and a releasable pool. These are required to explain the biphasic aspects of LH secretion. One pool appears to be affected positively by increasing levels of E_2, the other negatively. In general, E_2 exerts an inhibitory effect on the release of GnRH except at the mid-cycle surge release of LH which anticipates ovulation. The overall effect of the time constants of stimulation and inhibition is that once monthly a "window" is created in the wall of inhibition through which the accumulated LH can be released as a surge. A quantitative model of this more complex system is needed to describe the monthly variations in levels of LH release, and perhaps also the observed monthly changes in the rates and amplitudes of the short-term pulses occurring several times each day.

8.4 Use of a Threshold Discontinuity to Produce Cyclicity

Thompson et al. (1969) attempted to describe the female ovulatory cycle using a greatly simplified feedback model; the components included were FSH from the pituitary, oestradiol produced by the follicle and follicular size. Figure 8.5 shows the morphological structures and hormones relevant to this model. The authors propose linear differential equations (hormone production rate less hormone clearance rate). The negative feedback of plasma E_2 on the production rate of FSH is similar to that in Eq. (8.2) above. FSH concentration in plasma in turn stimulates follicular growth proportionally, and the follicle releases E_2 in proportion to its volume.

The cyclicity of the variations in hormone concentrations was achieved by a device used frequently in most of the other models described below. The variables are controlled by equations designed to drive the system towards unstable conditions at which an abrupt change in behaviour of the model occurs. This new behaviour requires description by a different set of equations; in mathematical terms there is a discontinuity in behaviour, a threshold is reached. Decision functions are used in computer programs to simulate thresholds. The levels and states of variables in the model are tested frequently and, depending on whether the threshold has been reached, one set of equations or another is used to calculate values of the variables. Sometimes it is possible to postulate a physiological mechanism or reason for the threshold event based on experimental studies. Otherwise, an empirical description of the observed changes is necessary in order to

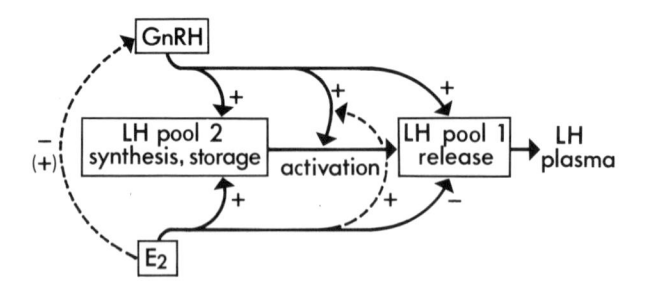

Fig. 8.4. A model of the feedback of oestradiol on LH release in the female. Details are given in the text. Redrawn from Yen, 1977, with kind permission

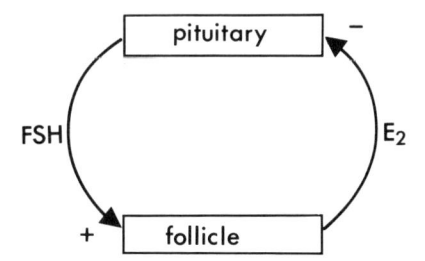

Fig. 8.5. Major components of the feedback model of the ovulatory cycle proposed by Thompson et al. (1969)

simulate the completed cycle; if the old equation becomes inadequate, an arbitrary change to a new one is made. In the necessary use of thresholds lacking physiological foundation lies a weakness in our understanding of the interactions of components causing the observed behaviour of the total system, and hence one of the deficiencies of these models.

In the case of Thompson's model, it is clear that positive stimulation of follicle growth described by the equation

$$d(\text{follicle volume})/dt = \text{positive rate constant} \times [\text{FSH}] \tag{8.7}$$

cannot continue indefinitely. When the physical limit of maximum follicle size is reached, this is postulated to cause ovulation. Over this threshold in the model, the newly defined state of the system retains the original equations but resets follicular volume to the minimum. Of course a different follicle responds to FSH in each cycle. The plasma level of E_2 is reduced after ovulation because it is dependent on follicular size; cyclic changes in E_2 levels maintain relative phase with follicular growth.

Thus cyclicity is generated not through the form of the differential equations describing a mechanism for negative feedback (as in the model of the male LH system of Sect. 8.3), but by stimulation to an unstable physical threshold which resets a variable. The negative feedback of E_2 on FSH in this model is superfluous both to cyclic ovulation and to cyclic changes in E_2 so long as adequate FSH is present for follicular growth. Negative feedback of E_2 is, however, necessary to produce cyclic changes in plasma FSH, but absence of such variations would not affect the cyclicity of the ovulation.

The form of the equations gives single peaks of FSH and E_2 in each cycle. The interaction of the variables is, however, too simple to yield the two major increases in plasma FSH and E_2 which appear to occur in the human menstrual cycle. A major failing of this model is that only interactions between FSH, E_2 and follicular growth are included. Other components, known to be required for cyclic ovulation, such as the cyclic surge of LH that occurs prior to ovulation, and the feedback loops involving LH and steroid hormones, are omitted.

8.5 A Physiologically Based Model of the Rat Oestrous Cycle

The LH surge is taken as a major cause of cyclic ovulation in a mathematical model describing the normal rat oestrous cycle (Schwartz and Waltz, 1970; Schwartz et al., 1977). The period of the rat cycle is either four or five days. This model, which is employed for numerical computations, makes use of a very small part of a more comprehensive descriptive model proposed earlier (Schwartz, 1969). The earlier model represents a useful graphical summary of the wealth of experimentally derived relationships then known between components of the female reproductive system in the rat but cannot be used for quantitative testing. Both models seem to have been useful in promoting clear definitions of time sequences, interactions and dependencies between components, and in inspiring further experiments.

The components of the quantitative model were selected because they, and their interactions, were known to be integral parts of the cycle, and nearly all the parameters were well characterized experimentally. Indeed. this is a distinctive feature of the model. The organs and hormones implicated are shown in Fig. 8.6. LH and FSH activities were not distinguished because, at the time, the control mechanism of the two hormones in the rat had not been shown to be separate.

The interactions of components were modelled by differential equations (including usually linear production and clearance rates of hormones), interrupted by several thresholds similar to the one described in the previous section. A brief verbal summary follows of some of the mathematical interpretations and devices used in the model.

Follicular development. The LH concentration in plasma is proposed to induce a proportional rate of growth in follicular radius; the rate constant was chosen to obtain a reasonable fit of the complete model to the experimental data. The follicle also regresses in size (becomes atretic) at a constant rate based on physiological considerations.

Secretion of oestradiol. Follicular surface area adds a positive proportional rate to the release of oestradiol into the plasma with a rate constant fitted to suit the performance of the model. Increases in follicular mass inhibit the release of E_2 owing to limited access of the blood supply. The concentration of E_2 in plasma is directly promoted by the level of LH, and clearance of E_2 occurs at a constant rate.

Secretion of LH. Ovarian E_2 generally adds a negative feedback term to the constant rate of LH production by the pituitary and proportional clearance of LH by other organs such as the liver and kidneys. A parabolic shaped function is used to describe this effect of E_2 on LH rather than a proportional one, in order to allow for the observed decrease in the influence of E_2 at higher concentrations. The LH surge is simulated in the following way. When the level of E_2 reaches a threshold determined from experimental data, and another threshold involving the time of day is passed (see below), an LH surge term is added to the equation describing the rate of change of the LH concentration. Its shape is predetermined to fit experimental data as a function of time only. Ovulation is then set to occur 6 h later.

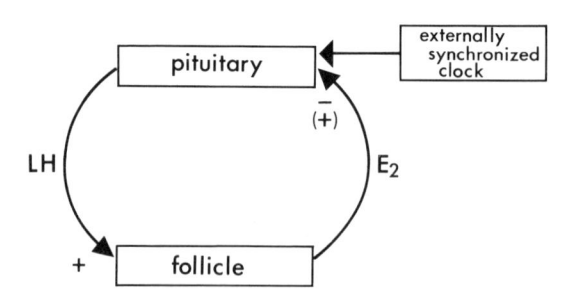

Fig. 8.6. Major components of the feedback cycle of the oestrous cycle of the rat, proposed by Schwartz and Waltz (1970)

In this model ovulation is not related to follicular maturity. As in the previous model, ovulation resets the calculated follicular size to its minimum so as to produce cyclicity in the system.

Timing of the LH surge in the rat is linked to lighting conditions; it is experimentally observed that LH surges can occur in rats only between 2 and 6 h after the mid-point of daily light periods. This externally synchronized clock cannot be said to control the cyclicity of the system in the same way as does the re-setting of follicle size. The influence of the clock on the pituitary merely controls the timing of ovulation, and interference with it can delay or prevent ovulation as occurs on exposure of the animal to constant light.

A CSMP language computer program of the model which describes equations (in terms of difference equations to allow the calculation of LH, E_2 and follicular radius at set intervals), threshold conditions, and values of parameters and variables set at the start of the calculation, have been published by Schwartz and Waltz (1970). A slightly modified program, written in the language APL, forms the basis of the description above (Schwartz et al., 1977). This latter publication provides a long account of the mathematical and physiological significance of the symbols used, and the terms required for instructing the computer.

Testing the model. The model simulates smoothed, averaged experimental data from normal cycling rats reasonably well, though it cannot, of course, mimic individual variability. It has been tested only in simulating the effects of ovariectomy in which it was qualitatively successful, although the level of LH rose too quickly in comparison with experiment. The performance of the model during other experimental manipulations or in pathological conditions remains untested. Without simple modification the model does not appear to be able to cope with the addition of exogenous E_2 to the system because follicular development has not been made a prerequisite for ovulation. Simulation of the addition of E_2 to the model would stimulate an LH surge resulting automatically in ovulation, regardless of follicular maturity.

8.6 An Empirical Model of the Rat Oestrous Cycle Controlled by Time

Inoué (Inoué et al., 1970; Inoué, 1973) has also devised qualitative and quantitative models for the oestrous cycle of the normal, mature, female rat. His qualitative model elaborates the neural aspects of the system.

The production in the hypothalamus of the releasing hormones FSH–RH and LH–RH, and prolactin inhibiting hormone, is suggested to be influenced by both positive and negative neural stimulation caused by steroid hormones, gonadotrophins, light and copulation. Differential equations are formulated for the neural stimulation, and the production, storage, release and transport of the hypothalamic releasing hormones. These processes in turn effect the production of FSH, LH and prolactin in the pituitary. It is proposed that oestradiol and progesterone rapidly activate the neural stimulus causing increased production and release of FSH–RH, LH–RH and ultimately FSH and LH from the pituitary, followed by activation of the neural inhibitory action with slower time constants and higher thresholds resulting in decreased production. This qualitative concept appears to explain a number of experimental observations on the effects of injecting steroid hormones by which both delay and advance of ovulation can be produced. [A limit cycle type model (Sect. 7.3.2.2) might perhaps also be appropriate.]

The ovarian component of Inoué's qualitative model is more complex than in the models described above. The developing follicle undergoes not just one functional change to drive the cycle, but two. After ovulation is achieved follicles are converted to corpora lutea secreting progesterone. These structures then decline and a new cycle begins with growth of more follicles.

This qualitative model expressed in terms of differential equations contains an unmanageably large number of parameters which are unknown and cannot be estimated nor reasonably deduced. Quantitative simulation and evaluation of the hypotheses are therefore impracticable.

The quantitative model actually tested by Inoué contains very few of the interactions elaborated in the descriptive model. It consists of difference equations giving the plasma levels of FSH, LH, E_2 and P, and continuous difference functions describing the progress of follicular maturation, ovulation, and the corpora lutea. In this model, the discontinuous event of ovulation is included in the calculations by means of a continuous curve like those describing the other variables. This ovulation function depends on the follicular morphology equations and on the concentration of LH; ovulation is presumed to occur when the function reaches a maximum value of 1. Negative feedback of steroid hormones on gonadotrophin production is ignored; positive feedback becomes active at defined phases of the cycle.

Several thresholds are used which are related to concentrations of variables. However, there are in addition six thresholds in which the forms of the equations describing the variables are changed at set intervals after the assigned beginning of the cycle. It is not difficult to generate a curve of any shape using a series of simple equations if the equation in use can be changed at arbitrary times selected to suit the data. A model showing changes of behaviour as a function of time only, says nothing about the conditions which are responsible for these changes. While levels of variables may be rigidly time-related in a normal averaged cycle, abnormal conditions or experimental changes in variables will surely change the time dependency of events; but the model with fixed time markers is unable to reflect this.

Inoué's model contains some confusing typographical errors. A further deficiency is apparent in the diagram of a model simulation. The equations do not describe a stable periodicity because the variables do not attain the same values at the beginning and end of the cycle illustrated.

Some disturbances to the rat oestrous cycle have been studied experimentally by Inoué, by linking the blood streams of two rats. After a few cycles, synchrony of phases between the two animals was established. The effects of similar mixing of phases in the mitotic cycle of slime moulds yielded interesting information on the behaviour of that rhythm (Sect. 7.3.4). Perhaps this technique could be used profitably for investigating phase resetting of the rat oestrous cycle.

8.7 An Attempt to Include More Variables

A more detailed model of the human menstrual cycle than that of Thompson et al. (1969) described in Sect. 8.4 has been put forward by Shack et al. (1971). Plasma concentrations of FSH, LH, E_2 and P are simulated and the ovary has two subcomponents, the growing follicle and the corpus luteum, into which the follicle is transformed at ovulation. Their model uses a number of thresholds and related decision functions choosing between suitable differential equations to simulate smoothed, averaged changes in plasma hormone concentrations. These decision functions incorporate the authors' hypotheses of what conditions are necessary to produce the events of the cycle. Nevertheless, some differential functions are used which, once initiated by thresholds, are dependent solely on time and cannot therefore be influenced by appropriate disturbances to the system.

Neither the parameter values for simulation of the model nor initial values are given, so that the strength of its physiological basis cannot be assessed. The equations describing production of steroid hormones use terms related to follicle size raised to the fourth and eighth powers without explanation. According to the authors, experimental data under normal conditions is simulated reasonably well; much of the data has, however, already been empirically fitted during construction of the model. Results of any other tests are not given in this publication. It is not, therefore, possible to judge the effectiveness of the model.

8.8 Eliminating the Differential Equations: A Finite Level Model

A suitable approach in modelling biological rhythms would appear to be the use of differential equations with cyclic solutions, as described above. At present it is not easy to verify experimentally interactions between components which yield such equations. The introduction of a decision function overcame the problem of cyclicity in a simple model of the menstrual cycle (Sect. 8.4). As more components were added to later models, thresholds and decision functions were relied upon more frequently to bring about changes in the behaviour of the variables. In effect, the content of each model is an hypothesis describing those levels of hormones and preceding events thought to be critically important in causing each observed change. The models are really complex maps of causality. The emphasis, however, was on output capable of being fitted to smoothed, average levels of plasma hormones. It was therefore necessary to devise, in addition, empirical differential or algebraic equations which were fitted piecewise between the observed events. To confine erratic experimental biological data which exhibits considerable variance to precise, smoothed, continuously varying curves for the purposes of modelling may be an unprofitable and misleading exercise.

In contrast, Seif and Gann (1972) use a direct approach in studying causality in their model of the menstrual cycle. By quantizing each variable to at most four levels (Sect. 1.2.4), they eliminate the need for smoothed continuous differential and algebraic equations to represent experimental data. The causal relationships between components of the system become the focus of the finite level model (Sect. 2.7). This removes the need for additional fallacy-prone hypotheses and interpretations concerning the detailed nature of the non-linearities of continuous interactions. Problems of non-linear interactions requiring description by complicated continuous equations or piecewise simplifications are dealt with easily by finite levels. This is because the possible range of values for a variable need not be divided into levels of equal size; instead, the sections can be related to important changes in the effect of the variable on other components. Furthermore, relatively sudden events such as the onset of menstruation and ovulation, which do not lend themselves naturally to description by differential equations, are readily included in the fabric of a finite level model.

Figure 8.7 shows the approximate experimental time dependencies of the variables included in the Seif and Gann model, namely E_2, P, FSH, LH, ovulation and menstruation. A finite level description of these data was set up as follows. Seven different states of the system were distinguished during the cycle; these were based on changes in hormone levels and events. The levels of hormones or occurrence of events in these states were chosen as shown in Fig. 8.8(a). Binary numbers were used to describe the levels; four levels of E_2 therefore required two binary digits, each with the value of 0 or 1. Eight binary digits, x_1 to x_8, each with two possible values, sufficed to describe all the experimental data shown when using this chosen form for the quantization.

Table 8.1(a) summarizes the values adopted by the x variables in each of the seven states of the quantized normal menstrual cycle shown in Fig. 8.8(a). The experimental values have thus been converted into finite level binary form. [The inverse transform is done simply using Table 8.1(a) and Figs. 8.8(a) and 8.7.]

An hypothesis was now advanced of how each experimental value in Table 8.1(a) is controlled by values of other variables in other states. This hypothesis described their understanding of causality in the menstrual cycle and included, as do other models, much information derived from experimentation.

The hypotheses of interactions significant to the control of the menstrual cycle used by Seif and Gann are shown in Fig. 8.9. In words, this diagram expresses the following. (1) Current FSH values are related to the values of E_2, P and FSH itself in

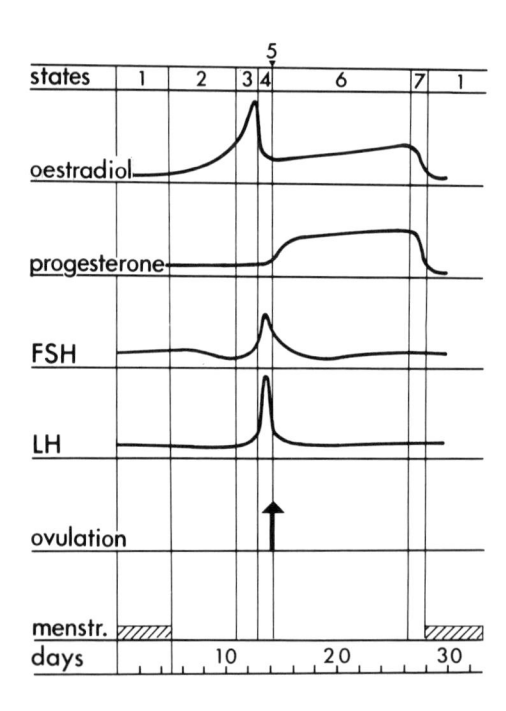

Fig. 8.7. Approximate experimental data on the menstrual cycle divided into seven states for use in the finite level model of Seif and Gann (1972). Redrawn with kind permission

Eliminating the Differential Equations: A Finite Level Model 215

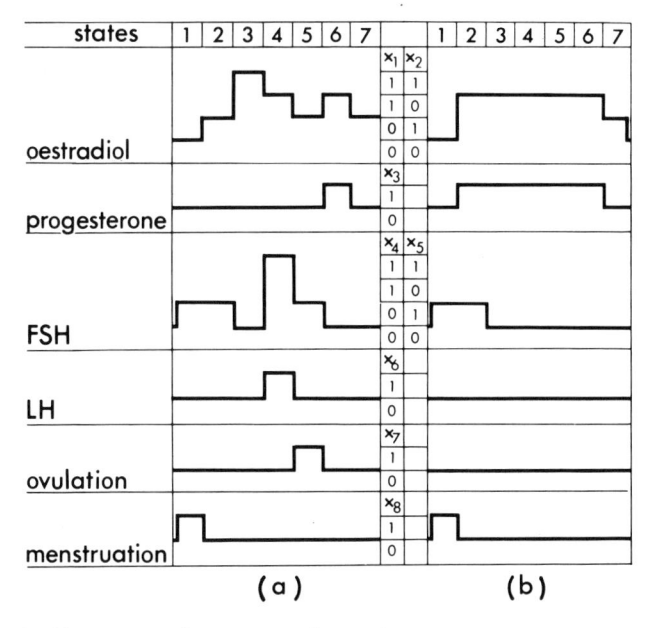

Fig. 8.8 a, b. Quantization of levels of hormones and occurrence of events in the menstrual cycle in the states of Fig. 8.7. **a** Normal cycle; **b** effects of contraceptive oestrogen and progesterone medication calculated by the model of Seif and Gann (1972). Redrawn with kind permission

the previous state. (2) Current LH values are related to the values of E_2 in the two previous states. (3) E_2 is dependent on all other values in the previous state, except menstruation. (4) P is dependent on the values of FSH, LH, P itself and ovulation in the previous state. (5) Ovulation is controlled by the values of FSH, LH, E_2 and P in the two previous states. (6) Menstruation is a function of E_2 and P in the two previous states.

Using these relationships, transfer functions $G_1, \ldots, G_8$ were formed which generated each x_i value in state t, $[x_i(t)]$ from the relevant x_i values in the previous

Table 8.1. Finite level values of variables describing the states of the menstrual cycle in Fig. 8.8 (a) and (b)[a]

a) Normal cycle							State	b) Simulation						
1	2	3	4	5	6	7		1	2	3	4	5	6	7
0	0	1	1	0	1	0	x_1	0	1	1	1	1	1	0
0	1	1	0	1	0	1	x_2	0	0	0	0	0	0	1
0	0	0	0	0	1	0	x_3	0	1	1	1	1	1	0
0	0	0	1	0	0	0	x_4	0	0	0	0	0	0	0
1	1	0	1	1	0	0	x_5	1	1	0	0	0	0	0
0	0	0	1	0	0	0	x_6	0	0	0	0	0	0	0
0	0	0	0	1	0	0	x_7	0	0	0	0	0	0	0
1	0	0	0	0	0	0	x_8	1	0	0	0	0	0	0

Source: Seif and Gann, 1972, with kind permission.
[a] (a) Description of a normal cycle; (b) values calculated from the model when oestrogen and progesterone were added to states 2 to 6.

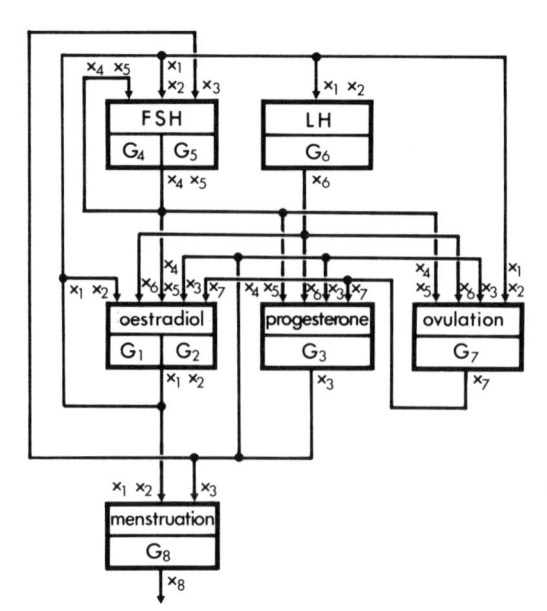

Fig. 8.9. Proposed model of causality in the menstrual cycle used by Seif and Gann (1972). See text for explanation. Redrawn with kind permission

state [$x_i(t-1)$] or two previous states [$x_i(t-1)$ and $x_i(t-2)$]. For example, the generalized form of the function required to describe menstruation at state t is the following

$$x_8(t) = f[x_1(t-1), x_1(t-2), x_2(t-1), x_2(t-2), x_3(t-1), x_3(t-2)]. \quad (8.8)$$

Seif and Gann describe a further transformation they used to assist the complex computations required to find transfer functions.

The derived functions obviously must reproduce the normal cycle if they have been correctly calculated. The model was tested by simulating the effects of contraceptive oestrogen and progesterone medication. The results are shown in Fig. 8.8(b) and Table 8.1(b). They are consistent with the biological findings of absent ovulation and surges of FSH and LH, while menstruation is maintained.

This model needs updating with more recent information concerning components, controls and time dependencies. Many more simulations and relevant experimental tests are required to elucidate whether the hypothesized interactions between components in the cycle are incorrect or inessential. For example, the cyclicity of menstruation may not be dependent on the occurrence of ovulation, nor therefore, presumably, the secretion of steroids by the resulting corpus luteum. It is difficult to determine which events drive the cycle and which are driven by it. The time intervals over which previous events influence current states is not known.

The purpose in devising the model was to illustrate the use of a mathematical technique rather than to initiate a thorough study of the menstrual cycle. Nevertheless, this approach appears to have freed the investigation of causality in the cycle from the hypothetical mechanistic details needed for description using differential equations. It is a particularly appropriate technique for studying complex systems, the postulated mechanisms of which lack strong experimental bases.

8.9 A "Complete" Description

The model of Bogumil et al. (1972 a; 1972 b) on the human menstrual cycle attempts a very much more detailed mathematical description than any discussed previously. The many hypotheses included in this model concern not only the direct causal connections between components as in the model of Seif and Gann (1972), but also endeavour to give detailed mathematical forms to these inter-relationships. The hypotheses are based on a wealth of experimental work described by Vande Wiele et al. (1970). Little attempt was made to distinguish the simplest representation compatible with data; as many experimental observations were included in the models as possible. The model equations were evaluated by computer.

The variables to be fitted by the model to the experimental data are E_2, P, A, LH and FSH concentrations in plasma, as was shown in Fig. 8.2. Differential and algebraic equations combined with multiple decision functions are used to describe their interactions. The three major components of the system included in the model correspond to morphological structures — the pituitary producing LH and FSH, the ovary secreting E_2, P and A, and the adrenal glands causing production of A and E_2 (see Fig. 8.10). Positive and negative feedback loops occur between the secretions of the ovary and those of the pituitary producing the cyclical changes in hormone concentrations and ovarian morphology. The hormones are also metabolized and removed from the circulation by organs such as the liver and kidney. The adrenal gland does not play a significant part in the model; it is assumed merely to add its secretions of E₂ and A to the general circulation at a constant rate.

Notice that in this model, as in the previous ones, GnRH produced in the hypothalamus is not included explicitly but is lumped into the pituitary behaviour. Bogumil (1976) later identifies the effect of GnRH on the cycle as being included in the equation describing the stimulus of LH release by E_2 and P. At present it is not possible to use this model to investigate the effects of any factors influencing the cycle through the hypothalamus other than E_2 and P. As in previous models, all other hormones, metabolites, environmental conditions and so on, are assumed to

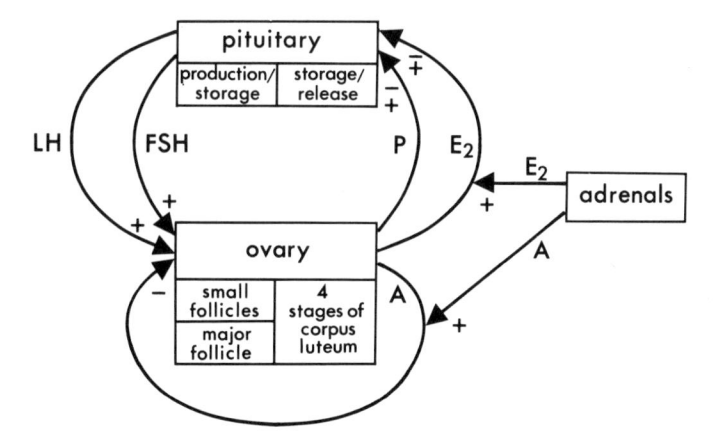

Fig. 8.10. Major components of the feedback model of the menstrual cycle proposed by Bogumil et al., 1972 a. The *arrows* represent transport by the general circulation

be constant or to vary in the same way throughout each cycle. The ovarian component is further divided into subcompartments to ease the mathematical description of its behaviour. Each subcompartment corresponds to an observed cyclic change in morphology. Different equations describe the development and transition from one stage to the next, and each stage contributes differently to the secretion of ovarian hormones. This greatly simplifies the description of the complex variations in secretions from the ovary and the varying effects of gonadotrophins and steroids on follicular development during the cycle. In the pre-ovulatory or follicular phase the behaviours of small and large follicles are distinguished, while after the LH surge and ovulation, four different stages of corpus luteum development are defined.

The pituitary is similarly divided into two compartments to describe the release of LH; these are probably not morphologically distinct but are dynamic pools necessary to reproduce two different kinds of effect of hormones on LH release.

The interactions between variables considered in this model are summarized schematically in Table 8.2. The equations for each output describe the transfer function of the inputs.

The following is a brief outline of a few of the mathematical interpretations made of physiological observations on interactions between the variables. Bogumil et al. (1972a) give a more complete description together with a useful list of many of the assumptions used in devising the 34 equations and the multiple decision functions included in them which together form the model. Speroff and Vande Wiele (1971) provide a helpful description of the background to the equations.

Gonadotrophins. Two mechanisms are postulated for the secretion of LH; in one E_2 and P inhibit LH release, in the other, active near mid-cycle, a large increase or surge in the release of LH occurs that is initiatied mostly by high levels of plasma E_2. Oestradiol in the latter situation has a positive feedback effect on LH release. This is terminated by the physical limit of depleted stores of LH, and a discontinuity caused by luteinization of the follicles which reduces the E_2 production, and hence its stimulus.

In previous models the rates of change of gonadotrophins in plasma were expressed as constant maximum rates from which were subtracted rates of clearance and a proportional or non-linear feedback term related to the level of E_2 in the plasma. That is,

Table 8.2. Summary of the interactions considered between components of the menstrual cycle in the model of Bogumil et al. 1972*a*

Inputs	Outputs						
	E_2	P	A	LH	FSH	Follicles	CL
E_2				+ −	−	+	
P				+ −			
A						−	
LH	+	+	+			+	+
FSH						+	
Follicles	+		+				+
CL	+	+	+				+

$$d[\text{FSH}]/dt = \text{constant maximum release}$$
$$-f([E_2]) - \text{clearance constant} \times [\text{FSH}]. \tag{8.9}$$

Bogumil and his colleagues derived instead an empirical equation describing experimental values of the steady state concentrations of FSH as a function of plasma levels of E_2. The steady state equations take the form of exponentials. In order to determine the dynamic aspects of gonadotrophin behaviour it was assumed that rates of change of FSH or LH are controlled only by plasma clearance rates. Therefore $d[\text{FSH}]/dt$ is expressed as the rate of clearance of a concentration of FSH represented by the difference between current total [FSH] and the steady state value determined by E_2 towards which the FSH level will move with time. That is,

$$d[\text{FSH}]/dt = \{[\text{FSH}]_{ss} - [\text{FSH}]\} \times \text{removal rate constant}. \tag{8.10}$$

This manoeuvre avoids the use of a parameter describing maximum FSH production, and bases the parameters of these equations on values that are measured directly. The release of gonadotrophins in response to plasma steroid levels is assumed to be instantaneous in these equations describing negative feedback.

The threshold concentration of E_2 at which the LH surge may occur is not a fixed value as in the previous models, nor is it a function only of the current E_2 level. It is made dependent also on previous concentrations of E_2 and P by use of a convolution integral (Sect. 2.3.3). The maximum contribution to the threshold is therefore the current E_2 value and less emphasis is given to previous E_2 values, the contributions of which decline exponentially as the time of their occurrence recedes. The stimulatory effect of E_2 levels on the release of LH is proposed to be a squared function of E_2 concentrations. This stimulation is delayed for 24 h to fit the experimental data and also incorporates a convolution integral so that the previous E_2 levels, and to a lesser extent P concentration, continue to be stimulatory. The recharging of totally depleted LH stores in the pituitary to a maximum value is postulated to take 14 days, because this is apparently required for correct performance of the model cycle. A number of parameters associated with the LH surge do not as yet have any physiological significance but are required to simulate experimental data from normal menstrual cycles.

Follicular growth. Growth is made dependent upon the surface area of the follicle which is influenced in turn by hormones while, as in the model of Schwartz (1969), the follicular mass inhibits growth because of reduced access to the blood supply. The rate of change of follicular radius is given in terms of a function of local (as opposed to plasma) ovarian E_2 concentration which saturates in physiological conditions, a non-linear function of FSH concentration in plasma, a proportional inhibition by androgens and inhibition by follicular mass. The number of growing follicles is determined by a convolution integral of present and previous concentrations of FSH, the decline in numbers with time representing atrophy of the follicles. A large set of decision functions based on follicular size and hormone levels is used to determine which of several equations describes various possible behaviours of the single follicle normally destined to ovulate.

The forms of the differential equations postulated to describe the appearance and decline of the four luteal phases of the follicles are empirical, and were designed to be consistent with observed morphological changes as well as the known influence of

LH on maintenance and transformation of these states. The parameters have no apparent physiological significance and the non-linear function describing the influence of plasma LH concentrations (approximated by a piecewise linearization) is arbitrary, but gives a good fit to the data.

Steroids. The equations representing steroid levels are also mathematical hypotheses designed to give results consistent with the measured response. There was insufficient physiological data to propose more precise forms of interaction. The secretory potential of active follicles is related to their surface areas and to an instantaneous response to a non-linear function of LH concentrations. The drop in the level of E_2 in plasma after the LH surge results from luteinization of follicles causing changes in the secretory patterns. To each steroid concentration, three luteal stages contribute a squared term related to surface area of the corpus luteum, and the fourth adds a cubic term related to mass. There is, in addition, a direct secretory response to LH levels. Because the metabolism and clearance rates of steroids are very rapid in comparison with the morphological changes controlling their production, plasma steroid concentrations are, in effect, always at the steady state and are therefore expressed as algebraic rather than differential equations.

In general, secretory responses to hormones are instantaneous (with the exception of the LH surge), while hormonally induced morphological changes produce the significant time-lags between events in the cycle (with the exception of the time lag caused by pituitary synthesis and storage of LH).

8.9.1 Testing the Model

This model has been investigated and tested more thoroughly than the others described, and partly for that reason has been more successful in showing important deficiencies in our understanding of the processes involved in the menstrual cycle. As we have seen in previous models, the ability of simulations to reproduce smoothed average cyclic changes in the variables is a basic requirement, but not a very discriminating one. Models with quite different simplifications, assumptions and forms seem to be able to accomplish this. (Yet another example is a model of Yates et al., 1971, based on different assumptions; its authors claim that it produces an excellent computer simulation of the normal cycle, although no mathematical details or results are given.)

Bogumil et al. (1972 b) divide the cycle into six stages exhibiting different behaviour of hormone levels and morphological changes (similar to the states used in the model of Seif and Gann shown in Fig. 8.7), for comparing the simulation of plasma hormone levels with experimental results. The model simulates the averaged experimental data acceptably well although a few details are inaccurate (see Sect. 8.9.1.1). It is claimed to simulate also effects of menopause, ovariectomy, treatment of hypophysectomized subjects by gonadotrophins, treatment with contraceptive steroids and other experiments reported in the literature, but no details are given.

8.9.1.1 The Effect of Short-Term Random Oscillations

One deficiency common to all the previous models is the invariance of the simulated cycle compared with the observed natural changes in timing and hormone levels from one cycle to the next. One of the most interesting aspects of this model was the testing of the effect of fluctuations in plasma concentrations of LH and FSH by the addition of small random changes in their levels. These could be caused naturally by such factors as neural responses or changes in the physiological parameters influenced by sleep, health, stress, metabolism and so on. The variations in concentration of LH and FSH tested were random, of low amplitude (between 10% and 40% root mean square), short-term (period of 0.5 to 12 h) and had zero mean value. The resulting cycles of this modified, stochastic model showed variation in length and hormone levels from one cycle to the next and even produced feasible anovulatory cycles. Thus the non-linearities built into the original deterministic model were such that simulations using this type of *short-term*, zero-averaged disturbance could successfully produce *long-term* functional variability of the menstrual cycle like that observed naturally. The structural stability properties of the model are therefore very similar to the real system with respect to these perturbations.

Many of the parameters assumed to be constant in Bogumil's model undoubtedly undergo variations which, if not related to the monthly cycle, may be at least circadian. One wonders if the non-linearities of the model would respond with the same structural stability to changes in factors such as the clearance rates of steroid hormones, the binding of hormones by plasma proteins, or rhythms in adrenal production of steroids.

The possible implications of hormonal oscillations, such as those observed in LH (and simulated above), for very sensitive control of the feedback system are discussed by Bogumil (1974), and have already been described (Sect. 7.4). To confirm such a hypothesis of control would be difficult. Detailed experiments on stimulus-response behaviour of ovarian tissues to gonadotrophins, and of the pituitary and hypothalamus to steroid hormones, would be needed to discover which aspects of hormone signals the receptors can detect and respond to in a discriminatory way. What time intervals, rates of change of hormone levels and concentrations are distinguishable? The smoothed daily measurements of hormones in plasma used in these models may not be the most relevant input for determining receptor response. Alternatively, our measurements of plasma hormone levels may detect much smaller changes than can be discerned by the target tissue itself. There is, however, evidence that the ovary of the sheep does detect individual pulses of LH because it responds to each of these by secreting increased amounts of E_2 and A at certain phases of the oestrous cycle (Baird et al., 1976).

8.9.1.2 Response to Infusions of Oestradiol and GnRH

A further test of the basic, deterministic model was made by Best (1975). He considered that it might be possible to find a single disturbance which would displace a limit cycle-type description of the menstrual model into or near to its steady state, as shown in other systems by Winfree (Sect. 7.3.2.2). The periodicity of the system would cease or become very slow so that ovulation would be indefinitely delayed, with obvious implications for contraception if the model was strongly physiologically based. He therefore tested Bogumil's model by simulating the effects of infusions of exogenous E_2 for 24 h on different days of the cycle. A discontinuity of the kind described in Sect. 7.3.2 was simulated with either delay or advance of ovulation occurring, depending on the day when the disturbance was applied. Long non-ovulatory cycles were produced in response to 24-h infusions of E_2 introduced between the 4th and 7th days of the cycle. However, according to Best some of these simulations do not agree with experimental results produced by the addition of large amounts of exogenous E_2 because such interference appears to invariably delay ovulation.

R. J. Bogumil (personal communication, 1978) has, however, found that there are fundamental problems which invalidate the use of Winfree's disturbance techniques in the menstrual cycle. More thorough tests simulating infusions of E_2 into his stochastic model on days 3 to 8 (Bogumil, 1976) showed behaviour of the system that is qualitatively in agreement with variations of some in vivo responses to this type of stimulus. Simulations of infusions of GnRH into the stochastic model produced interestingly varied responses of the system on which experimental data has yet to be reported.

8.9.2 Further Modifications

Feng et al. (1977) have made a few alterations to Bogumil's deterministic model. The changes relate to the pulsatile release of LH from the pituitary, and to the complex effect of both plasma E_2 levels and the rates of change of these levels on the release of LH and FSH. However, the hypothalamic hormone GnRH, important in the control of LH and FSH synthesis and release, is not explicitly included in this revised model. Several details in which the original deterministic model failed to describe the averaged normal cycle and to simulate some observed responses to E_2 infusions, were thereby altered.

Changes made to the description of secretion of gonadotrophins in the original deterministic model (see paragraph *Gonadotrophins*, Sect. 8.9) include the following. The simple instantaneous negative feedbacks of E_2 and P on LH release prior to the LH surge do not adequately describe details of averaged plasma increases in LH during the follicular phase. (Bogumil claims, however, that his stochastic model describes data from individuals well.) The follicular growth stage is divided therefore into four phases, the transition thresholds of which are determined by the levels of E_2 and P and the times spent at the previous stages. Each of these stages has associated with it a different curve describing the negative feedback effect of E_2 on LH release. These are designed to indicate desensitization of the pituitary to E_2 feedback with time. This allows a better fit of simulated plasma LH changes to data during the follicular phase, while maintaining the negative feedback effect of rapidly increased E_2 levels. The pituitary stores of LH and FSH vary in each follicular stage so that if the surge threshold is triggered prematurely by E_2 infusion, less LH and FSH are released than occurs in a normal cycle. The negative feedback effect of E_2 on LH levels is not only brought about instantaneously by current E_2 values as in Bogumil's model, but a convolution integral is used to allow an influence by the previous history of E_2 levels. Pulsatile secretion of LH and FSH is built into Feng's model empirically, but, in contrast to Bogumil's stochastic model, the pulses are deterministic, E_2 and P exerting negative feedback effects on the magnitudes and frequencies of the pulses, respectively. In the original model a high level of E_2 triggered the threshold to the LH surge and acted as a stimulus to it. In the modified model an abrupt drop in the level of E_2 after maintenance at a high value is hypothesized to trigger this threshold, thus accomodating some quoted observations on response to E_2 infusion. (Bogumil, 1976, mentions other experimental data to support the different hypothesis and performance of his stochastic model.) In order to correct the relative heights and timing of the FSH peaks simulated in the cycle by the original model, an FSH surge mechanism analogous to the LH behaviour was incorporated.

All these changes, assumptions and added parameters allow improved simulation of the behaviour of averaged natural systems. They also permit simulation of some of the available data on the complex stimulatory and inhibitory responses to disturbances on the addition of exogenous E_2 which depend on the manner in which it is administered. The forms chosen to describe the system are nevertheless arbitrary and empirical mathematical devices with very little physiological basis. This is because the relevant physiological information is not yet available.

8.10 Conclusions

The models of the ovulatory cycles described here range from the simplest to the highly detailed — from the use of three differential equations and a decision function to a computer program containing 1,000 statements and representing a mass of differential and algebraic equations, and decision functions. It is apparent that all of these models are far from "complete"; their construction leaves unanswered and untested very important questions. They highlight how the deficiencies in our knowledge of the behaviour of the components of the system preclude our understanding its behaviour as a whole and hinder construction of models which can be used for prediction. Even within the frame of these models (i.e. the ovulatory cycle of the healthy, mature female) a great deal of experimental investigation of mechanisms, parameters and variables is required. Recent knowledge needs also to be incorporated and to be tested.

Some suggestions indicating a few of the research areas that need investigation and modelling are as follows. Those properties of a hormonal signal to which receptor systems in the feedback cycle respond, need elucidation. The nonlinearities and time constants of receptor response to endogenous signals require clear definition. These statements represent a generalization of much of the following discussion (see also Sect. 7.4 and 8.9.1.1). For example, how far do previous cycles influence the form of the current cycle? The time constants used in the current models may be much too short. In the pituitary and hypothalamus mechanisms are required for the observed effects, both instantaneous and long term, of E_2 on LH, FSH and GnRH release by negative and positive feedback, and on the transition between these kinds of action.

The effects of progesterone on gonadotrophin secretion need clarifying. For example, during puberty, normal length anovular cycles exhibiting an LH surge can apparently occur regularly; this could imply that the cycle of LH surge release is little influenced by the luteal secretions of P and E_2. On the other hand, it has been proposed that progesterone, not oestradiol, plays the major role in negative feedback on LH secretion.

The cause of the pulsatile release of gonadotrophin is unknown. The effect of neural transmitters and feedback of the prolactin system on GnRH secretion is being investigated, as is the relationship between GnRH release and LH storage and release (see, for example, Yen, 1977; Turgeon and Barraclough, 1977; Knudsen and Barraclough, 1977; Knobil and Plant, 1978). The mechanism of action of gonadotrophins on both steroid production in the ovary and morphological changes needs further qualitative and quantitative definition (Moor et al., 1973; Seamark et al., 1974). How are follicles which ovulate selected from those which become atretic? The mechanism of ovulation remains unclear. [Rodbard (1968) has suggested an interesting theoretical, physical model for ovulation by treating the follicle as an elastic walled sphere like a balloon, containing a colloidal solution. His model has shown that within a critical range of parameter values rupture may occur by mechanical events alone caused by growth, pressure, volume or osmotic pressure, and stress–strain interactions. Variations in FSH, LH and E_2 levels would appear to affect different variables and parameters of this model.]

Effects of relaxin and inhibin during the cycle are not clearly understood. Relaxin may modify follicular collagen to trigger ovulation. What causes the corpora lutea to degenerate? There may well be significant rhythms in many of the parameters of the system such as clearance of hormones from plasma and hormone binding capacity of plasma proteins. Even circadian rhythms may show an unexpected influence through the non-linearities of the system. The significance to the menstrual cycle of levels and rhythms of adrenal output of steroid hormones and factors influencing this output needs investigation. For example, stress in rats can cause the elevation of plasma oestradiol arising from adrenal precursors.

These questions relate to the normal cycle. Many more can be asked about mechanisms in puberty, the menopause, pregnancy, seasonal breeding, pathological states and differences between species.

In conclusion, the most striking feature evident from studying these models is the variety of equations which give reasonable representations of the observed experimental data, namely the variation of steroid hormone and gonadotrophin concentrations in blood plasma. In each model these apparently appropriate equations have been derived from quite different assumptions and simplifications, and use different parameters. Finding equations to fit experimental data appears not to be the problem. As in all empirical modelling, the difficulty is to verify that the forms of the equations have captured the essence of the physiologically significant aspects of the mechanism involved. This can be investigated only by carefully designed experimental testing of predictions by manipulating variables and parameters. In general, this has not been done adequately on the models described. What little testing has been performed has been productive in revealing deficiencies in conceptual and experimental information. Such tests must, of course, be confined to situations within the frame of the model, which is in turn defined by the frame of the experimental results used in designing it. Whether or not investigations fall outside the frame of the model is sometimes difficult to determine; such is the case when administering synthetic hormones or using individuals showing pathological states. Another important aspect of testing, hardly considered in these models, is the determination of the sensitivity of the model's behaviour to the assumptions made. For instance, simulation of the response characteristics of the model to perturbation, which challenged the assumption of deterministic input of LH, was informative.

While none would argue with the statement

> If the equations accurately represent the performance of each component on an individual basis, then simultaneous solution of all the equations should yield results similar to the behaviour of the system as a whole (Bogumil et al., 1972 b),

the reverse of this is certainly fallacious. Because results obtained from mathematical formulations are similar to the behaviour of the system as a whole, then the detailed representation of components are *not* validated *unless* all assumptions and simplifications can be verified, and all parameters which were fitted to ensure coincidence of model and data have been shown to have accurate physiological meanings. Such a demand appears impossible in these complex systems. No model can be "proved"; every model eventually fails. But it is in this very failure that one of the major uses of modelling lies, for it shows that our experimental observations, concepts or mathematical techniques are inadequate, and gives guidelines for the remedy. In the meantime, our understanding of relationships in the system has been stated explicitly, and has been quantified, often requiring or suggesting new significant experiments.

9 Stochastic Models

This chapter presents examples of statistical mathematical models with applications in endocrinological research. They are models for dealing with stochastic, or random, processes (Sect. 1.2.6). A stochastic process is one in which the outcome is governed by chance; a probability is associated with the outcome of each event. This is in contrast to most of the models described elsewhere in this book which are deterministic—for any input, a particluar output is produced.

To make a statistical test involves comparing the characteristics of experimental samples with the predictions of an appropriate model. These predictions apply only if inherent assumptions are satisfied and it is therefore essential to ensure that the experimental data conform to the assumptions. For example, parametric statistical tests require that data be distributed in some defined way, usually normally. Most statistical tests are conveniently formulated in terms of a null hypothesis, stating that significant differences between model and data do not exist. Allowance for random variation is included in statistical models; if differences too great to have occurred by chance are found, the null hypothesis is rejected — the data do not have the properties predicted by the model. Appendix A gives a guide to the use of some statistical tests.

Here we outline how two different statistical concepts can be usefully applied in endocrinological research. In the first section we describe the use of the so-called non-parametric statistical methods, both to give these tests prominence and also to introduce them in a practical context to researchers who may be unfamiliar with their advantages.

The second section deals with certain aspects of the parametric technique known as multivariate analysis which have great potential usefulness in endocrinology. Different forms of this approach are used to analyse correlations between variables (principle component analysis, factor analysis) or to classify individual experimental units (cluster analysis, discriminant analysis). Endocrinological examples are given to illustrate these points.

Space does not permit us to describe other interesting examples of models based on probabilities, which have relevance in reproductive endocrinology. For instance, Sheps and Menken (1973) have developed and applied a variety of statistical models in their study of probability processes in conception and birth in populations. The models predict the effects of physiological constraints on the likelihood of these events, which must be understood before the more elusive cultural influences can be considered. Stewart and Stewart (1977) report the use of a statistical method for comparing the amino acid sequences of the beta-subunits of several gonadotrophins. This technique made it possible to draw quantitative conclusions regarding homology between hormones, and to identify individual amino acids and regions of the chains likely to be involved in the specificity of receptor interaction.

9.1 Non-Parametric Statistical Models

Non-parametric statistical tests do not require the estimation of parameters of statistical models such as means and standard deviations. Most are *randomization tests* because they can be used to determine the probability that a particular sample of observations could have been drawn entirely by chance from a given population. All these tests require only simple arithmetical manipulations. They are particularly useful for testing the significance of differences found in comparative experiments, which often merely classify responses qualitatively as being present or absent, high or low.

The tests we shall describe can all be done by hand. They are also almost all available in subprogram NPAR TESTS (Tuccy, 1977) which is part of the very useful package of computer programs known as SPSS (Nie et al., 1975), referred to in Sect. 11.18.1.

A simple example, hypothetical but typical, will help to clarify the differences between parametric and non-parametric tests of significance. Suppose we have measured the level of a certain steroid in the blood plasma of a group of women in the third trimester of pregnancy. For comparison, identical determinations have been made on a sample of non-pregnant women. The principles of the design of comparative experiments outlined in Chap. 4 were followed, with the intention of controlling for all factors except pregnancy. In particular, care was taken to select both groups of women randomly.

The intention is to discover whether the "average" level of the hormone in the blood of pregnant women is different from that of non-pregnant ones. Of course, if the results from the two groups are clearly different, there is no need for a statistical test. Assuming that there is some doubt, the parametric approach would be to calculate a mean and standard deviation (Sect. 10.1) for each group. But this requires that the data be distributed symmetrically; in fact the standard deviation cannot be interpreted if calculated for data that are not normally distributed. Thus the first step is to test the distribution of values in each group of data to see if they could have come from populations with normal distributions. This might be done by dividing each range of levels into about 15 equal subranges, and then assigning each measurement to the appropriate one. A graph of the frequency of occurrence of each subgroup should approximate to the shape of a normal distribution as determined from statistical tables. It would be preferable however, to test the samples quantitatively by means of the non-parametric Kolmogorov-Smirnov one-sample test. This test, described by Siegel (1956, pp. 47–52), can be carried out by hand or by using procedure K-S in the SPSS subprogram NPAR TESTS.

If the sample did not appear to come from a normally distributed population, then a transformation suitable for converting the distribution to a normal one would be sought. Probably a logarithmic transformation would be appropriate (Sect. 2.8.4). It is possible that no suitable transformation could be found, in which case one could proceed no further with a parametric analysis.

However, let us assume that the two samples of data have been found to be approximately normally distributed, or can be made so by transformation. The mean and standard deviation of each are then calculated, appropriate weighting being applied if necessary (Sect. 2.8.1). The mean is the parameter of a model defined by its method of calculation (Sect. 10.1) and required assumptions. Finally, the two mean levels of hormone are compared using the *t*-test if the standard deviations are similar (Sect. 10.9). This tests the null hypothesis (Sect. 10.5), namely that the two groups of women are samples from a single population.

The alternative, non-parametric approach would be as follows. The null hypothesis is again tested by making the initial assumption that the two samples were drawn from the same population. In this case, however, no mean or standard deviation is calculated. Therefore the form of the distribution of the samples is irrelevant, except that it is assumed to be the same for both groups. The probability of the two samples being from a single population is here tested directly. By calculating the number of ways in which all the permutations of the values found could be combined to yield two samples, it is possible to place a probability on the outcome observed. If the outcome is found to be unlikely to have occured by chance then it is inferred that the null hypothesis was in error and that the samples were not from the same population (Siegel, 1956, pp. 152–156; Colquhoun, 1971, pp. 116–124). In practice, this kind of randomization test requires no calculations because the values measured are first converted to ranks and the ranks, rather than the original data, are considered. Very little information is lost thereby and the tests are simplified to the point where it is necessary only to consult published tables.

The important assumption made in the use of such tests is that the original sampling is done strictly randomly.

9.1.1 Comparing Two Independent Samples

We shall illustrate the application of non-parametric methods by the following example. The effect of gonadotrophins on the production of cyclic adenosine monophosphate (cAMP) by tissues of the ovarian follicle was investigated by Weiss et al. (1978). Pooled theca and granulosa cells isolated from sheep ovarian follicles were treated with human chorionic gonadotrophin (hCG) or follicle stimulating hormone (FSH) in vitro, and the responsiveness of the tissues in terms of production of cAMP was measured.

In one of the experiments, the effect of hCG on the production of cAMP by theca and granulosa cells over a period of 40 min was compared in tissues isolated from both small and large follicles. The four groups of experimental results are shown in Table 9.1. We wish to test whether equal amounts of thecal tissue from small and large follicles produced equal amounts of cAMP in response to hCG.

Consider first the two samples of replicate results obtained from treating granulosa cells of small and large follicles shown on the left of Table 9.1. An "average" response for each sample is that of the median, which is 4.9 and 43.6 pmol cAMP/mg protein, respectively. Estimates of the 95 percent confidence intervals (Sect. 10.12), within which is expected to fall any other measurement on a member of the populations represented by the samples, were obtained by applying the useful non-parametric test due to Nair (Colquhoun, 1971, p.103). These were 0–16.2 and 11.4–268 pmol/mg protein, respectively.

The null hypothesis is tested by comparing the two samples using the *Wilcoxon* or *Mann-Whitney two-sample test*. This is a randomization test on ranks. That is, the values in the two samples are ordered together without regard to sample boundaries, and their ranks are recorded. This has been done in Table 9.1. Notice that where *ties* occur (replicates with the same value) the mean rank is assigned to

Table 9.1. Production of cAMP (pmol/mg protein in 40 min) by tissues from ovarian follicles after stimulation by hCG in vitro[a]

Granulosa cells				Theca cells			
Tissue from small follicles		Tissue from large follicles		Tissue from small follicles		Tissue from large follicles	
Response	Rank	Response	Rank	Response	Rank	Response	Rank
0	2	10.9	9	13.1	1	15.2	2
18.7	14	268	21.5	280	12.5	300	15
14.1	11	268	21.5	280	12.5	300	15
0	2	129	18	38.7	3	300	15
0	2	196	20	160	10	146	5
16.2	12	42.7	16	156	8	141	4
7.7	7.5	43.6	17	249	11	157	9
7.7	7.5	153	19	153	7	148	6
4.9	6	11.4	10				
3.6	5	17.2	13	$\sum R = 65$		$\sum R = 71$	
3.2	4	18.9	15				
$\sum R = 73$		$\sum R = 180$					

[a] Also shown are the ranks of the responses for use in the Wilcoxon (Mann-Whitney) randomization test. $\sum R$ equals a sum of ranks.

each. The sum of the ranks for each sample separately is then calculated and a table referred to which, for given sample sizes, shows the approximate probability of the two rank sums having been obtained purely by chance from a single population. This test assumes that sampling was done randomly. For our example, in which each sample contains 11 replicates, Colquhoun (1971, Table A3) lists an approximate probability of 0.01. There is thus a chance of only one in a hundred that the two samples came from the same population. Therefore we can, at this level of significance, assert that granulosa cells from small and large follicles differ in their response to hCG, as judged by cAMP production. When this test was repeated by computer using procedure M-W in the SPSS subprogram NPAR TESTS, the more accurate probability value of 0.0004 was obtained.

In contrast, the results for thecal tissue shown on the right of Table 9.1 were not significantly different.

The groups of replicates do not need to be the same size. The only requirement is that the samples be chosen randomly.

9.1.2 Comparing Two Samples Related by Pairs

It was assumed in the test described above that the individuals in the samples were independent, or unrelated to one another. If individuals are related, a different test should be used which will allow for the relationship, and provide a more sensitive measure. This is the case when, for example, a biological specimen is divided into two parts, so that one can serve as a control and the other measures the effect of treatment. This experimental approach reduces variance caused by uncontrolled differences between specimens, and should be analysed using a *paired* test. A suitable one is the *Wilcoxon matched-pairs signed-ranks test*, full descriptions of which are given by Siegel (1956, pp. 75–83) and Colquhoun (1971, 157–166).

9.1.3 Comparing More than Two Samples with Related Individuals

When there are more than two samples to be compared a different approach must be used. The following example describes what to do when individuals in the samples are related.

Consider the data of Weiss et al. (1978) shown in Table 9.2. In this experiment there were eleven samples of granulosa cells, each pooled from several large follicles. The responses in each row of the table were obtained using equal aliquots of pooled cells. That is, the effects of FSH and hCG on the production of cAMP by this tissue were compared with controls, comparison being made on fractions of the same sample. The individual responses in the rows of the table are therefore related, each row representing a separate sample chosen at random. We wish to concentrate our attention on the effect of gonadotrophins and disregard differences due to other variations between samples; therefore treatments and control are compared within each sample.

A suitable test is the *Friedman two-way analysis of variance* (Siegel, 1956, pp. 166–172, and Colquhoun, 1971, pp. 200–204). Ranks are again used, but this time the values are ordered separately within each row. The ranks (and their sums) are shown in Table 9.2. The number of treatments (columns), k, was 3 and the number of samples or blocks (rows), n, was 11. We define a quantity S

$$S = \sum_{j=1}^{k} R_j^2 - \left(\sum_{j=1}^{k} R_j \right)^2 / k \qquad (9.1)$$

where R_j is the rank sum of treatment j. In our example $S = 11^2 + 24^2 + 31^2 - (11 + 24 + 31)^2/3 = 206$. From Table A6 of Colquhoun (1971) it can be seen that when $k = 3$ and $n = 10$ (the maximum value listed) the probability of the value of S being as

Table 9.2. Production of cAMP (pmol/mg protein in 40 min) by granulosa cells from large follicles stimulated by FSH and hCG[a]

Sample	Control		FSH		hCG	
	Response	Rank	Response	Rank	Response	Rank
1	1.3	1	11.6	3	10.9	2
2	11	1	135	2	268	3
3	7.8	1	133	2	284	3
4	0	1	28.9	2	129	3
5	0	1	50.8	2	196	3
6	6.6	1	17.1	2	42.7	3
7	3.9	1	32.3	2	43.6	3
8	16.4	1	19.8	2	153	3
9	3.3	1	15.3	3	11.4	2
10	5.6	1	9.4	2	17.2	3
11	4.2	1	7.7	2	18.9	3
		$\sum R = 11$		$\sum R = 24$		$\sum R = 31$

[a] Eleven different samples of pooled granulosa cells were each divided into three parts. One part served as a control and the others were treated with FSH or hCG. Also shown are the ranks of the responses for use in the Friedman two-way analysis of variance. $\sum R$ equals a sum of ranks.

high as 206 by chance is less than about 0.001. When the test was repeated using the procedure FRIEDMAN in SPSS subprogram NPAR TESTS, a more accurate result of $p=0.0001$ was obtained. This is interpreted to mean that if the null hypothesis were true and there was no difference between the treatments, then the responses actually found would be expected to occur by chance only once in every 10,000 experiments. It is thus very probable that the null hypothesis was false and there is a significant effect of either or both gonadotrophins on the production in vitro of cAMP by granulosa cells from large ovarian follicles of sheep.

For large numbers of treatments or blocks, beyond the range of tables, an approximate method based on the χ^2 distribution can be used; this is described by Colquhoun (1971, p. 202).

9.1.4 Identifying the Difference: Critical Range Tests

It is fairly clear where the differences occur in this particular experiment; both FSH and hCG appear to have a stimulatory effect. In fact, this would have been apparent even if the differences between samples had not been controlled for, and the data had instead been tested using the Kruskal-Wallis one-way analysis for independent samples, referred to below. In many cases, however, it is not clear where the significant differences lie and then a critical range test must be used. It is not valid, for the reasons stated in Sect. 10.10, simply to test for significant differences between all possible pairs of rank sums as if they had all been obtained in isolation from the others.

The *critical range test* for comparing all possible pairs in the Friedman method is done very simply. When $k=3$ and $n=11$, Table A8 of Colquhoun (1971) shows that the probability of a difference as great as 11 in the sum of the ranks has a probability of 0.049 of occuring by chance if the null hypothesis is true. If the difference is 14, this probability is reduced to 0.008. Table 9.3 summarizes the differences in rank sums between all pairs. Thus it can be seen that the effects of both hCG and FSH were significant at the $p=0.01$ and 0.05 levels, respectively, but that there was no significant difference between the effects of the two gonadotrophins.

When there are more that 6 treatments or 20 replicates the table given by Colquhoun cannot be used and a calculation must be done instead. This is described by Hollander and Wolfe (1973, pp. 151–158).

Table 9.3. Critical range test applied to the rank sums calculated in Table 9.2[a]

	Control	FSH
FSH	13*	
hCG	20**	7

[a] The differences in rank sums are shown, together with the probabilities of their having occurred by chance in random samples drawn from a single population, as follows: *, $p=0.05$; **, $p=0.01$

9.1.5 Comparing More than Two Independent Samples

If, in contrast to the above example, the treatments are compared on *unrelated* samples then another test must be used. This is the *Kruskal-Wallis one-way analysis of variance by ranks* which is fully described by Siegel (1956, pp. 184–193) and Colquhoun (1971, pp. 191–195). Very much the same procedure is followed as in the Friedman test, and again a critical range test is required to identify significant differences. Details of the latter are provided by Colquhoun (1971, pp. 208–209). When the number of treatments is greater than 6, the number of replicates more than 20 or the samples are of unequal size, a calculation is performed as described by Hollander and Wolfe (1973, pp. 124–132).

9.1.6 Conclusions

It is hoped that this brief summary and examples of the use of non-parametric randomization tests have shown how they can be applied with advantage particularly when samples are small, the form of the distribution is not known and cannot be discovered, or the results are measured as ranks. An interesting description of the relative merits of non-parametric and parametric statistical models is given by Colquhoun (1971, Sect. 6.2).

9.2 Multivariate Analysis

Multivariate analysis comprises a variety of parametric statistical methods with the common aim of analysing the responses of systems in terms of more than one independent variable. Linear multivariate models, to which we shall confine our remarks, assume that a response can be described by a linear combination of terms. For example, if there are three independent variables in a system, the response or dependent variable y' is given by

$$y' = A'_1 x_1 + A'_2 x_2 + A'_3 x_3 + c \tag{9.2}$$

where A'_1 to A'_3 are parameters, x_1 to x_3 are values of the three independent variables, and c is a constant intercept. This equation is analogous to that of a straight line, except that there are contributions from three independent variables. The aim of a *multiple regression analysis* is to estimate the values of the three parameters yielding the best fit of this linear model to data, by the usual method of least squares.

It is convenient to standardize the values of the independent variables before analysis by expressing each as a z-score, or deviation from its group mean (Sect. 10.4). This normalizing transformation eliminates differences in scale of the independent variables and removes the constant intercept, Eq. (9.2) thus becoming

$$y = A_1 z_1 + A_2 z_2 + A_3 z_3. \tag{9.3}$$

Transforming the data in this way does not alter their statistical properties. What is more, the values of the parameters estimated from sets of z_1, z_2 and z_3 values measure the relative contributions of each z to the response, y. These normalized parameters are known as *standard partial regression coefficients*.

The techniques described below are all based on analysis of the covariance or correlation (Sect. 10.3) between several variables with the aim of simplifying their mathematical description so as to yield new, summary variables having convenient properties. It may thus be possible to identify a few underlying factors which are sufficient to explain the behaviour of many variables.

The following brief introduction to multivariate methods should be augmented by reference to standard works such as those by Lawley and Maxwell (1963) or Overall and Klett (1972). Davies (1971, Chap. 10) presents a biological point of view, and several computer programs.

9.2.1 Principal Component and Factor Analysis

Principal component analysis seeks to reduce the correlation (similarity) between observed variables by establishing, by linear transformation, a set of new variables, known as components or axes, which are at right angles to one another (orthogonal) and thus completely uncorrelated. Each variable is expressed as a sum of these uncorrelated components, as follows

$$z_i = \sum_{r=1}^{p} A_{ir} f_r \quad (i, r = 1, 2, \ldots, p) \tag{9.4}$$

where z_i is the value of the ith variable predicted by the model (expressed conveniently as a z-score) for comparison with the value measured on an individual of a sample, and A_{ir} is a parameter or loading measuring the contribution of the ith variable to the rth component, represented as f_r. That is, in these equations each of the original variables z is expressed as the sum of an equal number of uncorrelated components f each weighted by a loading A. The aim of the analysis is to estimate the values of the parameters in each equation so as to ensure the best fit to the data. No hypothesis is required concerning the new variables; the model is empirical and aims solely to express the data in terms of new, uncorrelated variables. Finally, a score characterizing each experimental unit in the sample can be calculated in terms of the components and appropriate loading parameters, so that comparisons between units can be made.

It is often found that one or more of the components has negligible effect in the calculation because its loadings are low. Such a component may be omitted from the calculation with negligible increase in the variance of the data about the fitted model, and a considerable simplification. This modification, known as *factor analysis* extends the above approach by attempting to account for or "explain" covariance or correlation between a large number of variables in terms of a minimum number of factors. Each factor is introduced so as to remove as much correlation as possible between variables. The minimum number of factors necessary to account for most of the correlation are added. Thus the factor model has the form

$$z_i = \sum_{r=1}^{k} A_{ir} f_r + e_i \quad (i = 1, \ldots, p) \tag{9.5}$$

where the number of factors f is restricted to k, as small a number as possible in comparison with p, the number of original variables. Notice the introduction of the error term e; unlike the case of principal component analysis, here the factors are fewer in number than the variables and thus cannot explain all the variance. The derived factors may be identified with one or more of the original variables if the relevent loadings are high. Scores for each experimental unit can then be calculated, as above.

A number of extensions of the method are possible. The set of axes (factors) may be "rotated" to strengthen the association between them and the original variables. Finally, the requirement that the factors be uncorrelated may be relaxed, thus allowing an oblique rotation and reintroducing some correlation between factors.

The problem is thus one of finding the minimum number of factors and estimating their loadings (parameters). It may be possible to associate a factor (which could represent several of the original variables if they all measure the same property of the system, thus being correlated) with some physical property of the system. Factor analysis can be used as a method of classification or clustering of variables (Sect. 9.2.2). For example, two factors may be found that are capable of replacing ten related variables. If the resulting factor scores for individuals fall into groups when plotted on a two-dimensional factor graph, a classification has been achieved.

It is not necessary that the measurements are normally distributed, although tests of significance carried out on the results may require this to be so. If the units of measurement of the different variables are not the same, then, for the results of the analysis to have physical meaning, the responses must be expressed in terms of z-scores. The following example illustrates these points.

9.2.1.1 Factor Analysis: Steroid Production by Ovarian Follicles

Factor analysis was used to find the minimum number of measurements necessary to characterize the steroid production of cultured follicles. Weiss (1978) measured steroid production by small (1–3 mm diameter) sheep ovarian follicles in vitro, using the culture techniques outlined by Weiss et al. (1978). Prior to culture, the follicles were divided into non-atretic, atretic and unclassified groups on the basis of their gross morphological appearance (Moor et al., 1978). Seventy-five follicles were maintained in vitro for 3 days and an extra 35 were removed from culture after the 1st day. The culture medium was changed daily and assayed for oestradiol, testosterone and progesterone. Results were expressed as ng steroid/mg wet wt. tissue per 24 h. Thus, there were 9 variables associated with each follicle. We are grateful to T. J. Weiss for permission to use his data for illustrative purposes.

In order for subsequent tests of significance to be applied, it was necessary to test the distributions of the results for normality using the Kolmogorov-Smirnov one-sample test (Sect. 10.8). That is, the distribution of the levels of oestradiol production by the normal follicles during the 1st day of culture was tested, as were each of the other sets of results. Several of the distributions were found to be significantly ($p < 0.05$) non-normal: after transformation by conversion to logarithms (Sect. 2.8.4) all were shown to be normal.

Factor analysis was applied to the results in an attempt to determine whether the steroid production of cultured follicles could be described reasonably accurately and precisely in terms of a small number of underlying factors, rather than in terms of the nine original variables. This was done using subprogram FACTOR of the SPSS package; details of the method and its interpretation are given by Nie et al. (1975). The input data were the logs of the concentrations of eight of the steroids in the culture medium from each follicle (the 9th, progesterone on the 1st day of culture, was negligible in every case and was omitted from the analysis). A principal factor solution was selected, followed by an oblique rotation of the factors to the terminal solution. A search was thus made for the smallest number of underlying factors to account for most of the variance; when this was found, the factors were rotated so as to further improve the fit. The fact that this rotation was oblique meant that the factors were no longer forced to be orthogonal (uncorrelated). This was logical because there was no reason to assume that any underlying factors should be completely unrelated.

The results of the analysis showed that three factors were sufficient to describe the data. The addition of extra factors did not significantly reduce the variance. Furthermore, 64% of the variance could be accounted for by the first two factors only and so the analysis was repeated with the number of factors limited to two.

The output of an oblique rotation analysis includes two matrices of coefficients relating the derived factors to the original variables. The first of these, the pattern matrix, provides a measure of the clustering or direct similarity of the variables to the derived factors. The second consists of correlation coefficients giving a measure of the total covariance between each factor and the original variables. The differences between these two matrices reflect the correlation between factors permitted in an oblique rotation in contrast to an orthogonal one.

Figure 9.1 (a) shows the results of the pattern matrix expressed as a graph of the correlation coefficients relating the two factors (the axes) to the variables. Thus the variable E2 (oestradiol output on the second day in culture) was correlated with Factor 1 to an extent of 0.886 (out of a possible maximum of 1) and with Factor 2 to an extent of only 0.065. Note that the results for oestradiol and testosterone were clustered together and all were associated with Factor 1, while the progesterone data were associated with Factor 2. Our hypothesis or model is, therefore, that one

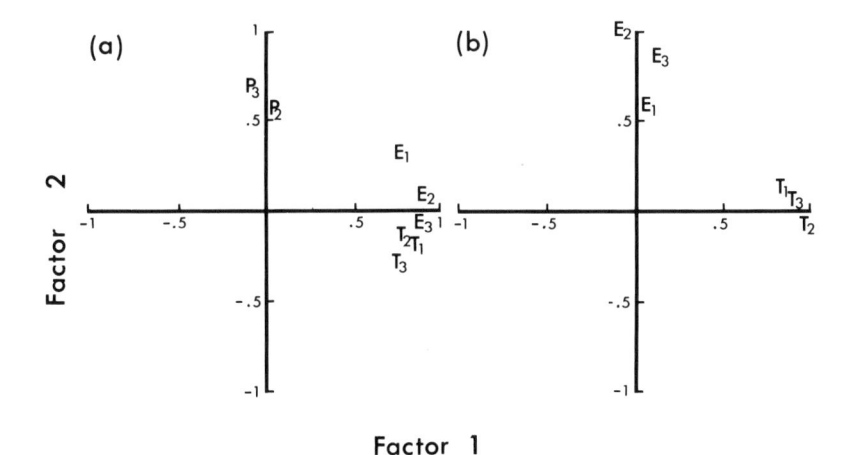

Fig. 9.1 a, b. Factor analysis applied to the steroid production of sheep ovarian follicles maintained in vitro for 3 days. The correlation coefficients between each variable and the hypothetical underlying factors are displayed graphically. E, oestradiol; T, testosterone; P, progesterone: the subscript numerals refer to the day of culture. **a** Variables E, T and P analysed; **b** variables E and T analysed. The first two factors only of each analysis are represented and their interpretation in **a** is different from that in **b**

property of the follicles in culture is related to the production of oestradiol and testosterone, and another to progesterone output. It is clear that there is little variation from day to day in either relationship, and a very similar result would be obtained by analysing the data from the first culture period only (the progesterone data then being omitted entirely).

It is possible to calculate a score for each follicle in terms of the new factors. This was also done by means of subprogram FACTOR, and the results are shown graphically in Fig. 9.2. Because there were two factors it was possible to draw a two-dimensional graph of the scores for each follicle. The two kinds of follicles, as judged by their gross morphology before culture, are differentiated on the graph. It can be seen clearly that the non-atretic and atretic follicles were generally fairly well distinguished in terms of the two underlying factors. Several of the follicles appeared to fall in the "wrong" section of the the graph; eight that were considered to be non-atretic morphologically produced steroids more characteristic of the atretic ones. This suggests that a number of the morphologically non-atretic follicles were in fact atretic (or partly so), as judged by their steroid production. There were also several atretic follicles which behaved similarly to non-atretic ones in their output of oestradiol and testosterone, but produced abnormally small amounts of progesterone.

A further simplification was possible. The results in Fig. 9.2 suggested that variation on the Factor 2 axis (related to progesterone production) was not very effective in distinguishing the non-atretic and atretic follicles. There was a tendency

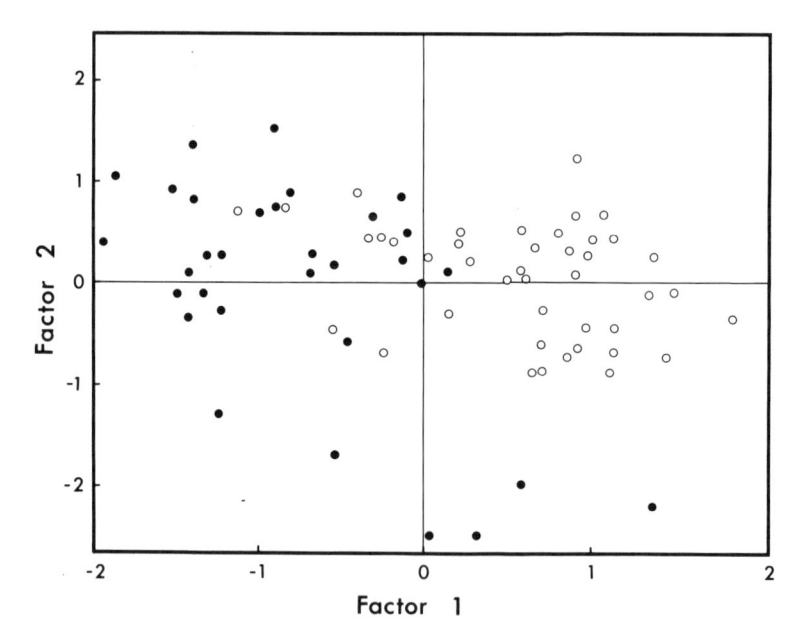

Fig. 9.2. Factor scores, expressed in standardized measure, for individual follicles. The two underlying factors were derived by factor analysis applied to the logs of measurements of oestradiol, testosterone and progesterone production by sheep ovarian follicles in vitro. Further details are given in the text. ○, Morphologically non-atretic; ●, morphologically atretic follicles

for atretic ones to produce more progesterone but the difference was small. The main distinguishing feature was that the non-atretic follicles produced relatively more oestradiol and testosterone. The analysis was therefore repeated with the progesterone data omitted. An even larger proportion (78%) of the (now reduced) variance was accounted for by the first two factors in the new analysis. A graph of the pattern matrix correlation coefficients is shown in Fig. 9.1 (b). The testosterone results on all three days were associated with a new Factor 1, and the oestradiol data with a new Factor 2. A two-dimensional plot of the individual scores showed that a clear distinction could again be drawn between the two groups in terms of oestradiol and testosterone production, the non-atretic follicles tending to produce high values of both steroids in comparison with atretic ones. This was exactly the same conclusion as before, but reached without the inclusion of the progesterone data. In fact, it would be possible to reduce the number of measurements required even further by omitting completely one or other of the sets of oestradiol or testosterone data because they were closely correlated. A distinction would then still be observed between the behaviours of the two groups of follicles.

This very simple example, in which the conclusions reached by way of the analysis were largely obvious from the raw data, was chosen for illustration so that the processes involved could be easily seen.

9.2.2 Cluster Analysis

Cluster analysis is a method for dividing individuals into two or more groups on the basis of a set of properties which they all share to some degree. Principal components or factors are examples of such properties. It is also possible to cluster on the basis of ranks rather than absolute measures, a technique which is known as *non-metrical multidimensional scaling*.

Cluster analysis may be divisive or agglomerative and hierarchical or nucleated. The *divisive* approach consists of assigning all individuals to a single group and then seeking to divide them into a larger number of groups. An *agglomerative* process is the reverse of this; one begins with a number of groups equal to the number of individuals and then by relaxing the criteria differentiating them, the groups are allowed progressively to coalesce. The pattern of this coalescence, as a function of increasing variance, may reveal distinct groups, or clusters.

Agglomeration methods may be *hierarchical* in which each group at a particular level of variance is condensed with another group at a higher level of variance. This forms a tree or divergent structure. Alternatively, the *nucleated* method of division is one in which the groups are regarded as being independent. In the absence of prior information suggesting a hierarchical structure, the latter model is more realistic.

Whatever method is used, the problem is to choose the most relevant measures of similarity. Because the techniques are applicable only to linear models they are often inappropriate when applied to highly non-linear biological systems. Consider the classification of individuals based on the absolute distance between their responses. when plotted on a graph. We often have no reason to assume that in a non-linear system two individuals that happen to fall far apart in terms of these particular measurements are more "different" than two other individuals which are closer together. Nevertheless, this is precisely what clustering assumes, based as it is on linear principles.

Clustering methods could be applied to the follicle scores represented graphically in Fig. 9.2. It might thus be possible to delineate quantitatively distinct clusters or groups in the data. This would be done without prior morphological or other knowledge. An attempt could then be made to associate these groups with the ones defined morphologically. Such, however, is the gradation in steroid production apparent between the non-atretic and atretic follicles that clear distinctions may not be possible. Another measure of similarity may possibly be found capable of providing a clearer separation. Details of clustering methods and suitable computer programs are given by Overall and Klett (1972), and Anderberg (1973).

Fowler et al. (1978) have used a hierarchical clustering method to analyse the steroid contents of the fluid of human ovarian follicles. Clustering was applied to minimize within-group variance in the results for each steroid from different groupings of follicles. A clear distinction could thus be made between preovulatory and ovulatory follicles.

9.2.3 Discriminant Analysis

Discriminant analysis is a technique for dividing individuals into previously defined groups on the basis of the values of a number of variables, not necessarily all measured in the same units. In this case a linear sum of variables, each multiplied by a discriminant coefficient, is sought which will provide the maximum numerical difference between two or more groups. The maximum number of discriminant functions that can be derived is one less than the number of groups to be separated. Thus a single discriminant function is generated to distinguish between two groups. This may be thought of as a process of maximizing between-group, and minimizing within-group, variance. Thus discriminant analysis, like the other multivariate techniques, depends on the reduction of multiple measurements to a single weighted composite. By finding appropriate weighting coefficients, several scores are reduced to a single one having the maximal capacity for distinguishing between members of two or more groups. It is possible to define a division point on the scale of scores which will minimize errors of misclassification. When the composite scores are normally distributed, means and variances for each group can be calculated, probabilities of misclassification determined and the likelihood of each individual belonging to a particular group calculated.

The parameters, or discriminant coefficients, are determined using a "training set" of individuals, previously defined as belonging to a certain group. Each "unknown", or individual with unknown characteristics, is then assigned to one of these groups on the basis of its score, calculated from the value of each variable and the previously determined discriminant coefficient. In this way one might, for example, separate individuals into two groups on the basis of their morphology and then compare this division with that obtained as a result of chemical analysis of the levels of several compounds. The following illustration using the follicle data does just this; an attempt is made to evolve a discriminant function based on steroid production in culture, capable of differentiating between atresia and non-atresia.

9.2.3.1 Application to Steroid Production by Ovarian Follicles

In Sect. 9.2.1.1 we used the technique of factor analysis to reveal simple factors underlying the steroid production of ovarian follicles in culture. There was also an indication that non-atretic and atretic follicles behaved differently and that analysis of the pattern of steroid output might provide a means of differentiating between these two groups. This would be a useful way of selecting groups of non-atretic follicles with homogeneous properties for experimental purposes. Ideally, one would want to make this selection after culture for a single day, or even shorter time, because follicles can be maintained for experimental purposes over a limited period only. Factor analysis suggested that this should be possible, and that only one or two steroids need be determined.

Discriminant analysis was applied to the follicle data after logarithmic transformation (see Sect. 9.2.1.1). The non-atretic and atretic groups (as judged by gross morphology) were used as the training groups to establish the discriminant coefficients. The follicles in the ungrouped set were then allocated to one or other of the non-atretic or atretic groups, depending on their behaviour in comparison with what were taken to be "genuine" members of these classes. The analysis was done using subprogram DISCRIMINANT of the SPSS package. Details of its use and the interpretation of results are given by Nie et al. (1975).

Initially, all eight variables were analysed. Stepwise entry of the eight variables into the analysis was done by selecting METHOD=WILKS. This procedure arranged the variables in order of their discriminating power. The relative importance of each variable in distinguishing between the groups is summarized in Table 9.4. The single discriminating function, which was a linear combination of the coefficients associated with each variable multiplied by the value measured (here the log of the value), was calculated for each follicle. The program then assigned each member of the training set to one or other group on the basis of the final score, and

Table 9.4. Relative abilities of variables to distinguish between non-atretic and atretic ovarian follicles in culture[a]

Variable	Wilks' lambda	Significance	Change in Rao's V on entry of each variable	Significance
E1	0.56	0	57	0
T2	0.46	0	27	0
P2	0.41	0	22	0
E3	0.38	0	12	0
T1	0.38	0	2	0.14
E2	0.38	0	0.5	0.49
T3	0.38	0	0.3	0.56
P3	0.38	0	0.2	0.69

[a] The variables were the logs of the steroid productions by the cultured follicles. E1, for example, refers to oestradiol output on the first day. Succeeding lines of the table show the improvement in the discriminating function as each variable is added to the analysis. Wilks' lambda measures the total discriminating power as the result of each addition; the smaller its final value the better. It is clear that only the first four variables are useful in the discrimination. The associated significances show that all the variables were capable of discriminating between the groups. The change in Rao's V shows the additional discrimination achieved as each variable is added to the discriminant function. The figures in the last column shows that that the first four variables only need be retained; the addition of each extra one beyond this number does not reduce the variance significantly.

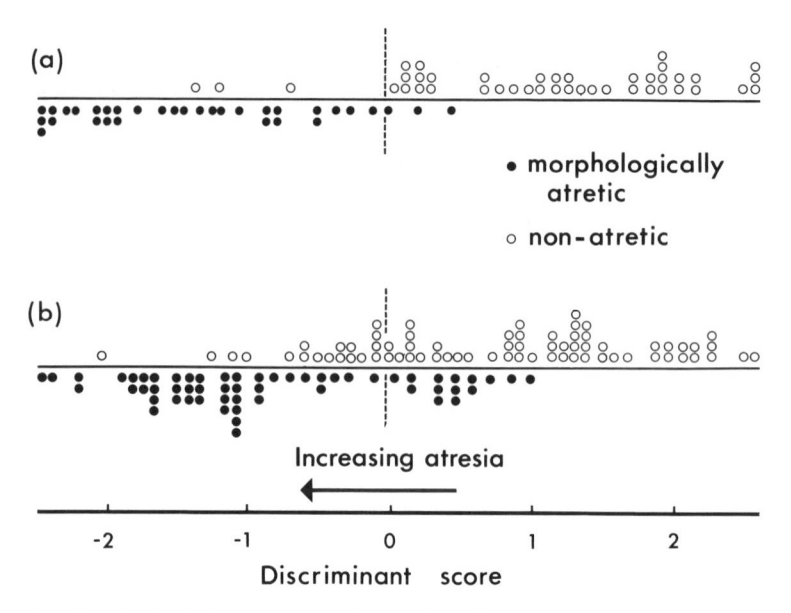

Fig. 9.3 a, b. Discriminant scores used to classify follicles on the basis of steroid production in culture. **a** Shows scores based on all variables (except progesterone on the first day). The classification was 92% correct in comparison with the results of gross morphological examination before culturing. **b** Shows scores based on oestradiol and testosterone output on the first day only. The discriminatory power, though reduced (74% "correct" assignment), is still valuable if borderline cases are excluded. The division point, which fell slightly below zero in the range of the scores, is shown by the *broken line*

compared the result with the actual group to which the follicle belonged. On the basis of the discriminant, 92.9 percent of the non-atretic and 90.9 percent of the atretic follicles were "correctly" classified. The results are shown in Fig. 9.3 (a). The classification could be improved by exchanging the more obviously misclassified individuals on the assumption that they were initially grouped wrongly. The analysis would then be repeated. There may, of course, be a gradation and some follicles will behave ambiguously. It is possible to associate a probability with the classification of each follicle. Table 9.5 lists a few of these. Follicles that were initially unclassified were assigned to one or other of the groups on the basis of their steroid productions, and a probability was associated with each of these assignments. It was then easy to select groups of follicles with memberships at any given level of probability of being correct. This was a great help in selecting homogeneous groups for further experimentation.

It would be advantageous to assign follicles on the basis of steroid production after only one day in culture. The analysis was therefore repeated using the data for oestradiol and testosterone on the first day. The resulting discriminant scores and classification achieved is shown in Fig. 9.3 (b). Only 74 percent of the follicles were then correctly classified but the results were still useful because a probability was associated with each and borderline individuals could be rejected. Once again the follicles could be ordered with respect to the degree of atresia displayed.

Table 9.5. Examples of the classification of ovarian follicles into non-atretic and atretic classes on the basis of steroid production in culture[a]

Follicle	Group on basis of morphology	Classification by steroid production	D^2	$p(G/X)$	Discriminant score
1	1	1	0.02	0.95	0.99
2	1	1	2.6	0.99	2.7
3	2	1	1.4	0.56	−0.06
4	2	2	1.2	0.61	−0.32

[a] D^2 is the distance (in standardized measure) of the result from the group centroid, squared. The value $p(G/X)$ is the probability of the predicted group membership being correct. The discriminant scores, in standardized measure, are the values plotted in Fig. 9.3.

10 Appendix A: A Summary of Relevant Statistics

Guidance is given here to statistical formulae and significance tests referred to in the text. A grasp of the basis of parametric statistics is essential both for understanding the method of least squares, and for applying many of the tests used in fitting models to data.

A set of experimental observations is considered to be a *sample* selected from a *population* of all possible measurements made under the same conditions. *Parametric* methods involve parameters estimated from a sample drawn from a population; it is necessary to establish that the measurements in the population are distributed (scattered) in a (usually) *normal* or *Gaussian* way (Colquhoun, 1971). If the data are not properly distributed, parametric methods will fail.

When no information is available about the characteristics of the population from which experimental data are drawn, it is preferable to employ *non-parametric* tests of significance. These tests do not depend upon the data being normally distributed. The importance and practical utility of certain non-parametric models are given special prominence in Chap. 9.

10.1 Variance, Standard Deviation and Weight

Let $x_1, \ldots, x_N$ be a sample of observations from a normally distributed population. The *variance* of this sample is equal to the sum of the squares of the differences between each observation and the sample mean, divided by the degrees of freedom. The *degrees of freedom* are the number of observations minus the number of parameters being estimated. In this case the mean is the only parameter, and thus the variance

$$V(x) = \sum_{i=1}^{N} (x_i - \bar{x})^2 / (N-1) \tag{10.1}$$

where N is the number of observations, and $\bar{x}$ is the mean. A quick way of calculating the variance is

$$V(x) = \sum_{i=1}^{N} x_i^2 - \left(\sum_{i=1}^{N} x_i \right)^2 / (N-1). \tag{10.2}$$

The *standard deviation of a sample* is the most common parametric measure of the scatter of observations about their mean. It equals the square root of the variance

$$s(x) = V(x)^{1/2}. \tag{10.3}$$

The *sample standard deviation of the mean*, (sometimes referred to as the *standard error of the mean*), is a parametric measure of the uncertainty in the *mean* of a sample, in contrast to the scatter in the members of the sample. It is the sample standard deviation divided by the square root of the number of observations

$$s(\bar{x}) = s(x)/N^{1/2} \tag{10.4}$$

where $s(\bar{x})$ is the sample standard deviation of the mean, $s(x)$ is the sample standard deviation, and N is the number of observations.

Standard deviations are measures of *uncertainty* or *error*, which, in statistical usage, has the meaning of chance variation between an observation and its true value. Mistakes or blunders are not encompassed by this term. Standard deviations have the same units as the variables they describe.

The *coefficient of variation* is a dimensionless quantity equal to the sample standard deviation divided by the mean, and is thus a measure of variation expressed in terms of the size of the expected value. It is often multiplied by 100 to give the *percentage coefficient of variation* (%CV).

A *weight* is a measure of the reliability of a mean. It is usually defined as

$$w(\bar{x}) = 1/V(\bar{x}) \tag{10.5}$$

where $w(\bar{x})$ is the weight and $V(\bar{x})$ the variance of the mean.

10.2 The Propagation of Variance

Uncertainties in variables are transferred to any combination of the variables, as follows. The variance of the *sum* or *difference* of two variables x and y is

$$V(x+y) = V(x) + V(y) \pm 2CoV(x,y) \tag{10.6}$$

where V is variance and CoV is covariance, defined as

$$CoV(x,y) = \sum_{i=1}^{N} (x_i - \bar{x})(y_i - \bar{y})/(N-1). \tag{10.7}$$

CoV can often be neglected (if x and y are uncorrelated CoV reduces to zero). It is omitted from the following definitions.

Adding (or subtracting) a *constant* does not affect variance

$$V(a \pm x) = V(x) \tag{10.8}$$

where a is a constant.

Multiplying by a *constant* does not affect variance

$$V(ax) = a^2 V(x). \tag{10.9}$$

Multiplying together two *variables*, each with variance

$$V(axy)/(xy)^2 = a^2 V(x)/x^2 + a^2 V(y)/y^2. \tag{10.10}$$

Dividing

$$V(ax/y)/(x/y)^2 = a^2 V(x)/x^2 + a^2 V(y)/y^2. \tag{10.11}$$

This last approximation is valid *only* if the denominator (y) is large in comparison with its standard deviation. An accurate estimate of the variance of the ratio of two variables with known variances can be made using Fieller's theorem (Colquhoun, 1971, pp 293–297). The difficulty arises because, although the sum or difference of two normally distributed variables is also normally distributed, their ratio is not. Other useful definitions are:

If $y = ax^{\pm b}$ then

$$V(y)/y^2 = b^2 V(x)/x^2. \tag{10.12}$$

If $y = ae^{\pm bx}$ then

$$V(y)/y^2 = b^2 V(x). \tag{10.13}$$

If $y = a \ln(\pm bx)$ then

$$V(y) = a^2 V(x)/x^2. \tag{10.14}$$

The approximate variance of *any function* $f(x_1, \ldots, x_N)$ of *uncorrelated* variables is

$$V(f) \cong (\delta f/\delta x_1)^2_{x=\bar{x}} V(x_1) + \ldots + (\delta f/\delta x_N)^2_{x=\bar{x}} V(x_N) \tag{10.15}$$

where the derivatives are evaluated at the mean of x.

Example: In Sect. 2.8.1 it is stated that the Lineweaver-Burk plot must be weighted by the fourth power of the substrate concentration if unbiased estimates of the parameters are to be obtained. This weighting factor is derived using Eq. (10.15)

$$V(1/x) = [d(1/x)/dx]^2_{x=\bar{x}} V(x)$$
$$= V(x)/\bar{x}^4.$$

10.3 Covariance and Correlation

The *correlation* between two variables is the ratio of their covariance to the square root of the product of their individual variances:

$$\text{correlation coefficient} = r = CoV(x, y)/[V(x) V(y)]^{1/2}. \tag{10.16}$$

Equivalently:

$$r = CoV(x, y)/[s(x)s(y)]. \tag{10.17}$$

Correlation equals covariance if the variables are in the form of z-scores (see below).

10.4 Z-Scores, or Standardized Measures

The normal or Gaussian distribution is an important concept and must be understood (Colquhoun, 1971). A useful manipulation based on it is the transformation of variables into *standard* form, or *z-scores*

$$z = (x - \bar{x})/s(x) \tag{10.18}$$

where z is the z-score, x is an observation in a normally distributed sample, $\bar{x}$ is the mean of the sample, and $s(x)$ is the standard deviation of the sample. Values of z are also normally distributed, with mean of zero and variance of 1. A graph of the standardized normal distribution of a large sample shows that about 68%, 95% and 99.7% of the area under the curve lie between $z = -1$ and 1, -2 and 2, and -3 and 3, respectively. If the sample is small (less that about 30), the t distribution is used instead. The program MODFIT calculates residuals and expresses them in the form of z-scores as an aid to detecting outliers.

10.5 Testing Hypotheses

A model cannot be proved to be a "correct" description of a phenomenon. A probability only can be placed on the match of a model with a sample of data, or the identity of two or more estimates of a parameter (Sect. 2.8.3).

It is standard practice to test the *null hypothesis*, which is that a model is adequate, or that there is no difference between parameter estimates. Because of the particular sample of data tested, the null hypothesis might be rejected when it is actually true; this is known as a *Type I error*. A *Type II error* occurs when a false hypothesis is accepted. Any attempt to decrease one type of error increases the change of the other. The *level of significance* is the maximum probability that one is willing to risk a Type I error. That is

$$\alpha = \text{size of Type I error}$$
$$= P \text{ (rejecting } H_0 | H_0 \text{ true)} \tag{10.19}$$

where P is the probability and H_0 is the null hypothesis.

Testing of a model requires knowledge of the uncertainty associated with the data (Sect. 3.5.1): similarly, if parameter estimates are to be compared, the uncertainty in each must be calculated (Sect. 3.5.6).

10.6 Runs-Test

The *one-sample runs-test* is a non-parametric technique for testing the hypothesis that a sample from a population has been taken randomly. It is suitable for testing the residuals (differences between fitted and experimental values in a model), and is intended to detect systematic divergence between the model and the data (Sect. 3.5.4). The runs-test is based on the sequence of positive and negative residuals in the range of the x values. A *run* is a succession of positive or negative residuals which are followed or preceded by those with opposite sign. The test consists of noting how many runs or changes in sign occur in the sample of residuals, and comparing this number with the entry in a table corresponding to the number of residuals. The probability is thus obtained of finding so few (or so many) runs in a random sample. Siegel (1956, pp. 52–58) gives further details.

10.7 Chi-Square Test

The non-parametric *chi-square* (χ^2) test can be used for testing the goodness of fit of a model to experimental data. It compares the differences between the model and data with the uncertainty (scatter) in the data at each point. That is

$$\chi^2 = \sum_{i=1}^{N} \{[\bar{y}_i - f(x_i)]/s(\bar{y}_i)\}^2 \tag{10.20}$$

where N is the number of observations, $\bar{y}_i$ is the mean of the values of a variable from a normal distribution, with standard deviation $s(\bar{y}_i)$, and $f(x_i)$ is the fitted value of y_i.

When χ^2 is divided by the degrees of freedom v the result is χ_v^2 or *reduced chi-square*. This is the statistic printed by the program MODFIT when MODE = 1, 11, −1 or 9, i.e. when standard deviation in the y values are supplied as part of the data. Reduced chi-square is the ratio of the observed spread to the expected spread of the observations, per degree of freedom. Tables of reduced chi-square (Bevington, 1969, pp. 314–315), or chi-square (Siegel, 1956, p. 249) which is then divided by v, imply that if the value of χ_v^2 is approximately equal to 1 the model is consistent with the sample of data points. This does not prove that the model is correct, only that it provides a plausible description of the data. Larger values of χ_v^2 mean either that the model is inappropriate or that the sample was not drawn randomly from a homogeneous population. This is the nearest we can approach to an absolute test of whether a model is appropriate. For more information see Bevington (1969, pp. 84–86) and Siegel (1956, pp. 42–47).

10.8 Tests of Normality of Distribution

Observations (or transformed observations) can be tested for normality of distribution in several ways. None is efficient if the sample is small. *Probit*, or for smaller samples *rankit*, plots are appropriate (Colquhoun, 1971). Alternatively, the chi-square (χ^2) test may be used to compare the data with the theoretical normal distribution (or any other distribution), and to calculate the probability of finding divergence between observation and expectation which is at least as large as that observed.

If it can be assumed that the variable has a continuous distribution, the *Kolmogorov-Smirnov one-sample test* is preferred. This is described by Siegel (1956, pp. 47–52).

10.9 Comparing Two Parameters: The *t*-Test

The *t*-test is suitable for determining whether two estimates of a parameter could have come from two samples of the same population. Tests for significant differences between more than two samples are discussed later.

For example, suppose we have used the program MODFIT to fit a straight line to two samples of data. We may want to test if the two lines have, within limits of experimental uncertainty, indistinguishable slopes and intercepts. This is equivalent to testing whether the two samples of data were drawn from the same population. The only suitable tests are the *t-test* or its equivalent in these circumstances, the *F*-test. Because they are equivalent we shall consider only the *t*-test.

The *t*-test can only be used to test pairs of parameters that have been derived from independent samples of data from *normally distributed* populations. Furthermore, the test is invalid unless the two groups have *homogeneous* or *approximately equal variances*. The test depends on the ratio between the difference in the parameters to the standard deviation in this difference. The statistic t is defined as

$$t = (\bar{x}_1 - \bar{x}_2)/s(\bar{x}) \tag{10.21}$$

where x is normally distributed, and $s(\bar{x})$ is the estimated standard deviation in the difference of the parameters. Thus an unbiased measure of the standard deviation in each parameter is essential. For this reason the test can strictly only be applied to the parameters of linear models, as it is only for these that unbiased uncertainties are guaranteed.

The t-test can also be applied to the parameters of non-linear models if the calculated uncertainties in the parameters have been shown to be accurate. This can be done by replicating the experiments many times with fresh, random samples of the two groups of data or, more conveniently, by means of Monte Carlo simulation (Sect. 2.8.2.1).

The t-test is applied as follows. It is required to test the null hypothesis that two parameter estimates are indistinguishable. The F-test (Sect. 10.11) must first be used to determine whether the variances in the two samples are homogeneous. The t-test is invalid if this is not the case, because the two samples are thus shown not to have been drawn from the same population. Assuming that the F-test shows no significant difference in the variances, the t-test is applied which, in the present case, has the form

$$t = |(A_{(1)} - A_{(2)}) - 0|/s(A_{(1)} - A_{(2)}) \tag{10.22}$$

where $A_{(1)}$, $A_{(2)}$ are the parameters being tested and $s(A_{(1)} - A_{(2)})$ is the standard deviation of the difference between the parameters. Zero is subtracted from the numerator because the null hypothesis is that the difference between the parameters is zero.

The value of $s(A_{(1)} - A_{(2)})$ is calculated using Eq. (10.6) with the assumption that covariance is zero. The calculated value of t is then compared with a table of the distribution of t for the particular number of degrees of freedom, which is the sum of the degrees of freedom for the two fits, as printed by MODFIT. The tabulated values of t depend also upon whether the hypothesis being examined requires a one or two-tailed test (Colquhoun, 1971, Sect. 6.1).

If one is interested in directly comparing two samples to see whether they could have come from the same population, rather than testing parameters estimated from the samples, it is generally preferable to use a non-parametric test. These depend neither on the data being normally distributed nor the variances being homogeneous (Sect. 9.1).

10.10 Comparing Any Number of Parameters: Analysis of Variance

A parametric test for determining if two or more samples are drawn from the same population is the *one-way analysis of variance*. Assumptions underlying the mathematical model of analysis of variance, and details of applying the test, are given by Colquhoun (1971, Sect. 11.2). In brief, the variance of replicates within a sample is compared with the variance between samples. If the variance between samples is significantly greater (by the F-test: Sect. 10.11) than the variance within samples, they cannot have all been drawn from the same population. This check must be made before applying the t-test.

Suppose ten different samples of a binding protein had been subjected to equilibrium dialysis, as described in Sect. 6.1.1.1. Suppose also that the model embodied in FUNCTN subprogram MASSACT with NTERMS set to 3 (thus modelling one specific, and one non-specific class of independent binding sites) was found to provide a satisfactory description of the data. Then, ten estimates of the three parameters would be obtained, each with a particular sample standard deviation, the square of which equals the within-sample variance. Analysis of variance could be used to determine whether all the estimates of, say, the association constant of the specific site, could have come from samples drawn from the same population. This would test whether the ten samples of protein differed in their association constants. It must be remembered that in order to apply parametric analysis of variance using the calculated uncertainties in the parameter estimates obtained from MODFIT, it is necessary to ensure that the model fitted to the data was not so non-linear as to invalidate the uncertainties. This could be checked by Monte Carlo simulation as illustrated in Sect. 6.2.2.2.

If analysis of variance indicated, at a given probability level, that significant differences did exist between the ten parameter estimates, one question remains − which sample or samples differ from the others? It is *not* possible to test all combinations of pairs by the *t*-test. When 100 samples are drawn from the *same* population, and all combinations of pairs of parameter estimates are tested in this way at the 5% level, there is almost complete certainty of finding at least one pair of values that is significantly different.

Instead, *critical range methods* must be used. A parametric one is Scheffé's test (Colquhoun, 1971, pp. 210–213). A non-parametric critical range test is illustrated in Sect. 9.1.4. The method consists of defining a *contrast* with which are compared the differences between all pairs.

10.11 The Variance Ratio of *F*-Test

The comparison of estimates of variance from two independent samples is called the *variance ratio test*, denoted by *F*. That is

$$F(v_1, v_2) = V_{v_1}(x)/V_{v_2}(x) = (\chi_1^2/v_1)/(\chi_2^2/v_2) \tag{10.23}$$

where v_1 and v_2 are the numbers of degrees of freedom in the estimates. That the *t*-test is a special case of the *F*-test, is shown clearly by Colquhoun (1971, pp. 179–180), who should also be consulted for further details of the *F*-test.

The *F*-test can be used to determine whether it is justifiable to add an extra parameter to a model. Its use is strictly limited to linear models, and only then if the parameters are *independent*, that is, their dependency values are low. But if a non-linear model can be shown to behave in an approximately linear way, then this test may be applied. It is probably more efficient to choose between models using the method described in Chap. 4.

To determine if variances of more than two samples are homogeneous, Bartlett's test should be applied (Snedecor and Cochran, 1967, pp. 296–298). Unfortunately, this test is very sensitive to non-normality of distributions and can only be used to compare distributions of proven normality.

10.12 Confidence Intervals

The *confidence interval* is a range within which the value of a parameter is expected to fall with a stated probability. The greater this probability, the wider must be the range. If an experiment is repeated many times, and confidence intervals at the 5 percent probability level computed for each experiment, then 95 percent of the calculated confidence intervals would include the true parameter values. See Colquhoun (1971, pp. 101–103) for an interesting and important discussion of the reliability of confidence intervals, the values of which must be regarded as optimistic.

The Gaussian confidence interval or range for the value of a parameter A is

$$A \pm ts(A) \qquad (10.24)$$

where A has been estimated from a sample of normally distributed observations, t is the statistic defined by the t distribution, and $s(A)$ is the standard deviation in the parameter estimate. The value of t depends on the degrees of freedom and the probability level required. Confidence limits on a *new observation*, which are wider than those on a parameter, are also readily calculated (Colquhoun, 1971, p. 107).

Details of the more lengthy calculation required for determining exact confidence limits on the *ratio* of two normally distributed variables using Fieller's theorem, are given by Colquhoun (1971, pp. 107–108).

The 5 percent level, or a chance of 1 in 20, popularized by R. A. Fisher, tends to be misused. He advocated regarding the probability of 0.05 as "suggestive", "rejection" being reserved for a probability of 0.01.

Non-parametric confidence limits are very easy to determine but cannot be applied to parameters determined by MODFIT, or any other model-fitting procedure based on parametric methods. Sect. 9.1.1 gives more information.

10.13 Control Charts

Control charts are graphical analyses for ensuring that a procedure (such as a radio-immunoassay) repeated over long periods of time, does not gradually change so as to cause bias in the results. Control charts are often constructed using constant, quality control samples, but other factors in an assay may also be controlled. The simplest control chart is a graph of the mean value of a quality control sample versus time, or assay number. Other more elaborate and useful methods have been described (Himmelblau, 1970, pp. 78–94).

One of the most informative and sensitive of these is the *cumulative sum* control chart, in which the cumulative sum of the response variable, or some function of it, is plotted. The advantage of cumulative sum control charts is that they minimize random fluctuations and accentuate moderate trends. A V-shaped template or overlay mask is used in conjunction with the chart to determine the slope of the chart over a particular region, because it is this that is of interest rather than absolute values. For an example of the use of a cumulative sum control chart to monitor the performance of a radio-immunoassay, see Kemp et al. (1978).

11 Appendix B: Computer Programs

The programs and subprograms listed and described here are referred to extensively throughout the text. It is hoped that they will give inspiration, and also a nucleus of useful techniques for getting started on modelling the results of analytical experiments.

Three main programs are provided. MODFIT is for fitting the equations of models to experimental data, SIMUL is for evaluating models and doing Monte Carlo simulations and DESIGN is for designing sequential experiments to discriminate between models and estimate parameters efficiently. These programs all have a similar structure and make use of common subprograms. The necessary subprograms describing the equations of the models (all called FUNCTN) are also provided. They are examples of model descriptions that should prove generally useful.

11.1 MODFIT: A General Model-Fitting Program

MODFIT is a computer program for fitting to experimental data equations of models that may be either linear or non-linear in their parameters. The general principles of this are the subject of Chap. 3; an outline of the mathematical basis of the program is given in Sect. 3.5. A listing of MODFIT appears in Table 11.1.

The working program consists of the main segment MODFIT and subprograms FIT, FUNCTN, FCHISQ and EIGEN, which are described below. The most flexible and convenient approach is to compile and load together all but FUNCTN. A suitable version of FUNCTN, which gives a mathematical description of the particular model being used in terms of the FORTRAN language, is then compiled and loaded with the rest of the program before running it. In order for FUNCTN to work correctly a number of its statements must take certain forms. The COMMON statement must be included, and array A declared. The current values of the parameters are stored in array A, the experimental values of the independent variable in array X, and the calculated values of the dependent variable must be left in array YFIT. Communication of these values between FUNCTN and FIT is by way of the BLANK COMMON block. Within subprogram FUNCTN a loop must be defined which calculates y values from x values and the current parameter estimates, according to the equation of the model, and deposits them in the corresponding elements of array YFIT. Arguments of FUNCTN are the number of experimental observations NPTS, the name of the array containing the current values of the parameters (A or B; up to fifteen values in each) and the number of parameters NTERMS in the particular model. Any of the examples of FUNCTN subprograms reproduced below illustrates these points.

MODFIT: A General Model-Fitting Program 251

Table 11.1. Program MODFIT[a]

```
      PROGRAM MODFIT (INPUT, OUTPUT, TAPE2, TAPE5=INPUT, TAPE6=OUTPUT)
C     **************
      COMMON X(100), Y(100), YFIT(100), SIGMAY(100), WEIGHT(100),
     1  SIGMAA(15), MODE
      COMMON /P/ AL1(15), AU1(15), DEPDCY(15)
      COMMON /D/ DV(100,15), AR(15,15), AP(15,15)
      REAL A(15), OLDA(15), PCV(15), RESID(100)
      EXTERNAL FUNCTN
      DATA AHEAD/1HA/, TERMPC/1./, ITLIM/20/
      TERM = TERMPC / 100.
      IFLAG = 0
      REWIND 2
      REWIND 5
C
C               READ MODE AND PARAMETERS
C
   10 READ(5,*) MODI
      IF (EOF(5)) 460,20
   20 IF (MODI .LT. 9) GOTO 30
      MODE = MODI - 10
      READ(5,*) NTERMS, (A(J), AL1(J), AU1(J), J = 1, NTERMS)
      IF (EOF(5)) 440,32
   30 READ(5,*) NTERMS, (A(J), J = 1, NTERMS)
      IF (EOF(5)) 440,31
   31 MODE = MODI
C
C               READ DATA
C
   32 I = 0
   50 READ(5,*) XX, YY
      IF (EOF(5)) 440,60
   60 IF (XX .EQ. 999.) GOTO 70
      I = I + 1
      X(I) = XX
      Y(I) = YY
      IF (MODE .LE. 0) GOTO 50
      READ(5,*) SIGMAY(I)
      IF (EOF(5)) 440,50
   70 CONTINUE
      NPTS = I
      NF = NPTS - NTERMS
C
C               SET WEIGHTS
C
      DO 130 I = 1, NPTS
      IF (MODE) 80,110,120
   80 IF (Y(I) .EQ. 0.) GOTO 110
      DUMMY = ABS(Y(I))
      WEIGHT(I) = 1. / DUMMY
      SIGMAY(I) = SQRT(DUMMY)
      GOTO 130
  110 WEIGHT(I) = 1.
      GOTO 130
  120 WEIGHT(I) = 1. / SIGMAY(I) ** 2
  130 CONTINUE
C
C               HEADING UP
C
      IF (MODE) 160,140,160
  140 WRITE(6,150)
  150 FORMAT(13H1RES VARIANCE)
      GOTO 180
```

Continued next page

[a] The basic program, used throughout this book, for fitting to data the equation of any model, linear or non-linear in its parameters. MODFIT calls subprograms FIT, FCHISQ, FUNCTN (the latter defines the model to be fitted) and EIGEN.

Table 11.1 (continued)

```
      160 WRITE(6,170)
      170 FORMAT(13H1R CHI SQUARE)
      180 WRITE(6,190) (AHEAD, J, J = 1, NTERMS)
      190 FORMAT(1H+, 18X, 9(A1, I2, 9X) / 19X, 6(A1, I2, 9X))
          FL = .001
C
C             FITTING LOOP
C
          DO 270 K = 1, ITLIM
            DO 230 J = 1, NTERMS
            OLDA(J) = A(J)
      230 CONTINUE
          CALL FIT (A, NPTS, NTERMS, FL, CHISQR, CHISQ1,
        1 FUNCTN, IFLAG, MODI)
          IF (K .EQ. 1) WRITE(6,240) CHISQ1, (OLDA(J), J = 1, NTERMS)
          WRITE(6,240) CHISQR, (A(J), J = 1, NTERMS)
      240 FORMAT(1X, 10G12.5 / 13X, 6G12.5)
          DO 250 J = 1, NTERMS
          IF (ABS(OLDA(J) - A(J)) .GT. ABS(TERM * OLDA(J))) GOTO 270
      250 CONTINUE
C
C             LAST CALL TO FIT WITH FL = 0
C
          CALL FIT (A, NPTS, NTERMS, 0., CHISQR, CHISQ1,
        1 FUNCTN, IFLAG, MODI)
          GOTO 300
      270 CONTINUE
          WRITE(6,290) ITLIM, TERMPC
      290 FORMAT(19H0*** STOPPING AFTER, I3, 16H ITERATIONS WITH /
        1 41H PARAMETER(S) STILL CHANGING BY MORE THAN, F5.1, 1H%)
C
C             WRITE FINAL PARAMETER VALUES AND THEIR STANDARD
C             DEVIATIONS, DEPENDENCIES, CONDITION NUMBER
C             AND CORRELATION COEFFICIENTS
C
      300 WRITE(6,240) CHISQR, (A(J), J = 1, NTERMS)
          WRITE(6,330) (SIGMAA(J), J = 1, NTERMS)
      330 FORMAT(13H0STD DEVS    , 9G12.5 / 13X, 6G12.5)
          DO 340 J = 1, NTERMS
          PCV(J) = SIGMAA(J) * 100. / A(J)
      340 CONTINUE
          WRITE(6,350) (PCV(J), J = 1, NTERMS)
      350 FORMAT(11X, 9(F11.1, 1H%) / 11X, 6(F11.1, 1H%))
          WRITE(6,351) (DEPDCY(J), J = 1, NTERMS)
      351 FORMAT(13H0DEPENDENCIES, 9G12.5 / 13X, 6G12.5)
          CALL EIGEN (NTERMS, EVRAT)
          WRITE(6,353) EVRAT
      353 FORMAT(17H0CONDITION NUMBER, F10.1)
          WRITE(6,354)
      354 FORMAT(25H0CORRELATION COEFFICIENTS)
          DO 355 J = 1, NTERMS
            DO 355 K = 1, J
            AR(J,K) = AR(J,K) / SQRT(AP(J,J) * AP(K,K))
      355 CONTINUE
          DO 358 J = 1, NTERMS
            DO 356 K = 1, J
            AP(J,K) = AR(J,K) / SQRT(AR(J,J) * AR(K,K))
      356 CONTINUE
          WRITE(6,357) AHEAD, J, (AP(J,L), L = 1, J)
      357 FORMAT(10X, A1, I2, 9G12.5 / 13X, 6G12.5)
      358 CONTINUE
C
C             WRITE OTHER RESULTS
C
          WRITE(6,360) MODI, NF, FL
      360 FORMAT(7H0MODE =, I3, 22H, DEGREES OF FREEDOM =, I4 /
        1 15H FINAL LAMBDA =, F21.16 //)
```

```
      2    8X, 1HX, 11X, 1HY, 9X, 4HYFIT, 6X, 8HRESIDUAL, 3X,
      3    10HZ-RESIDUAL)
           IF (MODE) 370,390,370
370   WRITE(6,380)
380   FORMAT(1H+, 63X, 6HSIGMAY)
390      DO 430 I = 1, NPTS
         RESID(I) = Y(I) - YFIT(I)
         SD = SIGMAY(I)
         IF (MODE .EQ. 0) SD = SQRT(CHISQR)
         ZRES = RESID(I) / SD
         WRITE(6,400) X(I), Y(I), YFIT(I), RESID(I), ZRES
400      FORMAT(1X, 5G12.5)
         IF (MODE) 410,430,410
410      WRITE(6,420) SIGMAY(I)
420      FORMAT(1H+, 60X, G12.5)
430      CONTINUE
      GOTO 10
440   WRITE(6,450)
450   FORMAT(36H0*** ERROR *** PREMATURE END OF DATA)
460   STOP
      END
```

Details of the way in which MODFIT and a FUNCTN subprogram are together loaded into any particular computer cannot be given here. A few minor changes will be required if MODFIT is run on a machine other than one manufactured by the Control Data Corporation. In most cases, these changes will be restricted to the first statement of the main program and the free-format READ statements, none of which is written in standard FORTRAN. Details will be given in the FORTRAN manual for your computer. In addition, it may be necessary to declare the variables AMAX and SAVE, and the array AR (all in FIT), to be double precision; consult an expert at your computing centre.

A slightly different procedure is followed if a model described in terms of differential equations is to be fitted. It is then necessary to load two extra subprograms into the computer. The first consists solely of a list of the differential equations to be integrated and the other is a subprogram for carrying out the integration. It is suggested that a subprogram suitable for integrating systems of stiff differential equations be used. A suitable one is D02AEF written by the Nottingham Algorithms Group, which is described in their Document No. 504 (1973). Owing to copyright restrictions it is not possible for us to reproduce the FORTRAN listing of this subprogram. You will have to obtain it (or something equivalent) from your computing centre. Details of exactly how D02AEF is used (it is referred to by the name STIFF hereafter) will be found in the description of the FUNCTN subprogram CA2 (Sect. 11.9).

MODFIT accepts data in free-format; i.e. without regard to its layout. Examples of input appear in Tables 11.2 and 11.15. The first number in Table 11.2, 0, is the value of MODE, a flag or switch that defines the type of error treatment to be followed. MODE set to 0 signifies that equal weighting is to be applied to all points, because estimates of the precision of the y measurements at each value of x are unavailable. Alternatively, MODE is set to 1 (Table 11.15) if estimates of precision (each expressed as a standard deviation of the mean) are included with the data; weighting according to the reciprocal of the variance will be applied. If MODE equals -1 this indicates that Poisson weightings will be used; the weights are set equal to the reciprocals of the y values.

Table 11.2. Example of input to MODFIT[a]

```
0     4    5   0.5   20   0.02
0    25
0.417 24
0.533 23
1.33  23
1.83  20
      .
      .
      .
110   2.5
117   1
999   999
```

[a] When FUNCTN subprogram RESERVR together with MODFIT and the necessary subprograms were loaded into the computer, and these input data were supplied on UNIT 5, the results shown in Table 3.1 and Fig. 5.1 were obtained. Notice that several lines of input have been omitted in order to save space.

If one wants to impose penalty functions (constraints) on the parameters during the fitting process for the reasons outlined in Sect. 3.5.3, the value of MODE is increased by 10 (i.e. becomes 9, 10 or 11).

The second number in the input data is NTERMS (4, in Table 11.2), the number of parameters in the model, and this is followed by the initial estimates of the parameters. These estimates can be very approximate in the case of a well-behaved linear function such as a polynomial, but should be as accurate as possible for more demanding non-linear models, such as those consisting of sums of exponentials. If the fitting process is to be constrained by penalty functions (i.e. if MODE is 9, 10 or 11) each initial parameter value is followed by a lower and upper bound, in that order.

Beginning at the next line is a list of the independent and dependent variables, in pairs, each pair followed by a value for the standard error in y if MODE is 1 or 11. The list is ended by 999   999. Further sets of input data may then follow (starting with MODE again).

MODFIT reads the input in statements labelled 10 to 70 of the listing in Table 11.1. The number of degrees of freedom (NF) is calculated and weightings are set in statements labelled 70 to 130. The variable controlling the progress of the Marquardt-Levenberg algorithm, FL, is set initially to 0.001. The first call to subprogram FIT begins the iterative process of optimization. On return from FIT the residual variance, RES VARIANCE, (calculated using the initial values of the parameters) is printed if MODE is 0 or 10. Otherwise, reduced chi-square (R CHI SQUARE) is given. At the same time the results of the first iteration are displayed.

Subprogram FIT (Table 11.3) is responsible for directing the path of the search. When far from the minimum the Marquardt-Levenberg algorithm approximates the method of steepest descent. As FL decreases (it is divided by 10 at the end of each call to FIT) the search becomes progressively more like a Gauss-Newton linearization. Each iteration of FIT may involve more than one subiteration within

Text continued page 257

Table 11.3. Subprogram FIT[a]

```
      SUBROUTINE FIT (A, NPTS, NTERMS, FL, CHISQR, CHISQ1,
C     **************
     1    FUNCTN, IFLAG, MODI)
      COMMON X(100), Y(100), YFIT(100), SIGMAY(100), WEIGHT(100),
     1    SIGMAA(15), MODE
      COMMON /P/ AL1(15), AU1(15), DEPDCY(15)
      COMMON /D/ DV(100,15), AR(15,15), AP(15,15)
      REAL BT(15), A(15), B(15), AJ(15), AL(15), AU(15)
      INTEGER IK(15), JK(15)
      NF = NPTS - NTERMS
      IF (NF) 10,10,30
10    WRITE(6,20)
20    FORMAT(52H0*** ERROR *** DEGREES OF FREEDOM ZERO OR NEGATIVE. /
     1    15X, 34HNO SOLUTION POSSIBLE. CHECK INPUT.)
      STOP
30    IF (IFLAG .EQ. 1) GO TO 45
      DO 40 J = 1, NTERMS
        BT(J) = 0.
          DO 40 K = 1, J
          AP(J,K) = 0.
40        CONTINUE
45    DO 70 J = 1, NTERMS
      AJJ = A(J)
      DELTA = .0001 * AJJ
      A(J) = AJJ + DELTA
      CALL FUNCTN (NPTS, A, NTERMS)
        DO 50 I = 1, NPTS
        DV(I,J) = YFIT(I)
50      CONTINUE
      A(J) = AJJ - DELTA
      CALL FUNCTN (NPTS, A, NTERMS)
        DO 60 I = 1, NPTS
        DV(I,J) = (DV(I,J) - YFIT(I)) / (2. * DELTA)
60      CONTINUE
      A(J) = AJJ
70    CONTINUE
      CALL FUNCTN (NPTS, A, NTERMS)
      IF (IFLAG .EQ. 1) RETURN
        DO 90 I = 1, NPTS
          DO 80 J = 1, NTERMS
          BT(J) = BT(J) + WEIGHT(I) * (Y(I) - YFIT(I)) *
     1      DV(I,J)
            DO 80 K = 1, J
            AP(J,K) = AP(J,K) + WEIGHT(I) * DV(I,J) *
     1        DV(I,K)
80          CONTINUE
90      CONTINUE
        DO 100 J = 1, NTERMS
          DO 100 K = 1, J
          AP(K,J) = AP(J,K)
100       CONTINUE
      CHISQ1 = FCHISQ (NPTS, NF)
102   IF (MODI .EQ. MODE .OR. FL .EQ. 0.) GO TO 108
      DO 106 J = 1, NTERMS
      AJ(J) = .0001 * A(J) * CHISQ1
      AL(J) = A(J) - AL1(J)
      IF (AL(J) .LE. 0.) AL(J) = 1.E-10
```

Continued next page

[a] Subprogram FIT is called by programs MODFIT, SIMUL and DESIGN. It is responsible for carrying out a least-squares fit of the model equation defined in subprogram FUNCTN to experimental data. This subprogram was based originally on the subprograms CURFIT and MATINV published by Bevington, 1969. Data reduction and error analysis for the physical sciences. Copyright by McGraw-Hill, New York, London. (Six statements identical to those used by Bevington are reproduced here with kind permission of McGraw-Hill Book Co.)

Table 11.3 (continued)

```
              AU(J) = AU1(J) - A(J)
              IF (AU(J) .LE. 0.) AU(J) = 1.E-10
              ALJSQ = AL(J) ** 2
              AUJSQ = AU(J) ** 2
              BT(J) = BT(J) - AJ(J) / ALJSQ - AJ(J) / AUJSQ
              AP(J,J) = AP(J,J) + 2. * AJ(J) / (ALJSQ * AL(J))
         1              + 2. * AJ(J) / (AUJSQ * AU(J))
   106    CONTINUE
   108    DO 120 J = 1, NTERMS
              DO 110 K = 1, NTERMS
              AR(J,K) = AP(J,K) / SQRT(AP(J,J) * AP(K,K))
   110        CONTINUE
              AR(J,J) = 1. + FL
   120    CONTINUE
          DO 310 K = 1, NTERMS
          AMAX = 0.
   130        DO 150 I = K, NTERMS
                  DO 150 J = K, NTERMS
                  IF (ABS(AMAX) - ABS(AR(I,J))) 140,140,150
   140            AMAX = AR(I,J)
                  IK(K) = I
                  JK(K) = J
   150        CONTINUE
          I = IK(K)
          IF (I - K) 130,200,180
   180        DO 190 J = 1, NTERMS
              SV = AR(K,J)
              AR(K,J) = AR(I,J)
              AR(I,J) = - SV
   190    CONTINUE
   200    J = JK(K)
          IF (J - K) 130,230,210
   210        DO 220 I = 1, NTERMS
              SV = AR(I,K)
              AR(I,K) = AR(I,J)
              AR(I,J) = - SV
   220    CONTINUE
   230    DO 250 I = 1, NTERMS
          IF (I - K) 240,250,240
   240     AR(I,K) = - AR(I,K) / AMAX
   250    CONTINUE
          DO 280 I = 1, NTERMS
              DO 280 J = 1, NTERMS
              IF (I - K) 260,280,260
   260        IF (J - K) 270,280,270
   270        AR(I,J) = AR(I,J) + AR(I,K) * AR(K,J)
   280        CONTINUE
          DO 300 J = 1, NTERMS
          IF (J - K) 290,300,290
   290     AR(K,J) = AR(K,J) / AMAX
   300    CONTINUE
          AR(K,K) = 1. / AMAX
   310    CONTINUE
          DO 370 L = 1, NTERMS
          K = NTERMS - L + 1
          J = IK(K)
          IF (J - K) 340,340,320
   320        DO 330 I = 1, NTERMS
              SV = AR(I,K)
              AR(I,K) = - AR(I,J)
              AR(I,J) = SV
   330    CONTINUE
   340    I = JK(K)
          IF (I - K) 370,370,350
   350        DO 360 J = 1, NTERMS
              SV = AR(K,J)
              AR(K,J) = - AR(I,J)
```

```
              AR(I,J) = SV
360        CONTINUE
370     CONTINUE
380     DO 390 J = 1, NTERMS
           B(J) = A(J)
              DO 390 K = 1, NTERMS
              B(J) = B(J) + BT(K) * AR(J,K) /
    1         SQRT (AP(J,J) * AP(K,K))
390     CONTINUE
        CALL FUNCTN (NPTS, B, NTERMS)
        CHISQR = FCHISQ (NPTS, NF)
        IF (FL .LT. 1.E-60) GOTO 410
        IF (CHISQ1 - CHISQR) 400,410,410
400     FL = 10. * FL
        GOTO 102
410     IF (MODE) 420,430,420
420     VARNCE = 1.
        GO TO 440
430     VARNCE = CHISQR
440     DEPVAR = VARNCE * FLOAT(NF) / FLOAT(NPTS - 1)
        DO 450 J = 1, NTERMS
           A(J) = B(J)
           VARA = VARNCE * AR(J,J) / AP(J,J)
           SIGMAA(J) = SQRT(VARA)
           DEPDCY(J) = 1. - DEPVAR / (VARA * AP(J,J))
450     CONTINUE
        FL = FL / 10.
        RETURN
        END
```

FIT if the algorithm finds that it must increase FL temporarily in order to reduce the value of the residual variance.

The operation of subprogram FIT is as follows. Partial derivatives of the model equation with respect to each parameter, the sensitivity coefficients, are calculated in statements labelled 45 to 70 by the approximate numerical method of central differences. This has been shown to be the most accurate of the approximate methods (Atkins, 1977). A final call to FUNCTN calculates the current fitted values of y (array YFIT). Next, the terms of vector BT and the curvature matrix AL are evaluated and AL is transposed. Chi-square is evaluated at the beginning of the current iteration by a call to FCHISQ. If required, penalty functions are evaluated and AL and BT are modified in statements labelled 102 to 106 according to the method outlined by Bard (1974, pp. 141-145 and pp. 160-162). AL is then normalized, its diagonal terms modified by the addition of the Marquardt-Levenberg coefficient FL, and inverted in statements labelled 108 to 370 to yield AR. The terms of the variance-covariance matrix (the un-normalized inverse of AL, recovered term by term from AR in statements labelled 380 to 390) are then used in conjunction with BT to calculate the new parameter values in array B. FUNCTN is called with these new values, chi-square is recalculated, and if no reduction in its value has occurred FL is increased and the process repeated. Usually, however, chi-square will have been reduced.

Dependencies and uncertainties in the parameters are calculated in statements labelled 410 to 450 using terms of the variance-covariance matrix. The *dependence* of each parameter is defined as 1 – (variance in the parameter, other parameters held constant)/(variance in the parameter allowing the others to change in the usual way). The variance in each parameter when all others are held constant is found by setting, in effect, all terms of AL other than the diagonal term corresponding to the particular parameter to zero before inversion. This is equivalent to finding the reciprocal of the relevant diagonal term.

FIT is called repeatedly and on every return each parameter is compared with its value at the previous return from FIT. If *all* the percentage changes in the parameters are less than the value of PCTERM (1% by default) the search for the minimum of the objective function is considered to have converged. If not, FIT is called again and the test repeated. If the number of iterations (separate calls to FIT), exceeds the value of ITLIM (20 by default) a message is printed and iteration stops. To continue, the data must be entered again with the latest values of the parameters as the initial estimates.

When the fitting terminates, a final call to FIT is made with the penalty functions and FL set to 0 to ensure that the uncertainties in the parameters are calculated correctly.

The final, optimized values of the parameters are printed together with either the corresponding residual variance or reduced chi-square (depending on the value of MODE), an estimate of the uncertainty in each parameter expressed as a standard deviation, and the ratio of this to the parameter estimate expressed as a percentage (percentage coefficient of variation). An example is given in Table 3.1.

The three related measures of parameter interaction are then printed: the dependencies, condition number and correlation coefficients (Sect. 3.5.8.1). The condition number is the ratio of the largest to the smallest eigenvalue of the unnormalized curvature matrix AL, and is a measure of the ill-conditioning of this matrix. High values are obtained if the model is over-parameterized, i.e. contains an excess of parameters. For further information concerning eigenvalues and ill-conditioning see Wilkinson (1965). The correlation coefficients are calculated in statements labelled 354 to 356, being placed in array AL in order to save computer memory space.

Then follows a list of each experimental x, y and fitted y value, as well as the residuals. Also printed are the residuals expressed as a fraction either of the mean residual standard deviation (square root of the residual variance) in the case of MODE equal to 0 or 10, or of the experimentally determined standard deviation when MODE is 1, $-1,11$ or 9. The program then seeks more data or, if there are none, stops.

Function FCHISQ (Table 11.4) is responsible for finding the current residual sum of squares, which is printed as RES VARIANCE if MODE is 0, or used in

Table 11.4. Function FCHISQ[a]

```
      FUNCTION FCHISQ (NPTS, NF)
C     ***************
      COMMON X(100), Y(100), YFIT(100), SIGMAY(100), WEIGHT(100),
     1   SIGMAA(15), MODE
      CHISQ = 0.
      DO 10 I = 1, NPTS
      CHISQ = CHISQ + WEIGHT(I) * (Y(I) - YFIT(I)) ** 2
   10 CONTINUE
      FCHISQ = CHISQ / FLOAT(NF)
      RETURN
      END
```

[a] For calculating the goodness of fit of a model equation to experimental data.

Table 11.5. Subprogram EIGEN[a]

```
        SUBROUTINE EIGEN (NTERMS, EVRAT)
C       ***************
C
C
C             FINDS EIGENVALUES OF A REAL SYMMETRIC MATRIX AND
C             RETURNS SQUARE ROOT OF RATIO OF LARGEST TO SMALLEST
C             EIGENVALUE AS EVRAT
C
        COMMON /D/ DV(100,15), AR(15,15), AP(15,15)
        INTEGER P, P1, P2, P3, Q, Q1, Q2, ROT
        REAL D(15), B(15), Z(15)
        IF (NTERMS .LT. 2) GOTO 270
           DO 40 P = 1, NTERMS
           B(P) = AP(P,P)
           D(P) = AP(P,P)
           Z(P) = 0.
 40        CONTINUE
        ROT = 0
           DO 240 I = 1, 50
           SM = 0.
           N1 = NTERMS - 1
              DO 60 P = 1, N1
              P1 = P + 1
              DO 60 Q = P1, NTERMS
              SM = SM + ABS(AP(Q,P))
 60           CONTINUE
           IF(SM .EQ. 0.) GOTO 250
           TRESH = 0.
           IF(I .LT. 4) TRESH = 0.2 * SM / NTERMS ** 2
              DO 200 P = 1, N1
              P2 = P + 1
                 DO 200 Q = P2, NTERMS
                 G = 100. * ABS(AP(Q,P))
                 IF ((I .LE. 4) .OR. (ABS(D(P)) + G .NE. ABS(D(P))) .OR.
   1                (ABS(D(Q)) + G .NE. ABS(D(Q)))) GOTO 80
                 AP(Q,P) = 0.
                 GO TO 200
 80              IF (ABS(AP(Q,P)) .LE. TRESH) GOTO 200
                 H = D(Q) - D(P)
                 IF (ABS(H) + G .NE. ABS(H)) GOTO 110
                 T = AP(Q,P) / H
                 GOTO 120
 110             THETA = 0.5 * H / AP(Q,P)
                 T = 1. / (ABS(THETA) + SQRT(1. + THETA ** 2))
                 IF (THETA .LT. 0.) T = -T
 120             C = 1. / SQRT(1. + T ** 2)
                 S = T * C
                 TAU = S / (1. + C)
                 H = T * AP(Q,P)
                 Z(P) = Z(P) - H
                 Z(Q) = Z(Q) + H
                 D(P) = D(P) - H
                 D(Q) = D(Q) + H
                 AP(Q,P) = 0.
                 P1 = P - 1
                 IF (P1 .LT. 1) GOTO 135
                    DO 130 J = 1, P1
                    G = AP(P,J)
                    H = AP(Q,J)
                    AP(P,J) = G - S * (H + G * TAU)
                    AP(Q,J) = H + S * (G - H * TAU)
 130                CONTINUE
 135             P3 = P + 1
                 Q1 = Q - 1
                 IF (Q1 .LT. P3) GOTO 145
                    DO 140 J = P3, Q1
                    G = AP(J,P)
```

Continued next page

Table 11.5 (continued)

```
               H = AP(Q,J)
               AP(J,P) = G - S * (H + G * TAU)
               AP(Q,J) = H + S * (G - H * TAU)
140         CONTINUE
145         Q2 = Q + 1
            IF (NTERMS .LT. Q2) GOTO 200
               DO 150 J = Q2, NTERMS
               G = AP(J,P)
               H = AP(J,Q)
               AP(J,P) = G - S * (H + G * TAU)
               AP(J,Q) = H + S * (G - H * TAU)
150         CONTINUE
200      CONTINUE
            DO 240 P = 1, NTERMS
            B(P) = B(P) + Z(P)
            D(P) = B(P)
            Z(P) = 0.
240      CONTINUE
250      EMAX = 1.E-30
         EMIN = 1.E30
            DO 260 J = 1, NTERMS
            IF (EMAX .LT. D(J)) EMAX = D(J)
            IF (EMIN .GT. D(J)) EMIN = D(J)
260      CONTINUE
         EVRAT = SQRT(EMAX / EMIN)
         GOTO 280
270      EVRAT = 0.
280      RETURN
         END
```

[a] EIGEN is called by programs MODFIT and SIMUL to calculate the ratio of the largest to smallest eigenvalues (known as the condition number) of the inverse of the un-normalized curvature matrix AL.

conjunction with the experimental uncertainty expressed as the standard deviation in the y values (SIGMAY) to calculate reduced chi-square (R CHI SQUARE).

Subprogram EIGEN (Table 11.5) calculates the eigenvalues of the un-normalized array AL, from which the condition number is found.

11.2 SIMUL: A Program for Monte Carlo Simulation

Program SIMUL is used either (1) for evaluating the response (dependent variable) of a model for given parameter values and range of the independent variable, or (2) for investigating the statistical properties of a model by means of Monte Carlo methods. The parameter estimates obtained on fitting a model to data can be tested for bias, and the calculated uncertainties evaluated. A listing of SIMUL, less the subprograms which it shares in common with MODFIT, appears in Table 11.6.

SIMUL has been designed to resemble MODFIT and to use the same subprograms. The working program consists of the main program SIMUL and subprograms FIT, EIGEN, a suitable version of FUNCTN, and GGNOF (see below). The description of MODFIT in Sect. 11.1 applies equally to SIMUL. SIMUL, too, can be used with dynamic models involving differential equations.

SIMUL accepts input in exactly the same form as does MODFIT. It must be noted, however, that optimized parameter estimates should be supplied, not initial guesses. Three, or sometimes four, extra pieces of information are also required if

Text continued page 265

Table 11.6. Program SIMUL[a]

```
            PROGRAM SIMUL (INPUT, OUTPUT, TAPE5=INPUT, TAPE6=OUTPUT, TAPE1,
C           *************
       1    TAPE2)
            COMMON X(100), Y(100), YFIT(100), SIGMAY(100), WEIGHT(100),
       1    SIGMAA(15), MODE
            COMMON /P/ AL1(15), AU1(15), DEPDCY(15)
            COMMON /D/ DV(100,15), AR(15,15), AP(15,15)
            REAL ASD(15), YTEMP(100), AMSD(15), OLDA(15), CHISQ(100),
       1    A(15), CASD(15,100), SUMA(15), SUMASQ(15), AM(15),
       2    CASDM(15), CASDME(15), AA(15), BIAS(15)
            EXTERNAL FUNCTN
            DATA AHEAD/1HA/, TERMPC/1./, ITLIM/20/
            TERM = TERMPC / 100.
            IFLAG = 0
            REWIND 1
            REWIND 2
            REWIND 5
C
C                 READ MODE AND PARAMETERS
C
      10    READ(5,*) MODI
            IF (EOF(5)) 580,20
      20    IF (MODI .LT. 9) GOTO 30
            MODE = MODI - 10
            READ(5,*) NTERMS, (A(J), AL1(J), AU1(J), J = 1, NTERMS)
            IF (EOF(5)) 540,32
      30    READ(5,*) NTERMS, (A(J), J = 1, NTERMS)
            IF (EOF(5)) 540,31
      31    MODE = MODI
      32    DO 45 J = 1, NTERMS
            AA(J) = A(J)
      45    CONTINUE
C
C                 READ DATA
C
            I = 0
      50    READ(5,*) XX, YY
            IF (EOF(5)) 540,60
      60    IF (XX .EQ. 999.) GOTO 70
            I = I + 1
            X(I) = XX
            Y(I) = YY
            IF (MODE .LE. 0) GOTO 50
            READ(5,*) SIGMAY(I)
            IF (EOF(5)) 540,50
      70    CONTINUE
            NPTS = I
            NF = NPTS - NTERMS
C
C                 READ CONTROL DATA FROM UNIT 1
C
            READ(1,*) NSETS, KEY, ISEED
            IF (EOF(1)) 71,72
      71    SDEV = 0.
            NSETS = 0
      72    IF (NSETS .EQ. 1) GOTO 590
            IF (NSETS .GT. 100) GOTO 560
            IF (MODE .NE. 0 .OR. NSETS .EQ. 0) GOTO 75
            READ(1,*) SDEV
            IF (EOF(1)) 610,75
C
C                 SET WEIGHTS
```

Continued next page

[a] This program, which can be used either for evaluating a model or for Monte Carlo simulation, calls subroutines FIT, FCHISQ, FUNCTN and EIGEN, and, in the second mode of operation, GGNOF.

Table 11.6 (continued)

```
C
   75      DO 130 I = 1, NPTS
            IF (MODE) 80,110,120
   80      IF (Y(I) .EQ. 0.) GOTO 110
            DUMMY = ABS(Y(I))
            WEIGHT(I) = 1. / DUMMY
            SIGMAY(I) = SQRT(DUMMY)
            GOTO 130
  110      WEIGHT(I) = 1.
            GOTO 130
  120      WEIGHT(I) = 1. / SIGMAY(I) ** 2
  130      CONTINUE
         CALL FUNCTN (NPTS, A, NTERMS)
            DO 135 I = 1, NPTS
            YTEMP(I) = YFIT(I)
  135      CONTINUE
         IF (NSETS .EQ. 0) GOTO 230
            DO 140 J = 1, NTERMS
            BIAS(J) = 0.
            CASDM(J) = 0.
            CASDME(J) = 0.
            SUMA(J) = 0.
            SUMASQ(J) = 0.
  140      CONTINUE
         RVM = 0.
         RMSM = 0.
         RVMSD = 0.
            DO 150 I = 1, 10
            DUMMY = GGNOF (ISEED)
  150      CONTINUE
         NRUN = 1
C
C              ADD NORMALLY DISTRIBUTED RANDOM ERROR WITH MEAN OF
C              ZERO, STANDARD DEVIATION OF SDEV IF MODE = 0 OR
C              SIGMAY(I) IF MODE DOES NOT EQUAL 0
C
  165      DO 170 I = 1, NPTS
            IF (MODE .NE. 0) SDEV = SIGMAY(I)
            Y(I) = YTEMP(I) + GGNOF (ISEED) * SDEV
  170      CONTINUE
            DO 180 J = 1, NTERMS
            A(J) = AA(J)
  180      CONTINUE
         FL = .001
C
C              FITTING LOOP
C
            DO 200 K = 1, ITLIM
               DO 195 J = 1, NTERMS
               OLDA(J) = A(J)
  195         CONTINUE
         CALL FIT (A, NPTS, NTERMS, FL, CHISQR, CHISQ1,
        1 FUNCTN, IFLAG, MODI)
               DO 190 J = 1, NTERMS
               IF (ABS(OLDA(J) - A(J)) .GT. ABS(TERM * OLDA(J))) GOTO 200
  190         CONTINUE
            ITERS = K
C
C              LAST CALL TO FIT WITH FL = 0
C
         CALL FIT (A, NPTS, NTERMS, 0., CHISQR, CHISQ1,
        1 FUNCTN, IFLAG, MODI)
            GOTO 210
  200      CONTINUE
         WRITE(6,205) ITLIM, TERMPC, NRUN
  205    FORMAT(21H0SIMDES HAS COMPLETED, I3,
```

```
      1 27H ITERATIONS WITH PARAMETERS / 23H STILL CHANGING BY MORE
      2    5H THAN, F4.1, 19H% IN SIMULATION RUN, I3)
        STOP
  210 DO 220 J = 1, NTERMS
        BIAS(J) = BIAS(J) + AA(J) - A(J)
        CASD(J,NRUN) = SIGMAA(J)
        CHISQ(NRUN) = CHISQR
        SUMA(J) = SUMA(J) + A(J)
        SUMASQ(J) = SUMASQ(J) + A(J) * A(J)
  220 CONTINUE
        RVM = RVM + CHISQR
        RVMSD = RVMSD + CHISQR * CHISQR
        RMSM = RMSM + SQRT (CHISQR)
        IF (NRUN .EQ. NSETS) GOTO 230
        NRUN = NRUN + 1
        GOTO 165
C
C            END SIMULATION - OUTPUT
C
  230 WRITE(6,240) NSETS, NF, MODE
  240 FORMAT(29H1NUMBER OF SIMULATION RUNS = , I3 /
      1    22H DEGREES OF FREEDOM = , I3 /
      2    7H MODE = , I2)
        IF (MODE .EQ. 0 .AND. NSETS .NE. 0) WRITE(6,250) SDEV
  250 FORMAT(44H CONSTANT EXPERIMENTAL STANDARD DEVIATION = , G12.5)
        WRITE(6,260) (AHEAD, J, J = 1, NTERMS)
  260 FORMAT(11H0PARAMETERS, 8X, 9(A1, I2, 9X) / (19X, 6(A1, I2, 9X)))
        WRITE(6,270) (AA(J), J = 1, NTERMS)
  270 FORMAT(13X, 9G12.5 / 6G12.5)
        WRITE(6,280)
  280 FORMAT(1H0, 12X, 1HX, 9X, 4HYFIT)
        IF (MODE .NE. 0) WRITE(6,290)
  290 FORMAT(1H+, 33X, 6HSIGMAY)
        DO 320 I = 1, NPTS
        WRITE(6,300) X(I), YTEMP(I)
  300 FORMAT(7X, 2G12.5)
        IF (MODE .NE. 0) WRITE(6,310) SIGMAY(I)
  310 FORMAT(1H+, 30X, G12.5)
  320 CONTINUE
        IF (NSETS .EQ. 0) GOTO 10
        ANSETS = NSETS
        SQRTN = SQRT (ANSETS)
        DO 330 J = 1, NTERMS
        AM(J) = SUMA(J) / ANSETS
        ASD(J) = SQRT ((SUMASQ(J) - SUMA(J) * SUMA(J) / ANSETS) /
      1              (ANSETS - 1.))
        AMSD(J) = ASD(J) / SQRTN
        BIAS(J) = BIAS(J) / ANSETS
  330 CONTINUE
        IF (KEY .NE. 1) GOTO 410
        IF (MODE) 360,340,360
  340 WRITE(6,350)
  350 FORMAT(13H0RES VARIANCE)
        GOTO 380
  360 WRITE(6,370)
  370 FORMAT(13H0R CHI SQUARE)
  380 WRITE(6,390)
  390 FORMAT(1H+, 15X, 30HCALCULATED STANDARD DEVIATIONS)
        DO 405 K = 1, NSETS
        WRITE(6,400) CHISQ(K), (CASD(J,K), J = 1, NTERMS)
  400 FORMAT(1X, 10G12.5 / 6G12.5)
  405 CONTINUE
  410 WRITE(6,420) (AM(J), J = 1, NTERMS)
  420 FORMAT(35H0MEAN VALUES OF PARAMETER ESTIMATES / 13X, 9G12.5 /
      1    13X, 6G12.5)
        WRITE(6,430) (AMSD(J), J = 1, NTERMS)
  430 FORMAT(13H STD DEVS    , 9G12.5 / 13X, 6G12.5)
        WRITE(6,432) (BIAS(J), J = 1, NTERMS)
```

Continued next page

Table 11.6 (continued)

```
    432   FORMAT(13H0MEAN BIAS      , 9G12.5 / 13X, 6G12.5)
          WRITE(6,435) (ASD(J), J = 1, NTERMS)
    435   FORMAT(43H0STANDARD DEVIATIONS OF PARAMETER ESTIMATES /
         1   13X, 9G12.5 / 13X, 6G12.5)
C
C                     CALCULATE VARIOUS STATISTICS
C
          DO 440 K = 1, NSETS
            DO 440 J = 1, NTERMS
            CASDM(J) = CASDM(J) + CASD(J,K)
            CASDME(J) = CASDME(J) + CASD(J,K) * CASD(J,K)
    440   CONTINUE
          RVMSD = SQRT ((RVMSD - RVM * RVM / ANSETS) / (ANSETS - 1.)) /
         1          SQRTN
          RMSM = RMSM / ANSETS
          RVM = RVM / ANSETS
          DO 450 J = 1, NTERMS
          CASDME(J) = SQRT((CASDME(J) - CASDM(J) * CASDM(J) / ANSETS) /
         1            (ANSETS - 1.)) / SQRTN
          CASDM(J) = CASDM(J) / ANSETS
    450   CONTINUE
          WRITE(6,460) (CASDM(J), J = 1, NTERMS)
    460   FORMAT(46H0MEAN VALUES OF CALCULATED STANDARD DEVIATIONS /
         1   13X, 9G12.5 / 13X, G12.5)
          WRITE(6,470) (CASDME(J), J = 1, NTERMS)
    470   FORMAT(13H STD DEVS     , 9G12.5 / 13X, 6G12.5)
          WRITE(6,472) (DEPDCY(J), J = 1, NTERMS)
    472   FORMAT(13H0DEPENDENCIES, 9G12.5 / 13X, 6G12.5)
          CALL EIGEN (NTERMS, EVRAT)
          WRITE(6,473) EVRAT
    473   FORMAT(17H0CONDITION NUMBER, F10.1)
          WRITE(6,474)
    474   FORMAT(25H0CORRELATION COEFFICIENTS)
          DO 475 J = 1, NTERMS
            DO 475 K = 1, J
            AR(J,K) = AR(J,K) / SQRT(AP(J,J) * AP(K,K))
    475   CONTINUE
          DO 478 J = 1, NTERMS
            DO 476 K = 1, J
            AP(J,K) = AR(J,K) / SQRT(AR(J,J) * AR(K,K))
    476     CONTINUE
          WRITE(6,477) AHEAD, J, (AP(J,L), L = 1, J)
    477     FORMAT(10X, A1, I2, 9G12.5 / 13X, 6G12.5)
    478   CONTINUE
          IF (MODE) 500,480,500
    480   WRITE(6,490) RVM
    490   FORMAT(19H0MEAN RES VARIANCE , G12.5)
          GOTO 520
    500   WRITE(6,510) RVM
    510   FORMAT(19H0MEAN R CHI SQUARE , G12.5)
    520   WRITE(6,530) RVMSD, RMSM
    530   FORMAT(8H STD DEV, 11X, G12.5 / 19H MEAN ROOT MEAN SQR, G12.5)
          GOTO 10
    540   WRITE(6,550)
    550   FORMAT(36H0*** ERROR *** PREMATURE END OF DATA)
          STOP
    560   WRITE(6,570)
    570   FORMAT(38H0*** ERROR *** TOO MANY RUNS REQUESTED)
    580   STOP
    590   WRITE(6,600)
    600   FORMAT(43H0*** ERROR *** MUST REQUEST MORE THAN 1 RUN)
          STOP
    610   WRITE(6,620)
    620   FORMAT(46H0*** ERROR *** PREMATURE END OF DATA ON UNIT 1)
          STOP
          END
```

Monte Carlo simulations, option (2), are to be performed. These are provided on input file 1, referred to as UNIT 1. The first is NSETS, the number of simulations required, up to a maximum of 100. Alternatively, if NSETS is 0 or if there is no input on UNIT 1, SIMUL merely calculates the values of the response variable [option (1)] and then stops. Next is KEY. If KEY is 1, each simulation run produces printed values of the residual variance or reduced chi-square, and the calculated uncertainties in the parameters. The third value is ISEED, an integer greater than 1 which initiates the pseudo-random number generator used to provide simulated standard deviations. The ability to set ISEED allows a simulation to be repeated with an identical selection of pseudo-random deviates. If MODE is 0 or 10 a fourth value must be supplied, SDEV, the standard deviation in each simulated experimental measurement. Otherwise, the standard deviation of the simulated y value is taken from the corresponding value of SIGMAY supplied with the data.

SIMUL reads the input and assigns weights as does MODFIT. The experimental y values are not used but some values, if necessary dummy ones, must be supplied to complete the input format. All that is required are optimized parameter estimates and a particular set of x values. These, together with the equation of the model (described by subprogram FUNCTN) completely define the experimental frame and model.

The statements following label 130 generate fitted y values; these are retained in array YTEMP. Statements labelled 165 to 170 generate the first set of simulated y values in array Y by adding deviates supplied by subprogram GGNOF. A listing of GGNOF is not supplied because of copyright restrictions. This subprogram is available in the International Mathematical and Statistical Library which is supplied at most computing centres. It returns a single pseudo-random deviate from a normal distribution with a mean of 0 and a standard deviation of 1. Subroutine GGNOF or its equivalent will have to be obtained elsewhere. Alternatively, Davies (1971, pp. 396–400) provides short FORTRAN subprograms suitable as replacements for GGNOF.

For each cycle through the loop ending at label 200, least squares fitting is done as in MODFIT. A new set of simulated data is then generated and the fitting is repeated, until the required number of data sets have been processed.

Results are printed beginning at statement labelled 230 (see Table 3.2). The input is reproduced and, if KEY is 1, the sets of calculated parameter uncertainties follow. Then come the mean parameter estimates, the standard deviations in these means and the mean bias values. Ideally, the latter should be small in comparison with the standard deviation in the parameter estimates.

Next are printed the standard deviations of the parameter estimates for direct comparison with the means of the calculated values for which standard deviations are included as a measure of precision.

If MODE is 0 or 10, *approximate* values of the dependencies, condition number and correlation coefficients are printed. In order to save time and space, these are calculated once at the end of the simulation runs using the results of the last simulation. If MODE is other than 0 or 10, however, they are correct. Finally, the mean residual variance or reduced chi-square is shown, together with its standard deviation. Also printed is the mean of the root mean squares for comparison with the constant experimental standard deviation, SDEV, if used, as evidence that the random deviates had yielded the requested residuals.

Note that if MODE is neither 0 or 10, and KEY was set to 1, the printed values of the calculated standard deviations in the parameter estimates will all be equal. This is because they do not, in this case, depend on the particular experimental y values but only on the model and the parameter and x values supplied. Also in this case, because the program constructs data to correspond accurately with the model supplied, the value of mean reduced chi-square will always be close to 1, the value expected if the model provides a good description of the data. Examples of the use of SIMUL will be found in Sects. 3.7.1.1 and 6.2.2.2.

11.3 FUNCTN Subprogram RESERVR: Exponential Decay

Subprogram RESERVR (Table 11.7) is capable of fitting to data a sum of up to seven exponential decay terms as defined by Eq. (2.6). It is, for example, suitable for describing the decrease in specific radioactivity in a reservoir compartment after injection of tracer. Illustrations of its use will be found in Sects. 3.7.1, 5.1.1 and 5.2.2.1. The number of exponential terms summed is equal to NTERMS/2. The multiplier parameters are odd-numbered values of array A and the exponential ones are even-valued.

Table 11.7. FUNCTN subprogram RESERVR[a]

```
      SUBROUTINE FUNCTN (NPTS, A, NTERMS)
C
C         *** RESERVR ***
C
      COMMON X(100), Y(100), YFIT(100), SIGMAY(100), WEIGHT(100),
     1 SIGMAA(15), MODE
      REAL A(15)
        DO 2 I = 1, NPTS
        SUM = 0.
          DO 1 J = 1, NTERMS, 2
          SUM = SUM + A(J) * EXP(-A(J+1) * X(I))
    1     CONTINUE
        YFIT(I) = SUM
    2   CONTINUE
      RETURN
      END
```

[a] For describing the disappearance of a substance from a reservoir compartment according to the sum of a number of exponential decay terms with the form of Eq. (2.7).

11.4 FUNCTN Subprogram EXPCUBE: Growth of Organisms

Subprogram EXPCUBE (Table 11.8, see next page), embodying the analytical model of Eq. (3.7), is suitable for describing the patterns of growth of a surprisingly wide range of organisms. It has been applied in Sect. 3.7.2 to measurements of the increase in weight with age of African elephants, where details of the parameters are given. A slightly more general version of this sigmoidal or logistic model, given by FUNCTN subprogram RIAH (Sect. 11.15), is described in Sect. 6.2.2.1 in connection with the empirical modelling of competitive protein-binding assays.

Table 11.8. FUNCTN subprogram EXPCUBE[a]

```
      SUBROUTINE FUNCTN (NPTS, A, NTERMS)
C
C               *** EXPCUBE ***
C
      COMMON X(100), Y(100), YFIT(100), SIGMAY(100), WEIGHT(100),
     1 SIGMAA(15), MODE
      REAL A(15)
        DO 20 I = 1, NPTS
        YFIT(I) = A(1) * (1. - EXP(-A(2) * (X(I) - A(3)))) ** 3
  20    CONTINUE
      RETURN
      END
```

[a] For fitting the model of Eq. (3.7) to data on the growth of organisms.

11.5 FUNCTN Subprogram POLYNOM: General Polynomial

This subprogram (Table 11.9) may be used for fitting any model consisting of a sum of terms in x raised to successive interger powers. The form of the model is determined by the value of NTERMS. For example, when NTERMS is 2 the model is a straight line; parameter A1 is the intercept and A2 is the gradient. When MODE is 1 and standard deviations in each value of the response or dependent variable y are included, a weighted least squares fit to a straight line is obtained, If NTERMS is 3, the model is a quadratic (parameter A3 is then the term in x^2) and the coefficient in x is retained as well. A1 is always the value of the constant. Polynomials of the nth degree are obtained by setting the value of NTERMS to $(n+1)$. Notice how the polynomial model is formed by means of the inner loop ending at statement labelled 10.

A special case occurs if NTERMS equals 1. The program then searches for a single constant fitting the data which is, of course, the mean. In this case the x variable has no meaning and any dummy values may be given. A weighted mean is obtained by setting MODE to 1 and supplying standard deviations with the data.

Table 11.9. FUNCTN subprogram POLYNOM[a]

```
      SUBROUTINE FUNCTN (NPTS, A, NTERMS)
C
C               *** POLYNOM ***
C
      COMMON X(100), Y(100), YFIT(100), SIGMAY(100), WEIGHT(100),
     1 SIGMAA(15), MODE
      REAL A(15)
        DO 20 I = 1, NPTS
        SUM = 0.
        IF (NTERMS .EQ. 1) GO TO 15
        PROD = 1.
          DO 10 J = 2, NTERMS
          PROD = PROD * X(I)
          SUM = SUM + A(J) * PROD
  10      CONTINUE
  15    YFIT(I) = A(1) + SUM
  20    CONTINUE
      RETURN
      END
```

[a] For fitting to data a polynomial up to, and including, any integer power of $x \leqslant 14$ [Eq. (2.6)].

11.6 FUNCTN Subprogram FOLL: Growth of Ovarian Follicles

This subprogram (Table 11.10) embodies the theoretical mathematical model of Eq. (3.9) corresponding to the physical model of an ovarian follicle shown in Fig. 3.6. The single parameter A1 represents a constant wall thickness (Sect. 3.7.3).

Table 11.10. FUNCTN subprogram FOLL[a]

```
      SUBROUTINE FUNCTN (NPTS, A, NTERMS)
C
C              *** FOLL ***
C
      COMMON X(100), Y(100), YFIT(100), SIGMAY(100), WEIGHT(100),
     1 SIGMAA(15), MODE
      REAL A(15)
        DO 20 I = 1, NPTS
        D = X(I)
        YFIT(I) = .52359 * (D ** 3 - (D - 2. * A(1)) ** 3)
   20   CONTINUE
      RETURN
      END
```

[a] For fitting the analytical model of Eq. (3.9) to measurements of the mass of ovarian follicular wall tissue as a function of diameter.

11.7 DESIGN: A Program for Efficient Experimental Design

DESIGN (Table 11.11) is a program for implementing the methods of sequential experimental design described in Chap. 4. It may be used for designing experiments to differentiate efficiently between contending models or, when a particular model has been chosen, to define experiments most likely to improve the precision of the parameter estimates. Alternatively, an automatic transition can be made from one mode to the other, in order to achieve a compromise. DESIGN is similar to MODFIT and SIMUL in that it is capable of fitting models linear or non-linear in their parameters to data, and it makes use of the same subprograms.

DESIGN is run each time a new experimental point or "experiment" becomes available. Instructions to the program are supplied on UNIT 1 in the form of answers to prompts. The initial priming data is provided on UNIT 5, and output appears on UNIT 6. After each run the current data are written to UNIT 16 and should be retained as a file in the computer until the results of the next experiment become available. DESIGN is written in standard FORTRAN with the exceptions already noted for MODFIT and SIMUL. In particular, if the program is to be run on a machine other than one manufactured by the Control Data Corporation it will be necessary only to change the program header statement, the free format input and output statements, and the statements which detect the end of file condition.

DESIGN calls subprograms FIT, FCHISQ, SERDES and TCALC. It also needs between two and five FUNCTN subprograms to define the required models. These must be renamed FUNC1 to FUNC5. In general terms, the program reads data from initial experiments, fits up to five different models, and determines the two most likely ones, on the basis of both the residual variance and the number of

Text continued page 275

Table 11.11. Program DESIGN[a]

```
      PROGRAM DESIGN (INPUT, OUTPUT, TAPE5 = /80, TAPE6 = OUTPUT,
C     **************
     1 TAPE16 = /500, TAPE1 = /80, TAPE2)
      EXTERNAL FUNC1, FUNC2, FUNC3, FUNC4, FUNC5
      COMMON X(100), Y(100), YFIT(100), SIGMAY(100), WEIGHT(100),
     1   SIGMAA(15), MODE
      COMMON /T/ T(5,100), TMAX(5), INDTMX(5), SDMOD(5), VARMOD(5),
     1   L(5), YF(5,100), ALMAX, INDLMX, D0MAX, IND0MX, YFSIG(100),
     2   EMAX, INDEMX, W1, W2, CMAX, INDCMX, MODELS, NFITS, XF(100)
      COMMON /P/ AL1(15), AU1(15), DEPDCY(15)
      COMMON /D/ DV(100,15), AR(15,15), AP(15,15)
      REAL L, LAMDA, ALX(15,5), AUX(15,5)
      DIMENSION A(15,5), AA(15), NTERMS(5), PCENTS(15),
     1   XTEMP(100), ITERS(5), FLAM(5),
     2   MODD(5), SIGMA(15,5), MODI(5), VAR(5), DEP(15,5)
      DATA MODDLE / 5HMODEL /
      TERMPC = 1.
      ITLIM = 200
      NFITS = 100
      LAMDA = .2
      TERM = TERMPC / 100.
      WRITE(6,10)
   10 FORMAT(23H TYPE 5 FOR 1ST ENTRY, / 23H      16 FOR RE-ENTRY... )
      READ(1,*) N
      REWIND N
      REWIND 2
      IF (N .EQ. 5) GO TO 20
      READ(16,*) MODELS, NSTART
      GO TO 35
   20 WRITE(6,30)
   30 FORMAT(37H+TYPE IN NUMBER OF MODELS, UP TO 5... )
      READ(1,*) MODELS
C
C           READ INITIAL PARAMETERS AND DATA POINTS
C
   35 DO 40 I = 1, MODELS
      READ(N,*) MODI(I)
      IF (MODI(I) .LT. 9) GO TO 32
      MODD(I) = MODI(I) - 9
      READ(N,*) NT, (A(J,I), ALX(J,I), AUX(J,I), J = 1, NT)
      GO TO 39
   32 MODD(I) = MODI(I)
      READ(N,*) NT, (A(J,I), J = 1, NT)
   39 NTERMS(I) = NT
   40 CONTINUE
      IF (N .EQ. 16) GO TO 75
      K = MODELS - 1
      DO 70 I = 1, K
      J = I + 1
      DO 70 LL = J, MODELS
      IF (MODD(I) .EQ. MODD(LL)) GO TO 70
      WRITE(6,60)
   60 FORMAT(50H0*** ERROR *** MODES MUST BE THE SAME FOR ALL MODE
     1   ,2HLS)
      STOP
   70 CONTINUE
   75 MODE = MODD(1)
      MDI = MODI(1)
C
C           INPUT EXPERIMENTAL POINTS
C
```

Continued next page

[a] A program for designing sequential experiments so as to differentiate between models, or estimate parameters efficiently. It calls subprograms FIT, FCHISQ, TCALC, SERDES, and between two and five FUNCTN subprograms.

Table 11.11 (continued)

```
      100   DO 140 I = 1, 101
            I1 = I
            READ(N,*) XX, YY
            IF (EOF(N)) 110,130
      110   WRITE(6,120)
      120   FORMAT(41H0*** ERROR *** END-OF-DATA MARKER MISSING)
            STOP
      130   IF (XX .EQ. 999.) GO TO 160
            X(I) = XX
            Y(I) = YY
            IF (MODE .LE. 0) GO TO 140
            READ(N,*) SIGMAY(I)
      140   CONTINUE
            WRITE(6,150)
      150   FORMAT(48H0*** ERROR *** TOO MANY DATA POINTS. MAXIMUM 100)
            STOP
      160   NPTS = I1 - 1
            IF (N .EQ. 16) GO TO 162
            NSTART = NPTS
            IF (NSTART .LE. NFITS) GO TO 180
            WRITE(6,161)
      161   FORMAT(42H0*** ERROR *** MORE THAN NFITS DATA POINTS)
            STOP
      162   IF (NPTS .LE. 100) GO TO 165
            WRITE(6,163)
      163   FORMAT(47H0*** ERROR *** NEW DATA POINT CANNOT BE ENTERED /
         1    14X, 48H YOU ALREADY HAVE MAXIMUM NUMBER ALLOWABLE (100) )
            STOP
      165   WRITE(6,170)
      170   FORMAT(43H TYPE IN NEW EXPERIMENTAL X AND Y VALUES...)
            NPTS = NPTS + 1
      172   READ(1,*) X(NPTS), Y(NPTS)
            IF (MODE .NE. 1) GO TO 174
            WRITE(6,173)
      173   FORMAT(52H TYPE IN SD AT NEW POINT - IF UNKNOWN ENTER ZERO... )
            READ(1,*) SIGMAY(NPTS)
      174   IF (X(NPTS) .GE. X(1) .AND. X(NPTS) .LE. X(NSTART)) GO TO 178
            WRITE(6,175) X(1), X(NSTART)
      175   FORMAT(32H NEW X OUTSIDE INITIAL X-RANGE :, G12.4, 1H-, G12.4 /
         1    13H TYPE 1 IF OK/
         2    27H           2 TO REREAD NEW POINT/
         3    18H           3 TO STOP...)
            READ(1,*) IFLAG
            IF (IFLAG - 2) 178,172,177
      177   STOP
C
C
C                 ESTIMATE SD AT NEW X IF ENTERED ABOVE AS ZERO, AND IF MODE
C                 = 1, ALLOWING NEW X TO BE WITHIN OR OUTSIDE INITIAL X-RANGE
C
      178   IF (MODE .EQ. 0) GOTO 180
            IF (SIGMAY(NPTS) .NE. 0.) GO TO 180
            DO 179 J = 2, NSTART
            IF (X(NPTS) .GT. X(J) .AND. J .LT. NSTART) GO TO 179
            SIGMAY(NPTS) = SIGMAY(J) - (X(J) - X(NPTS)) / (X(J) - X(J - 1))
         1    * (SIGMAY(J) - SIGMAY(J - 1))
            GO TO 180
      179   CONTINUE
C
C                 SET WEIGHTS
C
      180   DO 192 I = 1, NPTS
            IF (MODE) 182, 188, 190
      182   IF (Y(I) .EQ. 0.) GO TO 188
            DUMMY = ABS(Y(I))
            WEIGHT(I) = 1. / DUMMY
            SIGMAY(I) = SQRT(DUMMY)
            GO TO 192
```

DESIGN: A Program for Efficient Experimental Design

```
      188     WEIGHT(I) = 1.
              GO TO 192
      190     WEIGHT(I) = 1. / SIGMAY(I) ** 2
      192     CONTINUE
C
C                   IF RE-ENTRY READ XF, AND YFSIG IF MODE NE 0, FROM UNIT 16
C
              IF (N .EQ. 5) GO TO 199
              READ(16,*) (XF(I), I = 1, NFITS)
              IF (MODE .EQ. 0) GO TO 270
              READ(16,*) (YFSIG(I), I= 1, NFITS)
              GO TO 270
C
C                   ON INITIAL ENTRY ONLY SET UP XF, AND ALSO YFSIG IF MODE
C                   NE 0, DIVIDING RANGES BETWEN EXPERIMENTAL POINTS SO AS TO
C                   ALLOW FOR FUNNY INCREMENTS
C
      199     DIV = FLOAT (NFITS) / FLOAT (NPTS - 1)
              XF(1) = X(1)
              IF (MODE .NE. 0) YFSIG(1) = SIGMAY(1)
              N = 2
              K = NPTS - 1
                DO 210 J = 1, K
                Z = FLOAT (J) * DIV
                NDIV = Z
                IF (FLOAT (NDIV) .LT. Z) NDIV = NDIV + 1
                XINT = (X(J + 1) - X(J)) / FLOAT (NDIV - N + 1)
                IF (MODE .NE. 0) SDINT = (SIGMAY(J + 1) - SIGMAY(J)) /
     1                                   FLOAT(NDIV - N + 1)
                  DO 200 I = N, NDIV
                  XF(I) = XF(I - 1) + XINT
                  IF (MODE .NE. 0) YFSIG(I) = YFSIG(I - 1) + SDINT
      200       CONTINUE
                N = NDIV + 1
      210     CONTINUE
C
C                   NOW FIT EACH MODEL IN TURN, ITERATING THROUGH FIT
C
      270   I = 1
      280   IFLAG = 0
              NT = NTERMS(I)
                DO 285 J = 1, NT
                IF (MDI .EQ. MODE) GO TO 283
                AL1(J) = ALX(J,I)
                AU1(J) = AUX(J,I)
      283       AA(J) = A(J,I)
      285     CONTINUE
              FL = .001
              IFL = 1
      287   J = 1
      288     DO 290 JJ = 1, NT
              PCENTS(JJ) = AA(JJ)
      290   CONTINUE
C
C                   CHANGING PARAMETERS FOR CURRENT MODEL IN AA, PREVIOUS
C                   VALUES FROM LAST FITTING RUN IN PCENTS
C
      295   GO TO (300, 310, 320, 330, 340) I
C
C                   THIS SECTION TO FIT EACH MODEL IS USED 4 TIMES,
C                   FIRSTLY IN THE ITERATION LOOP, SECONDLY FOR THE FINAL FIT
C                   SETTING FL = 0, THIRDLY WHEN CALCULATING THE FITTED
C                   VALUES OF Y AT THE NFITS X-POINTS AND DERIVATIVES NEEDED
C                   BY TCALC, LASTLY WHEN CALCULATING YFITS FOR BEST MODEL.
C                   IFL IS THE FLAG POINTING TO THE NEXT STATEMENT.
C
      300 CALL FIT (AA, NPTS, NTERMS(1), FL, VAR(1), DUMMY,
```

Continued next page

Table 11.11 (continued)

```
        1  FUNC1, IFLAG, MDI)
           GO TO 350
      310 CALL FIT (AA, NPTS, NTERMS(2), FL, VAR(2), DUMMY,
        1  FUNC2, IFLAG, MDI)
           GO TO 350
      320 CALL FIT (AA, NPTS, NTERMS(3), FL, VAR(3), DUMMY,
        1  FUNC3, IFLAG, MDI)
           GO TO 350
      330 CALL FIT (AA, NPTS, NTERMS(4), FL, VAR(4), DUMMY,
        1  FUNC4, IFLAG, MDI)
           GO TO 350
      340 CALL FIT (AA, NPTS, NTERMS(5), FL, VAR(5), DUMMY,
        1  FUNC5, IFLAG, MDI)
      350 GO TO (355, 370, 410, 475) IFL
      355    DO 360 JJ = 1, NT
             IF (ABS (PCENTS(JJ) - AA(JJ)) .GT. ABS (TERM * PCENTS(JJ)))
        1      GO TO 362
C
C                TEST EACH PARAMETER FOR HAVING CHANGED BY LESS THAN
C                TERM DURING LAST ITERATION
C
      360    CONTINUE
             GO TO 366
      362 J = J + 1
           IF (J .LE. ITLIM) GO TO 288
           WRITE(6,364) ITLIM, I, TERMPC
      364 FORMAT(/23H PROGRAM HAS COMPLETED ,I3, 22H ITERATIONS USING MODE
        1   , 2HL ,I1/47H WITH PARAMETER(S) STILL CHANGING BY MORE THAN ,
        2    F4.1,1H%/49H TYPE IN 1 TO CONTINUE, 2 TO EXIT AT THIS POINT..
        3   , 1H.)
           READ(1,*) NN
           IF (NN .EQ. 2) STOP 4
           GO TO 287
C
C                COME HERE AFTER SATISFACTORY FITTING OF I-TH MODEL
C
      366 ITERS(I) = J
           IFL = 2
           FLAM(I) = FL
           FL = 0.
           GO TO 295
C
C                LAST CALL TO FIT WITH FL SET EQUAL 0
C
      370 VARMOD(I) = VAR(I)
           IF (MODE .EQ. 0) GO TO 375
C
C                IF MODE NE 0 VAR IS REDUCED CHI SQUARE, NOT RESIDUAL
C                VARIANCE. MUST RECALCULATE RESIDUAL VARIANCE FOR SERDES.
C
           DUMMY = 0.
             DO 372 JJ = 1, NPTS
             DUMMY = DUMMY + (Y(JJ) - YFIT(JJ)) ** 2
      372    CONTINUE
           VARMOD(I) = DUMMY / FLOAT(NPTS - NTERMS(I))
      375    DO 380 JJ = 1, NT
             A(JJ,I) = AA(JJ)
             SIGMA(JJ,I) = SIGMAA(JJ)
             DEP(JJ,I) = DEPDCY(JJ)
      380    CONTINUE
             DO 383 JJ = 1, NPTS
             XTEMP(JJ) = X(JJ)
      383    CONTINUE
             DO 386 JJ = 1, NFITS
             X(JJ) = XF(JJ)
      386    CONTINUE
           IFL = 3
```

```
            IFLAG = 1
            NPTS1 = NPTS
            NPTS = NFITS
            GO TO 295
C
C               CALL TO FIT TO CALCULATE FITTED Y S FOR NFITS X-VALUES
C               AND DERIVATIVES FOR ENTRY TO TCALC
C
  410       DO 420 JJ = 1, NFITS
            YF(I,JJ) = YFIT(JJ)
  420       CONTINUE
            NPTS = NPTS1
  430       DO 440 JJ = 1, NPTS
            X(JJ) = XTEMP(JJ)
  440       CONTINUE
            CALL TCALC (NTERMS(I), I)
            IF (I .EQ. MODELS) GO TO 450
            I = I + 1
            GO TO 280
C
C               FIND X POSITION WITH MAXIMUM VALUE OF C
C
  450   CALL SERDES (NPTS, 1, LAMDA, MODEL2)
            RMU = L(INDLMX) / L(MODEL2)
            ALOGRM = ALOG (RMU)
            CMU = RMU * 100. / (1. + RMU)
C
C               WRITE RESULTS
C
            WRITE(6,460) NPTS
  460       FORMAT(/ 17H EXPERIMENTS 1 - , I2 / 19H ***************** )
C
C               WRITE PARAMETERS AND DEPENDENCIES FOR EACH MODEL
C
            IFL = 4
            DO 510 I = 1, MODELS
            NT = NTERMS(I)
              DO 470 J = 1, NT
              AA(J) = A(J,I)
              PCENTS(J) = SIGMA(J,I) * 100. / AA(J)
  470         CONTINUE
            IF (I .NE. INDLMX) GO TO 475
            FL = 0.
            GO TO 295
  475       NF = NPTS - NT
            IF (MODE .EQ. 0) WRITE(6,480) I, I
            IF (MODE .NE. 0) WRITE(6,485) I, I
  480       FORMAT(/ 11H RESID VAR , I1, 4X, 21HPARAMETERS FOR MODEL , I1)
  485       FORMAT(/ 10H R CHI SQ , I1, 5X, 21HPARAMETERS FOR MODEL , I1)
            WRITE(6,488) VAR(I), (AA(J), J = 1, NT)
  488       FORMAT(1X, 10G12.5 / 13X, 6G12.5)
            WRITE(6,490) (SIGMA(J,I), J=1,NT)
  490       FORMAT(13H STD. DEVS. =, 9G12.5 / 13X, 6G12.5)
            WRITE(6,500) (PCENTS(J), J=1,NT)
  500       FORMAT(11X, 9(F11.1, 1H%) / 11X, 6(F11.1, 1H%))
            WRITE(6,505) (DEP(J,I), J = 1, NT)
  505       FORMAT(13H DEPENDENCIES, 9G12.5 / 13X, 6G12.5)
            WRITE(6,506) FLAM(I), NF, ITERS(I)
  506       FORMAT(15H FINAL LAMBDA =, F14.10, 23H  DEGREES OF FREEDOM = ,
     1          I2, 14H  ITERATIONS =, I3)
  510       CONTINUE
C
C               WRITE INFORMATION ON CURRENT BEST MODEL
C
            WRITE(6,511) INDLMX, MODEL2
  511       FORMAT(/42H FIT DETAILS FOR CURRENT BEST MODEL: MODEL, I2,
     A          20H (NEXT BEST IS MODEL, I2, 1H),
```

Table 11.11 (continued)

```
      1    / 8X, 1HX, 11X, 1HY, 9X, 4HYFIT, 6X, 8HRESIDUAL, 3X,
      2    10HZ-RESIDUAL)
           IF (MODE .NE. 0) WRITE(6,512)
  512     FORMAT(1H+, 63X, 6HSIGMAY)
           IF (MODE .EQ. 0) SD = SQRT(VARMOD(INDLMX))
           DO 515 I = 1, NPTS
             RESID = Y(I) - YFIT(I)
             IF (MODE .NE. 0) SD = SIGMAY(I)
             ZRES = RESID / SD
             WRITE(6,513) X(I), Y(I), YFIT(I), RESID, ZRES
  513       FORMAT(1X, 5G12.5)
             IF (MODE .NE. 0) WRITE(6,514) SIGMAY(I)
  514       FORMAT(1H+, 60X, G12.5)
  515     CONTINUE
C
C                 WRITE DESIGN RESULTS
C
           WRITE(6,525) (MODDLE, K, K = 1, MODELS)
  525     FORMAT(/ 16H LIKELIHOODS:       ,5(A6, I1, 5X))
           WRITE(6,526) (L(K), K = 1, MODELS)
  526     FORMAT(15X, 5(F8.6, 4X))
           I = INDLMX
           J = MODEL2
           WRITE(6,530) I, J, RMU, I, J, ALOGRM, I, CMU, I, TMAX(I),
      1    XF(INDTMX(I)), J, TMAX(J), XF(INDTMX(J)), D0MAX, XF(IND0MX),
      2    EMAX, XF(INDEMX), W1, W2, CMAX, XF(INDCMX)
  530     FORMAT(/ 3H L(, I1,   4H)/L(, I1, 1H),  T24, 2H= , G12.4/
      3    6H LN(L(, I1, 4H)/L(, I1, 2H)),  T24, 2H= , G12.4/
      4    21H CONFIDENCE IN MODEL , I1, 2H =, T27, F6.1, 1H% ,
      4    18X, 28HPERFORM NEXT EXPERIMENT AT X /
      5    14H T(MAX) MODEL , I1, 2H =, T20, G12.4, 8H  AT X =, T41,G12.4,
      5    27H VALUE INDICATED BELOW FOR: /
      6    14H T(MAX) MODEL , I1, 2H =, T20, G12.4, 8H   AT X =, T41,G12.4/
      7    8H D0(MAX), 8X, 1H=,   T20, G12.4, 8H   AT X =, T41, G12.4,
      7    24H -- MODEL DISCRIMINATION /
      8    7H E(MAX), 9X, 1H=,    T20, G12.4, 8H   AT X =, T41, G12.4,
      8    24H -- PARAMETER ESTIMATION /
      9    5H W1 =, F6.4, 6H  W2 =, F6.4 /
      A    7H C(MAX), 9X, 1H=, T20, G12.4, 8H   AT X = , T41, G12.4,
      B    24H -- COMBINED REQUIREMENT)
C
C                 WRITE CURRENT DATA TO UNIT 16
C
           REWIND 16
           WRITE(16,*) MODELS,NSTART
           DO 550 I = 1, MODELS
             NT = NTERMS(I)
             WRITE(16,*) MODI(I), NTERMS(I)
             IF (MODI(I) .LE. 1) GO TO 540
             WRITE(16,*) (A(J,I), ALX(J,I), AUX(J,I), J = 1, NT)
             GO TO 550
  540       WRITE(16,*) (A(J,I), J=1, NT)
  550     CONTINUE
           DO 560 I = 1, NPTS
             WRITE(16,*) X(I), Y(I)
             IF (MODE .EQ. 1) WRITE(16,*) SIGMAY(I)
  560     CONTINUE
           WRITE(16,*) XX, YY
           WRITE(16,*) (XF(I), I = 1, NFITS)
           IF (MODE .NE. 0) WRITE(16,*) (YFSIG(I), I = 1, NFITS)
           STOP
           END
```

DESIGN: A Program for Efficient Experimental Design

experimental points. It then compares the responses of these two models as functions of the *x* varaible to find the value of *x* at which they diverge maximally, and recommends that the next experiment be done at that point. The complementary processes of analysis and experiment are repeated until probabilities or precisons of the desired magnitude are obtained.

The program begins by inquiring whether an initial or subsequent run is to be made. It then requests the number of models. The FUNCTN subprograms describing the required models will have already been loaded. The initial data is provided in the same format as for MODFIT or SIMUL except that values of MODE, NTERMS and initial parameter estimates are given for each model, in the correct order. On subsequent runs the program reads the previous data from UNIT 16 and requests the new experimental result. If MODE is 1, an estimate of the sample standard deviation of the mean response at that point is also required. The new point is normally expected to lie within the original experimental frame, but it need not. Weights are set and the range of the independent variable is divided into steps by the algorithm in statements labelled 199 to 210. Each model is fitted, using penalty functions if required, following the same procedure as MODFIT. An extra call is made to FIT to calculate the derivatives of the model with respect to each parameter (sensitivity coefficients) and then subprogram TCALC is entered.

TCALC (Table 11.12) calculates values of T as defined by Eq. (4.1), which are measures of the total uncertainty in the parameters of a model as a function of the

Table 11.12. Subprogram TCALC[a]

```
      SUBROUTINE TCALC (NTERMS, MODEL)
C     ****************
C
C           THIS ROUTINE FINDS T VALUES FOR UP TO 5 MODELS, 1 FOR EACH
C           CALL. THE CALCULATION IS DONE FOR NFITS X VALUES.
C
      COMMON X(100), Y(100), YFIT(100), SIGMAY(100), WEIGHT(100),
     1 SIGMAA(15), MODE
      COMMON /D/ DV(100,15), AR(15,15), AP(15,15)
      COMMON /T/ T(5,100), TMAX(5), INDTMX(5), SDMOD(5), VARMOD(5),
     1 L(5), YF(5,100), ALMAX, INDLMX, DOMAX, INDOMX, YFSIG(100),
     2 EMAX, INDEMX, W1, W2, CMAX, INDCMX, MODELS, NFITS, XF(100)
      TTMAX = 0.
        DO 30 N = 1, NFITS
        C = 0.
          DO 10 I = 1, NTERMS
          C = C + (DV(N,I) * SIGMAA(I)) ** 2
10        CONTINUE
        IF (MODE .NE. 0) TT = YFSIG(N) * YFSIG(N) + C
        IF (MODE .EQ. 0) TT = VARMOD(MODEL) + C
        IF (TTMAX .GT. TT) GO TO 20
        TMAX(MODEL) = TT
        TTMAX = TT
        INDTMX(MODEL) = N
20      T(MODEL,N) = TT
30      CONTINUE
      RETURN
      END
```

[a] Calculates the value of the independent variable at which the response of each of up to five models has the greatest variance. Varying experimental standard deviations are taken into account if MODE is not 0 or 10.

independent variable. If the uncertainty in the dependent variable is not constant, that is, if MODE is not 0, the calculation is modified to allow for this. The maximum value of T, and the point in the range of the x variable at which it occurs, are returned to DESIGN.

Control then passes to SERDES (Table 11.13), the algorithms of which are described in Sect. 4.2.2. Briefly, the likelihood associated with each model is calculated. Then a T-weighted difference between the responses of all pairs of models, $D0$, is calculated in such a way that most weight is given to the differences between the two models currently having the greatest likelihood. If MODE is not 0, variation in the local estimates of experimental standard deviation is taken into account. A summary value, E, which is the likelihood-weighted T value as a function of x, is then calculated and the combined discriminatory measure, C, is determined. The latter allows the selection of a design in which progressively more weight is given to experiments that will increase the precision in the parameters once the most suitable model has emerged. Some control over the progression can be gained by altering the value of the variable LAMDA (see Hill et al., 1968).

The likelihood ratio and the confidence in the current "best" model are then calculated. The fitted parameters and other summary data are printed for each model, followed by the experimental measurements and the fitted values for the best model. The likelihoods and confidence, and maximum values of T, $D0$, E and C, are also printed (see Table 4.1). DESIGN then writes a record of the current data to UNIT 16 for retention until the next run.

Table 11.13. Subprogram SERDES[a]

```
      SUBROUTINE SERDES (NPTS, NDES, LAMDA, MODEL2)
C     ******************
C
C           USING SETS OF Y VALUES FITTED BY THE VARIOUS MODELS,
C           AND THE OPTION OF NON-CONSTANT EXPERIMENTAL SD, (SIGMAY),
C           DERIVES MODEL DISCRIMINATION AND PARAMETER ESTIMATION
C           CRITERIA AND COMBINES THEM ACCORDING TO WEIGHTS.
C
      COMMON X(100), Y(100), YFIT(100), SIGMAY(100), WEIGHT(100),
     1  SIGMAA(15), MODE
      COMMON /T/ T(5,100), TMAX(5), INDTMX(5), SDMOD(5), VARMOD(5),
     1  L(5), YF(5,100), ALMAX, INDLMX, D0MAX, IND0MX, YFSIG(100),
     2  EMAX, INDEMX, W1, W2, CMAX, INDCMX, MODELS, NFITS, XF(100)
      REAL LAMDA, L, D0(100), E(100)
C
C           CALCULATION OF PROBABILITIES ASSOCIATED WITH EACH MODEL,
C           L S. ALSO FIND MODEL SD S
C
      INDLMX = 1
      ALMAX = 0.
      SUML = 0.
      DO 10 M = 1, MODELS
      SDMOD(M) = SQRT (VARMOD(M))
      L(M) = (SDMOD(M) ** (-NPTS))
      SUML = SUML + L(M)
   10 CONTINUE
      DO 30 M = 1, MODELS
      L(M) = L(M) / SUML
```

[a] Calculates the likelihoods of up to five alternative models as descriptions of the current data, and then finds the value of the independent variable at which the responses of the two most likely models diverge maximally. Varying experimental standard deviations are taken into account if MODE is not 0 or 10.

```
              IF (ALMAX .GT. L(M)) GO TO 20
              AL2 = ALMAX
              MODEL2 = INDLMX
              ALMAX = L(M)
              INDLMX = M
              GO TO 30
      20      IF (AL2 .GT. L(M)) GO TO 30
              AL2 = L(M)
              MODEL2 = M
      30      CONTINUE
              IF (NDES .GT. 1) RETURN
              D0MAX = 0.
              MODM1 = MODELS - 1
              EMAX = - 1.E90
              CMAX = 0.
C
C
C                   FIND WEIGHTS :    W1 = MODEL DISCRIMINATION
C                                     W2 = PARAMETER ESTIMATION
C
              AM = FLOAT(MODELS)
              W1 = (AM * (1. - ALMAX) / (AM - 1.)) ** LAMDA
              W2 = 1. - W1
                DO 80 N = 1, NFITS
C
C                   CALCULATE T-WEIGHTED DIFF. BETWEEN FITTED Y S OF MODELS.
C                   WEIGHTING BY L S PUTS DISCRIMINATING EMPHASIS BETWEEN BEST
C                   PAIR OF MODELS. SETS D0
C
              D0(N) = 0.
                DO 40 I = 1, MODM1
                I1 = I + 1
                  DO 40 J = I1, MODELS
                  SI = T(I,N) * T(I,N)
                  SJ = T(J,N) * T(J,N)
                  YDIFF = YF(J,N) - YF(I,N)
                  T1= - 1. + 0.5 * (SI * SI + SJ * SJ + YDIFF * YDIFF *
     1               (SI + SJ)) / (SI * SJ)
                  D0(N) = D0(N) + L(I) * L(J) * T1
      40      CONTINUE
C
C                   CALCULATE E S FROM L S AND T S
C
              E(N) = 0.
                DO 50 M = 1, MODELS
                E(N) = E(N) + L(M) * T(M,N) / TMAX(M)
      50      CONTINUE
C
C                   FIND MAX VALUE OF C (COMBINED DISCRIM FACTOR) D0MAX EMAX
C
              IF (D0MAX .GT. D0(N)) GO TO 70
              D0MAX = D0(N)
              IND0MX = N
      70      IF (EMAX .GT. E(N)) GO TO 80
              EMAX = E(N)
              INDEMX = N
      80      CONTINUE
              DO 90 N = 1, NFITS
              C = W1 * D0(N) / D0MAX + W2 * E(N) / EMAX
              IF (CMAX .GT. C) GO TO 90
              CMAX = C
              INDCMX = N
      90      CONTINUE
              RETURN
              END
```

11.8 FUNCTN Subprogram CA1: Compartmental Analysis

This subprogram (Table 11.14) embodies mathematical models of both the two-compartment and three-compartment systems shown in Figs. 5.4(a) and (b). The derivation of the equation describing the former model is given in Appendix C as an illustration of integration by means of Laplace transforms.

CA1 is supplied with pairs of parameters describing the forcing function representing the variation of specific activity in the reservoir compartment as a function of time. That is, RESERVR is previously fitted to data showing the variation with time of the specific activity of a substance in a reservoir compartment (such as in blood plasma after an injection of tracer), and the estimated values are read into CA1. In this way a mathematical description of the reservoir compartment is transferred to the model of the compartment with which it exchanges.

CA1 deals with up to six pairs of forcing function parameters. They are added in order on the input file UNIT 2. The total number of parameters to be read is

Table 11.14. FUNCTN subprogram CA1[a]

```
      SUBROUTINE FUNCTN (NPTS, A, NTERMS)
C
C           *** CA1 ***
C
      COMMON X(100), Y(100), YFIT(100), SIGMAY(100), WEIGHT(100),
     1  SIGMAA(15), MODE
      COMMON /CA1/ M, K, Q(12)
      REAL A(15), P(2)
      IF (M .EQ. 1) GOTO 30
      M = 1
      READ(2,*) K, (Q(I), I = 1, K)
      IF(EOF(5)) 70,5
    5 WRITE(6,10)
   10 FORMAT(28H ------------------------- )
      WRITE(6,20) (Q(I), I = 1, K)
   20 FORMAT(28H CA1 - RESERVOIR PARAMETERS: /
     1  26H MULTIPLIER   EXPONENTIAL / 6(1X, 2G12.5 /))
      WRITE(6,10)
   30 L1 = 1
      IF (NTERMS .EQ. 3) L1 = 2
         DO 60 I = 1, NPTS
         P(1) = 0.
         P(2) = 0.
            DO 40 J = 1, K, 2
            DO 40 L = 1, L1
            P(L) = P(L) + (A(L) * Q(J) / (A(L) - Q(J+1))) *
     1             (EXP(-Q(J+1) * X(I)) - EXP(-A(L) * X(I)))
   40       CONTINUE
         IF (NTERMS .EQ. 3) GOTO 50
         YFIT(I) = P(1)
         GOTO 60
   50    YFIT(I) = A(3) * P(1) + (1. - A(3)) * P(2)
   60    CONTINUE
      RETURN
   70 WRITE(6,80)
   80 FORMAT(39H0*** ERROR *** ERROR IN INPUT TO FUNCTN)
      STOP
      END
```

[a] For modelling the exchange between a reservoir compartment and either a single peripheral compartment (NTERMS = 1) or two peripheral compartments in parallel sampled together (NTERMS = 3). Parameters of the forcing function representing the time course of specific radioactivity in the reservoir compartment are read from UNIT 2.

indicated by the value of the variable preceding this list. An example of input data is shown in Table 11.15 and the corresponding output is reproduced in Table 5.2.

Subprogram CA1 works as follows. On the first call the value of variable M is unset, and the statements at the beginning are activated causing the input parameters to be read. On subsequent calls this section is by-passed. The value of NTERMS controls the form of the model. The number of cycles through the loop ending at statement labelled 40 is equal to the number of exponential terms required to describe the disappearance of specific activity from the reservoir compartment. The calculated distribution of specific activity between the two peripheral compartments sampled simultaneously is carried out in the statement labelled 50.

To fit the two-compartment model, NTERMS is set to 1. The single parameter A1 then represents the rate constant k_{12}. To fit the three-compartment model NTERMS is set to 3. Again, A1 is k_{12}, A2 is k_{13} and A3 is the mass of compartment 2 of the model of Fig. 5.4(b) expressed as a fraction of the combined masses of compartments 2 and 3. The third parameter is required because of the assumption that in model (b) compartments 2 and 3 are both in the same tissue and are sampled simultaneously. Optimizing the value of A3 is a way of estimating what proportion of the total tissue mass is in compartment 2 and what proportion is in compartment 3.

Table 11.15. Example of input to MODFIT and subprogram CA1[a].

UNIT 5:–			UNIT 2:–	
1	1	0.1	4	
0.4167	76.4	10	1687.7	0.62963
0.75	151	11	212.87	.012433
4	291	15		
16	209	19		
48	163	18		
999	999			

[a] The data represent the means (and sample standard deviations of the means) of the specific radioactivity of zinc in endometrial tissue from non-pregnant rabbits at five time intervals after injection of labelled zinc. The values of K and array Q are read from UNIT 2 by CA1; K is the number of parameters and array Q contains the parameter estimates of the forcing function obtained from fitting subprogram RESERVR to the blood plasma data (Table 5.1).

11.9 FUNCTN Subprogram CA2: Compartmental Analysis

This subprogram (Table 11.16) describes the physical model shown in Fig. 5.4(b) in which remote compartments 2 and 3 both exchange material reversibly with the reservoir compartment, but do not themselves interact directly, even though they are in the same tissue. It is equivalent to subprogram CA1 but, whereas CA1 represents integrated equations, CA2 is couched in terms of differential equations which must be integrated numerically.

Table 11.16. FUNCTN subprogram CA2[a]

```
      SUBROUTINE FUNCTN (NPTS, A, NTERMS)
C
C             *** CA2 ***
C
      COMMON X(100), Y(100), YFIT(100), SIGMAY(100), WEIGHT(100),
     1   SIGMAA(15), MODE
      COMMON /CA2/ M, K, Q(12), AB(15)
      INTEGER IP(2)
      REAL A(15), F(2), W(2), B(2), G(2), X0, H, H0, A1(9,2), A2(9,2),
     1   D(2,2)
      EXTERNAL AUX
      DATA G / 2 * 0.01 /
          DO 10 J = 1, NTERMS
          AB(J) = A(J)
   10     CONTINUE
      IF (M .EQ. 1) GOTO 60
      M = 1
      READ(2,*) K, (Q(I), I = 1, K)
      IF(EOF(5)) 100,30
   30 WRITE(6,40)
   40 FORMAT(28H -------------------------- )
      WRITE(6,50) (Q(I), I = 1, K)
   50 FORMAT(28H CA2 - RESERVOIR PARAMETERS: /
     1   26H MULTIPLIER    EXPONENTIAL / 6(1X, 2G12.5 /))
      WRITE(6,40)
   60 W(1) = 0.
      W(2) = 0.
      N = 2
      IFAIL = 0
      IT = 1
      X0 = 0.
      H = 0.
          DO 90 I = 1, NPTS
   70     H0 = X(I) - X0
        CALL STIFF (X0, W, G, IT, N, H0, H, AUX, A1, A2, D, IP, B, F, K1,
     1       IFAIL)
          IF (IFAIL .EQ. 0) GOTO 80
          H = H * 0.1
          IFAIL = 0
          GOTO 70
   80     YFIT(I) = A(3) * W(1) + (1. - A(3)) * W(2)
   90     CONTINUE
      RETURN
  100 WRITE(6,110)
  110 FORMAT(39H0*** ERROR *** ERROR IN INPUT TO FUNCTN)
      STOP
      END
      SUBROUTINE AUX (F, W, X0)
C     **************
      COMMON X(100), Y(100), YFIT(100), SIGMAY(100), WEIGHT(100),
     1   SIGMAA(15), MODE
      COMMON /CA2/ M, K, Q(12), AB(15)
      REAL F(2), W(2)
      W1 = 0.
          DO 10 I = 1, K, 2
          W1 = W1 + Q(I) * EXP(-Q(I+1) * X0)
   10     CONTINUE
      F(1) = AB(1) * (W1 - W(1))
      F(2) = AB(2) * (W1 - W(2))
      RETURN
      END
```

[a] For modelling (by numerical integration) the separate exchange between two peripheral compartments sampled together and a reservoir compartment, according to the model of Fig. 5.4(b). The additional subprogram AUX defines the model in terms of differential equations.

The first part of the subprogram, in which the input parameters are read, is identical in action to CA1. The following part is concerned with initializing variables for entry to the integration subprogram, which, for the reason explained in Sect. 11.1, is not listed here. We shall, however, describe the arguments of this subprogram, here named STIFF, in detail.

Variable X0 is the initial value of the x or independent variable. Array W contains the initial values of the variables expressed as differentials in the equations representing the mathematical model [in the present case Eqs. (5.14) and 5.16)]. If $dy/dx = f(A, x)$, W(1), on entry to STIFF, equals the initial value of y. (Array F contains the values of the differentials themselves, dy/dx, but they are not referenced in CA2.) Array G contains values equal to the maximum errors to be tolerated in the integration, one for each differential equation. The value of IT controls the way in which errors are handled. N is the number of differential equations to be integrated. The interval in the range of the independent variable over which the current integration will be carried out is set by the value of H0. Each time through the loop ending at statement 90, H0 is made equal to the difference between the current value of x and the previous one. Note that STIFF returns the incremented value of x at the end of the integration step. The step length for the integration is controlled by H. A value of 0 indicates that automatic selection of step length will be carried out by STIFF.

AUX is the name of an auxillary subprogram the sole purpose of which is to describe the mathematical model, expressed as N differential equations, to subprogram STIFF. More details will be found below.

The remaining arguments are variables used by STIFF internally. IFAIL is set by STIFF and its value on return indicates if integration was successful. In particular, if IFAIL is not 0, the automatic step length has become too large: it is reduced and STIFF is re-entered.

The statement labelled 80 assigns the required proportion of the specific activity of each peripheral compartment to the current value of YFIT.

Subroutine AUX defines the model in terms of differential equations. W1 is set to the current value of the specific activity in the reservoir compartment. The values of the differentials (array F), are then set. These two statements are all that are required to define the model.

11.10 FUNCTN Subprogram CA2A: Compartmental Analysis

This subprogram (section AUX of which is listed in Table 11.17) is similar to CA2 but describes instead the physical model shown in Fig. 5.4(c) in which exchange occurs between compartments 2 and 3, and compartment 2 alone communicates with the reservoir. This is known as a series configuration in contrast with the model described by FUNCTN CA2 which represents a parallel model.

FUNCTN CA2A is identical to CA2 and is not listed. The only difference required to describe the series model is to change slightly the equations defined in the AUX subroutine.

Table 11.17. AUX subprogram for use with subprogram CA2A[a]

```
       SUBROUTINE AUX (F, W, X0)
C      **************
       COMMON X(100), Y(100), YFIT(100), SIGMAY(100), WEIGHT(100),
     1   SIGMAA(15), MODE
       COMMON /CA2A/ M, K, Q(12), AB(15)
       REAL F(2), W(2)
       W1 = 0.
         DO 10 I = 1, K, 2
         W1 = W1 + Q(I) * EXP(-Q(I+1) * X0)
  10   CONTINUE
       F(1) = AB(1) * (W1 - W(1)) + AB(2) * (1. - AB(3))
     1        * (W(2) - W(1)) / AB(3)
       F(2) = AB(2) * (W(1) - W(2))
       RETURN
       END
```

[a] In conjunction with CA2A, this subprogram is suitable for modelling serial exchange between two peripheral compartments (sampled together) and a reservoir compartment, according to the model of Fig. 5.4(c).

11.11 FUNCTN Subprogram CA3: Compartmental Analysis

This subprogram (Table 11.18) embodies a mathematical model of the physical one shown in Fig. 5.7. It is suitable for modelling any number of peripheral compartments exchanging a substance with a reservoir compartment, the one into which either a labelled substance or drug is injected. It may be convenient to express the concentration of tracer at time t in terms of the fraction of dose administered, which, in the labelled compartment (the reservoir) at time zero, equals 1. Note that the sizes of the peripheral compartments are not estimated.

The exact form of the model is controlled by the value of NTERMS. If NTERMS (which must be equal to at least 3) is *odd* it is assumed that the specific activity or concentration of the substance at time zero in the reservoir compartment is known, and that the data have all been normalized to this figure (which will itself therefore be equal to 1). Parameter A1 is then the rate constant of irreversible loss of substance from the compartment and A2 and A3, A4 and A5, and so on, are the pairs of rate constants of exchange of substance into and out of the reservoir, respectively. If the value of NTERMS is *even* (which means that it must be at least 4), there will also be included a parameter representing the specific activity or concentration of the substance in the reservoir at time zero. This is a case where an initial condition appears as a parameter to be optimized (Sects. 2.1.3 and 3.6). Parameter A1 is then the estimated initial specific activity or concentration, and A2 equals the irreversible rate of loss from the reservoir compartment: A3 and A4, A5 and A6, and so on, correspond to the pairs of rate constants described above.

Notice the way in which the differential equations are formed by the loop in subroutine AUX. If it is desired to fit a model with more than five peripheral compartments the sizes of all the arrays with the present length of six must be increased.

If experimental observations on one or more of the peripheral compartments are available, this information can be taken into account in the fitting process. The calculated levels of substance in each compartment are available for comparison

Table 11.18. FUNCTN subprogram CA3[a]

```
      SUBROUTINE FUNCTN (NPTS, A, NTERMS)
C
C              *** CA3 ***
C
      COMMON X(100), Y(100), YFIT(100), SIGMAY(100), WEIGHT(100),
     1   SIGMAA(15), MODE
      COMMON /CA3/ AB(15), N1, IFLG
      INTEGER IP(6)
      REAL A(15), F(6), W(6), B(6), G(6), X0, H, H0, A1(9,6), A2(9,6),
     1   D(6,6)
      EXTERNAL AUX
      IF (NTERMS - 2 * (NTERMS / 2)) 2,2,3
    2 N = NTERMS / 2
      IFLG = 2
      GOTO 4
    3 N = NTERMS / 2 + 1
      IFLG = 1
    4 N1 = N
      DO 5 J = 1, N
      G(J) = 0.1
      W(J) = 0.
    5   CONTINUE
      IF (IFLG .EQ. 1) W(1) = 1.
      IF (IFLG .EQ. 2) W(1) = A(1)
      DO 10 J = 1, NTERMS
      AB(J) = A(J)
   10   CONTINUE
      IFAIL = 0
      IT = 1
      X0 = 0.
      H = 0.
      DO 90 I = 1, NPTS
   70   H0 = X(I) - X0
      CALL STIFF (X0, W, G, IT, N, H0, H, AUX, A1, A2, D, IP, B, F, K1,
     1   IFAIL)
      IF (IFAIL .EQ. 0) GOTO 80
      H = H * 0.1
      IFAIL = 0
      GOTO 70
   80   YFIT(I) = W(1)
   90   CONTINUE
      RETURN
      END
      SUBROUTINE AUX (F, W, X0)
C     **************
      COMMON X(100), Y(100), YFIT(100), SIGMAY(100), WEIGHT(100),
     1   SIGMAA(15), MODE
      COMMON /CA3/ AB(15), N1, IFLG
      REAL F(6), W(6)
      Z1 = 0.
      Z2 = 0.
      DO 10 I = 2, N1
      J = 2 * I - 2
      IF (IFLG .EQ. 1) J = J - 1
      Z1 = Z1 + AB(J+1) * W(I)
      Z2 = Z2 + AB(J+2)
      F(I) = AB(J+2) * W(1) - AB(J+1) * W(I)
   10   CONTINUE
      F(1) = Z1 - (AB(IFLG) + Z2) * W(1)
      RETURN
      END
```

[a] For fitting to data a model consisting of a number of peripheral compartments exchanging in parallel with a reservoir compartment. The initial specific activity or concentration in the reservoir may be chosen to be estimated as a parameter. The additional AUX subprogram defines the model in terms of differential equations.

with the data. All that is required are one or more extra statements after the one labelled 80; the calculated level in compartment 2 is in W(2), and so on. The input data would be modified slightly. For example, if measurements had been made on compartments 1 and 2 then these results could be input alternately, and a switch in the program would ensure that first one calculated value and then the other would be inserted into the correct element of array YFIT, for later comparison with Y in subprogram FIT. The model is thus fitted to the data from both compartments simultaneously, i.e. there would be two dependent variables. See Sect. 11.17 for an example of this.

11.12 FUNCTN Subprogram MASSACT: Ligand Binding

MASSACT will deal with the results from any ligand-macromolecule binding experiment in which an independent-site model is appropriate, up to and including the case of two specific binding sites plus a non-specific one (Fig. 11.19). Choice is made by selection of a value for NTERMS of between 1 and 5, as described below. The simpler forms are obtained by deleting terms from the general expression which is a cubic in the y variable B/T, the ratio of bound to total ligand. The terms of this equation were obtained by expansion and rearrangement of Eq. (6.12). Rodbard et al. (1978, Appendix B) have derived the same relationships.

Table 11.19. FUNCTN subprogram MASSACT[a]

```
      SUBROUTINE FUNCTN(NPTS,A,NTERMS)
C
C              *** MASSACT ***
C
      COMMON X(100),Y(100),YFIT(100),SIGMAY(100),WEIGHT(100),
     1 SIGMAA(15),MODE
      REAL A(15),K1,K2,K3,K1K2
      GOTO(10,20,30,40,50)NTERMS
C
C              SET-UP FOR 1 NON-SPECIFIC SITE
C
10    K3=A(1)
      K1=0.
      Q1=0.
      K2=0.
      Q2=0.
      GOTO 60
C
C              SET UP FOR 1 SPECIFIC SITE
C
20    K1=A(1)
      Q1=A(2)
      K2=0.
      Q2=0.
      K3=0.
      GOTO 60
C
C              SET-UP FOR 1 SPECIFIC + 1 NON-SPECIFIC SITES
C
```

[a] For fitting to data a number of different models of specific and/or non-specific (low affinity) classes of independent binding sites.

FUNCTN Subprogram MASSACT: Ligand Binding

```
30      K1=A(1)
        Q1=A(2)
        K3=A(3)
        K2=0.
        Q2=0.
        GOTO 60
C
C               SET-UP FOR 2 SPECIFIC SITES
C
40      K1=A(1)
        Q1=A(2)
        K2=A(3)
        Q2=A(4)
        K3=0.
        GOTO 60
C
C               SET-UP FOR 2 SPECIFIC + 1 NON-SPECIFIC SITES
C
50      K1=A(1)
        Q1=A(2)
        K2=A(3)
        Q2=A(4)
        K3=A(5)
60      K1K2=K1*K2
        DO 110 I=1,NPTS
           XI=X(I)
           X2=XI*XI
           X2K1K2=X2*K1K2
           A0=X2K1K2*(K3+1.)
           A1=-X2K1K2*(3.*K3+2.)
     1        -XI*(K1K2*(Q1+Q2)+(K1+K2)*(K3+1.))
           A2=X2K1K2*(3.*K3+1.)
     1        +XI*(2.*K1K2*(Q1+Q2)+(K1+K2)*(2.*K3+1.))
     2        +K1*Q1+K2*Q2+K3+1.
           A3=-X2K1K2*K3-XI*(K1K2*(Q1+Q2)
     1        +(K1+K2)*K3)-(K1*Q1+K2*Q2+K3)
        GOTO(100,70,70,80,80)NTERMS
70      IF(XI.EQ.0.)GOTO 100
        YFIT(I)=(-A2+SQRT(A2*A2-4.*A1*A3))/(2.*A1)
        GOTO 110
80      IF(XI.EQ.0.)GOTO 100
           CALL CUBIC(A0,A1,A2,A3,IT,ROOT1,ROOT2,ROOT3,IRR)
        IF(IT.EQ.1)GOTO 90
C
C               SAVE ROOT 2 AS THE ONE WANTED
C
        IF(IT.EQ.3)YFIT(I)=ROOT2
        GOTO 110
C
C               DON'T OFTEN EXPECT TO GET ONLY ONE REAL ROOT
C
90      YFIT(I)=ROOT1
        GOTO 110
100     YFIT(I)=-A3/A2
110     CONTINUE
        RETURN
        END
```

If NTERMS is 1, MASSACT models a single class of non-specific (low affinity or unsaturable) binding sites. A single class of specific or saturable sites is represented when NTERMS is 2; when it is 3 the model consists of one class of specific and one of non-specific sites. NTERMS set to 4 defines a model in which there are two classes of specific sites with different association constants. When NTERMS equals 5 the complete model consisting of two classes of specific and one of non-specific sites is obtained. The way in which this choice is achieved will be clear from following the logical path controlled by the value of NTERMS.

Subprogram CUBIC (Table 11.20) is called only if NTERMS is greater than 3, when it is necessary to calculate the roots of a cubic equation. The roots of cubic equations are found using Cardan's method; this subprogram will find roots whether they are real or complex, but here real roots only will be considered (signalled by IRR=3). The one required is the value returned by the variable ROOT2. Arguments for CUBIC consist of the four coefficients of the cubic equation defined in Eq. (6.13). Alternatively, the well-known formula for solving a quadratic equation is used for the case of a single specific site (NTERMS equal to 2 or 3).

Table 11.20. Subprogram CUBIC[a]

```
        SUBROUTINE CUBIC(A0,A1,A2,A3,IT,ROOT1,ROOT2,ROOT3,IRR)
        IF(.NOT.(ABS(A0).LT.1.0E-90)) GOTO 10
        IRR=0
        GOTO 110
10      IRR=1
        B1=A1/A0
        B2=A2/A0
        B3=A3/A0
C
C          REMOVE QUADRATIC TERM
C
        ALPHA=-B1/3.
        Q=B2+ALPHA*(2.*B1+3.*ALPHA)
        R=B3+ALPHA*(B2+ALPHA*(B1+ALPHA))
        Q=-Q
        R=-R
        IF(.NOT.(ABS(Q).LE.1.0E-50)) GOTO 50
        IT=1
        IF(ABS(R).LE.1.0E-9) GOTO 30
        IF(R) 20,30,40
20      ROOT1=-R**0.33333333
        GOTO 90
30      IT=3
        ROOT3=ALPHA
        ROOT2=ROOT3
        ROOT1=ROOT2
        GOTO 110
40      ROOT1=R**0.33333333
        GOTO 90
50      CONTINUE
        DELTA=0.25*R*R-Q*Q*Q/27.
        IF(DELTA) 100,100,60
60      CONTINUE
C
C          CUBIC HAS ONE REAL ROOT AND TWO COMPLEX ROOTS
C
        IT=1
        EPS2=1.
        EPS1=EPS2
        DELTA=SQRT(DELTA)
        X1=0.5*R+DELTA
        IF(.NOT.(X1.LT.0.)) GOTO 70
        EPS1=-1.
        X1=-X1
70      X2=0.5*R-DELTA
        IF(.NOT.(X2.LT.0.)) GOTO 80
        EPS2=-1.
        X2=-X2
```

[a] Uses Cardan's method to find the roots of the general cubic equation defined by Eq. (6.13).

```
80      CONTINUE
        ROOT1=EPS1*X1**0.33333333+EPS2*X2**0.33333333
C
C               EVALUATE COMPLEX ROOTS
C
90      ROOT1=ROOT1+ALPHA
        X1=-0.5*(B1+ROOT1)
        X2=B2+ROOT1*B1+ROOT1*ROOT1
        X2=SQRT(X2-X1*X1)
        ROOT2=X1
        ROOT3=X2
        GOTO 110
C
C               EVALUATE REAL ROOTS
C
100     IT=3
        PHI=ACOS(2.59807622*R/Q**1.5)
        PHI=PHI/3.
        RM=1.1547006*SQRT(Q)
        PI3=1.04719754
        ROOT1=RM*COS(PHI)+ALPHA
        ROOT2=-RM*COS(PI3-PHI)+ALPHA
        ROOT3=-RM*COS(PI3+PHI)+ALPHA
110     RETURN
        END
```

11.13 FUNCTN Subprogram GEN BIND: Ligand Binding

This subprogram (Table 11.21, see next page) embodies the theoretical, general binding model represented by Eq. (6.16). The exact form of the model is determined by the values of NTERMS, P, M and N. NTERMS sets the total number of parameters, and the variables P and M define them. The value of P represents the number of compound terms [the first term in Eq. (6.16)]. For each increment in P two more parameters are added to the model. The value of M gives the number of factor terms in Eq. (6.16) to be summed (the second term). Each of these adds a further parameter to the model. The integer number of sites associated with each class defined by the value of M is given by a list of values read into array N.

For instance, in the example given in Sect. 6.1.2.1, the total number of adjustable parameters was chosen by setting NTERMS to 3. One compound term was selected by setting P to 1, one factor term by setting M to 1, and the number of sites to be described by the latter term, N(1), was 2; these values were supplied on input UNIT 2. (If M had been 3, for example, N(2) and N(3) would also have been required: when no compound terms are needed, P is set to 0.) Thus the total number of parameters (NTERMS) equals 2P+M and the total number of binding sites is

$$2P + \sum_{I=1}^{M} N(I).$$

Table 11.21. Subprogram GENBIND[a]

```
            SUBROUTINE FUNCTN (NPTS, A, NTERMS)
C
C                  *** GENBIND ***
C
            COMMON X(100), Y(100), YFIT(100), SIGMAY(100), WEIGHT(100),
          1    SIGMAA(15), MODE
            COMMON /GENBIND/ MM, M, P, N(10)
            REAL A(15)
            INTEGER P
            IF (MM .EQ. 1) GOTO 40
            MM = 1
            READ(2,*) P, M, (N(I), I = 1, M)
            IF(EOF(2)) 90,10
       10   WRITE(6,20)
       20   FORMAT(28H -------------------------- )
            WRITE(6,30) P, (N(I), I = 1, M)
       30   FORMAT(24H GENBIND -    P      SITES /
          1    I14, 3X, 10I4)
            WRITE(6,20)
       40   NP = 2 * P
              DO 80 I = 1, NPTS
              F = X(I)
              SUM = 0.
              IF (P .EQ. 0) GOTO 60
                DO 50 IP = 1, NP, 2
                SUM = SUM + (F * (2. * F - A(IP))) / (F * F - A(IP) * F +
          1            A(IP+1))
       50     CONTINUE
       60   IF (M .EQ. 0) GOTO 75
            IN = NP + 1
            K = 1
              DO 70 IM = IN, NTERMS
              SUM = SUM + FLOAT(N(K)) * F / (F - A(IM))
              K = K + 1
       70     CONTINUE
       75   YFIT(I) = SUM
       80   CONTINUE
            RETURN
       90   WRITE(6,100)
      100   FORMAT(39H0*** ERROR *** ERROR IN INPUT TO FUNCTN)
            STOP
            END
```

[a] For fitting the general binding model of Eq. (6.16) to experimental data.

11.14 FUNCTN Subprogram RIA: Competitive Protein-Binding

This subprogram (Table 11.22) embodies the theoretical model of competitive protein-binding described by Eq. (6.17) in which ligand or hormone binds to a single class of sites with an association constant K (A1) in competition with labelled ligand having a differnt association constant K' (A2). Parameter A3 is equal to the concentration of sites expressed in the same units as the concentration of ligand.

Also involved is the concentration of tracer in the solution at equilibrium (again expressed in the same units). This value, preceded by 1, is entered from UNIT 2 directly into the subprogram by the first few statements which, controlled by the value of the varaible M, are read once only on the first call.

Subprogram CUBIC (Table 11.20) is used to calculate the roots of Eq. (6.17) (which is actually a cubic equation in $R_{F/B}$) by the method described in Sect. 11.13. The required real root is returned as the variable ROOT1.

FUNCTN Subprogram RIAH: Competitive Protein-Binding

Table 11.22. FUNCTN subprogram RIA[a]

```
      SUBROUTINE FUNCTN (NPTS, A, NTERMS)
C
C               *** RIA ***
C
      COMMON X(100), Y(100), YFIT(100), SIGMAY(100), WEIGHT(100),
     1  SIGMAA(15), MODE
      COMMON /RIA/ M, K, Q(12)
      REAL A(15)
      IF (M .EQ. 1) GOTO 8
      M = 1
      READ(2,*) K, (Q(I), I = 1, K)
      IF(EOF(2)) 70,4
    4 WRITE(6,6)
    6 FORMAT(28H ------------------------- )
      WRITE(6,7) (Q(I), I = 1, K)
    7 FORMAT(28H RIA - TRACER CONCENTRATION: /
     1    8X, G12.5, 6H UNITS )
      WRITE(6,6)
    8 Z1 = 1. / A(3)
      DO 10 I = 1, NPTS
      A0 = A(2) / A(1)
      A1 = 1. + A0 * (1. - Q(1) / A(3)) - Z1 * (X(I) + 1. / A(1))
      A2 = 1. - Z1 * (1. / A(1) + Q(1) + X(I) + 1. / A(2))
      A3 = -1. / (A(2) * A(3))
      CALL CUBIC (A0, A1, A2, A3, IT, ROOT1, ROOT2, ROOT3, IRR)
      YFIT(I) = ROOT1
   10 CONTINUE
      RETURN
   70 WRITE(6,80)
   80 FORMAT(39H0*** ERROR *** ERROR IN INPUT TO FUNCTN)
      STOP
      END
```

[a] For fitting to data the analytical model of competitive protein-binding described by Eq. (6.17).

11.15 FUNCTN Subprogram RIAH: Competitive Protein-Binding

This subprogram (Table 11.23) embodies the empirical model (Healey's model) described by Eq. (6.18). The response or dependent varaible is either counts bound B or the ratio B/T. A1 is the response at infinite dose, A2 is the response at zero dose, A3 is ln(dose) at a response midway between the zero and infinite dose responses, and A4 is the Hill coefficient.

Table 11.23. FUNCTN subprogram RIAH[a]

```
      SUBROUTINE FUNCTN (NPTS, A, NTERMS)
C
C               *** RIAH ***
C
      COMMON X(100), Y(100), YFIT(100), SIGMAY(100), WEIGHT(100),
     1  SIGMAA(15), MODE
      REAL A(15)
      DO 10 I = 1, NPTS
      XI = X(I)
      IF (XI .EQ. 0.) XI = 1.E-30
      Z = EXP(A(3) - A(4) * ALOG(XI))
      YFIT(I) = A(1) + A(2) * (Z / (1. + Z))
   10 CONTINUE
      RETURN
      END
```

[a] For fitting to data the empirical model of Eq. (6.18).

11.16 FUNCTN Subprogram SIN: Rhythmical Data

This subprogram (Table 11.24) embodies the model of a single sine curve described by Eq. (7.3). It is suitable for providing an empirical description of any rhythmical data for which estimates are required of the period. The independent variable is commonly time; parameter A1 represents the amplitude, A2 the phase (in units of time), A3 the period (also in units of time) and A4 the mean response.

Table 11.24. FUNCTN subprogram SIN[a]

```
      SUBROUTINE FUNCTN(NPTS,A,NTERMS)
C
C            *** SIN ***
C
      COMMON X(100),Y(100),YFIT(100),SIGMAY(100),WEIGHT(100),
     1       SIGMAA(15),MODE
      REAL A(15)
      DO 1 I=1,NPTS
    1 YFIT(I)=A(1)*SIN((A(2)+X(I))*6.283185/A(3))+A(4)
      RETURN
      END
```

[a] For fitting the model of Eq. (7.3), a single sine curve, to a time-series.

11.17 FUNCTN Subprogram LIMIT: Limit Cycles

LIMIT (Table 11.25) is a subprogram suitable for solving a set of differential equations describing a non-linear system giving rise to limit cycle behaviour [Eqs. (2.19) and (2.20)]. The equations can conveniently be solved by numerical integration.

This representation of Eqs. (2.19) and (2.20) does not include the diffusion terms (the first terms on the right-hand sides). It is assumed instead that diffusion is instantaneous and can be neglected. Thus the cyclical behaviour of the solution of the equations results solely from the dynamic relationship between them.

Parameters A1 and A2 equal A and B, respectively, in Eqs. (2.19) and (2.20). They represent the steady state concentrations of two substances to which the system described by the equations is open. Parameters A3 and A4 are the initial conditions of the variables y and z.

This subprogram illustrates how to deal with two dependent variables arising from two equations describing the model. Notice how a switch (statement labelled 75) ensures that the first and subsequent odd-numbered elements of array YFIT are filled with values of W(1), while even-numbered ones receive values of W(2). W(1) is equivalent to y in Eqs. (2.19) and (2.20), W(2) to z. F(1) and F(2) represent dy/dt and dz/dt, respectively.

To fit this model to data, values of time (the independent variable) alternating with values of first y and then z are provided as input, and both equations of the model are fitted simultaneously (see also the comments at the end of Sect. 11.11).

Examples of the use of this subprogram in conjunction with program SIMUL are shown in Figs. (2.13) and (2.14).

Table 11.25. FUNCTN subprogram LIMIT[a]

```
      SUBROUTINE FUNCTN (NPTS, A, NTERMS)
C
C            *** LIMIT ***
C
      COMMON X(100), Y(100), YFIT(100), SIGMAY(100), WEIGHT(100),
     1  SIGMAA(15), MODE
      COMMON /LIMIT/ AB(15)
      INTEGER IP(2)
      REAL A(15), F(2), W(2), B(2), G(2), X0, H, H0, A1(9,2), A2(9,2),
     1  D(2,2)
      EXTERNAL AUX
      DATA G / 2 * 0.01 /
      DO 10 J = 1, NTERMS
      AB(J) = A(J)
  10  CONTINUE
      W(1) = AB(3)
      W(2) = AB(4)
      N = 2
      IFAIL = 0
      IT = 1
      X0 = 0.
      H = 0.
      DO 90 I = 1, NPTS
  70  H0 = X(I) - X0
      CALL STIFF (X0, W, G, IT, N, H0, H, AUX, A1, A2, D, IP, B, F, K1,
     1  IFAIL)
      IF (IFAIL .EQ. 0) GOTO 75
      H = H * 0.1
      IFAIL = 0
      GOTO 70
  75  IF((I/2) * 2 - I) 80,85,85
  80  YFIT(I) = W(1)
      GOTO 90
  85  YFIT(I) = W(2)
  90  CONTINUE
      RETURN
      END
      SUBROUTINE AUX (F, W, X0)
C     **************
      COMMON X(100), Y(100), YFIT(100), SIGMAY(100), WEIGHT(100),
     1  SIGMAA(15), MODE
      COMMON /LIMIT/ AB(15)
      REAL F(2), W(2)
      W1SQW2 = W(1) * W(1) * W(2)
      F(1) = AB(1) - (AB(2) + 1.) * W(1) + W1SQW2
      F(2) = AB(2) * W(1) - W1SQW2
      RETURN
      END
```

[a] Embodies the model defined by Eqs. (2.19) and (2.20), which describe limit cycle behaviour.

11.18 Other Programs for Fitting Non-Linear Models to Data

These notes provide a brief introduction to several other programs for fitting linear or non-linear models to data. They are all much larger and more complicated than MODFIT, the comparable program provided above. They have more facilities because they are contained within large packages designed for versatility. They are available, or may be suitable for installation, at many computing centres.

11.18.1 SPSS NONLINEAR

This is one of a large and very efficient set of programs known as the Statistical Package for the Social Sciences (Nie et al., 1975). NONLINEAR, described by Robinson (1977), is fully integrated into the SPSS system and is particularly convenient to use, especially for those familiar with SPSS. NONLINEAR will deal with any model, including those having several independent or dependent variables. The Marquardt-Levenberg method is used to direct the search. It is the responsibility of the user to supply FORTRAN statements defining the model, equivalent to the FUNCTN subprogram required by MODFIT. Bounds may be applied to the parameters and the effect of holding constant any of the parameter values is easily investigated. Versions of SPSS are available for a variety of large computers and the package is provided at many computing centres.

11.18.2 MLAB: An Online Modelling Laboratory

MLAB is a comprehensive and powerful program package designed to facilitate the description, manipulation and evaluation of models of any degree of complexity, including those consisting of differential equations. It is suitable for simulation or fitting models to data. Full details of this program and a list of references to the literature where it has been used are given by its author (Knott, 1977). An endocrinological application is described by Ketelslegers et al. (1975). MLAB is best used from a display terminal because the program has excellent facilities for drawing two- and three-dimensional diagrams. The ease with which a model can be modified and the results depicted graphically is most impressive. The program is, unfortunately, very large and can at present be installed only on a Digital Equipment Corporation PDP-10 or PDP-20 computer.

11.18.3 SAAM: Simulation, Analysis and Modelling

This large program has been developed over a long period with the particular aim of modelling kinetic systems such as those encountered in compartmental analysis. It is introduced by Berman (1965) and fully described in the instruction manual provided by its authors (Berman and Weiss, 1977). Many standard kinetic models are available within this package, which can be used for both simulation and fitting to data. A list of references to a wide range of publications in which the program has been used is provided in the manual. A typical application is in the study of thyroxine and iodide transport in sheep (McGuire and Berman, 1978).

11.18.4 Other Programs

The following programs are also available, but we have little experience of them.
  NON-LIN (Metzler, C.). Kalamazoo, Mich.: Upjohn Chemical Co., 1969.
  BMDX85 Biomedical Computer Package (Sampson, P. F.). Los Angeles, Calif.: University of California at Los Angeles, 1970.
  NLIN IBM Share Program No. 360D-13.2.003. Least Squares Estimation of Non-Linear Parameters. New York: IBM Corp., 1969.
  A short parameter-fitting routine for compartmental models (Feldman, H. A.). Comput. Prog. Biomed. 7, 135–144 (1977).

Optimization Techniques with FORTRAN (Kuester, J. L., Mize, J. H.). New York-London: McGraw-Hill, 1973. Algorithms for searching for minima and estimating parameters by a variety of methods.

See also the survey provided by Johnson (1974).

12 Appendix C: Analytical Integration by Laplace Transform

The following is an example of the use of an analytical method to integrate a differential equation in compartmental analysis. The integration is necessary in order to convert an equation in terms of the rate of change of specific activity, da/dt, into an equation in specific activity, a, to allow comparison with experimental values of a. Integration is here carried out by means of Laplace transforms (Sect. 2.2), but any of the other standard analytical or numerical methods suggested, e. g. by Riggs (1970), would be suitable. Numerical integration of similar compartmental models by computer is illustrated in Sects. 5.2.3–5.2.5.

A differential equation [Eq. (5.14)] describing the rate of change with time of a_2, the specific activity of tracer in compartment 2 of model (a) in Fig. 5.4, is derived in Sect. 5.2.3.1. In this equation the value of a_1, the specific activity of tracer in the reservoir compartment, can be calculated at any time t from an empirical forcing function previously fitted to experimental data obtained from the reservoir compartment. We shall assume that the empirical function consists of the sum of two exponential terms (see the example in Sect. 5.2.2.1). That is

$$a_1 = A_1 e^{-A_2 t} + A_3 e^{-A_4 t}. \tag{12.1}$$

From Eq. (5.14),

$$da_2/dt = k_{12}(a_1 - a_2).$$

Substituting for a_1,

$$da_2/dt = k_{12}(A_1 e^{-A_2 t} + A_3 e^{-A_4 t} - a_2). \tag{12.2}$$

From tables of Laplace transforms (see, for example, Table A1 of Atkins, 1969) we find the transforms

$$\mathscr{L}[f(t)] = \check{f}(s), \tag{12.3}$$

$$\mathscr{L}[df(t)/dt] = s\check{f}(s) - f(0), \tag{12.4}$$

and

$$\mathscr{L}[me^{-nt}] = m/(s+n) \tag{12.5}$$

where $f(0)$ is the initial condition in the time domain. Setting $a_2 = f(t)$ and taking Laplace transforms term by term in Eq. (12.2),

$$s\check{f}(s) - f(0) = k_{12}[A_1/(s+A_2) + A_3/(s+A_4) - \check{f}(s)]. \tag{12.6}$$

At zero time there is no tracer in compartment 2; hence $f(0) = 0$. Rearranging,

$$\check{f}(s) = k_{12} A_1 / [(s+A_2)(s+k_{12})] + k_{12} A_3 / [(s+A_4)(s+k_{12})]. \tag{12.7}$$

Appendix C: Analytical Integration by Laplace Transform

Eq. (12.4) must now be expressed as the sum of partial fractions to allow the application of reverse Laplace transforms. Consider the first term on the right-hand side of Eq. (12.7). Let u and v be two constants such that

$$k_{12}A_1/[(s+A_2)(s+k_{12})] = u/(s+A_2) + v/(s+k_{12})$$
$$= [s(u+v) + (uk_{12} + vA_2)]/(s+A_2)(s+k_{12}). \quad (12.8)$$

Comparing terms in Eq. (12.8),

$$v = -u, \quad (12.9)$$
$$u = k_{12}A_1/(k_{12} - A_2). \quad (12.10)$$

Thus

$$k_{12}A_1/[(s+A_2)(s+k_{12})] = k_{12}A_1/[(k_{12}-A_2)(s+A_2)] \\ - k_{12}A_1/[(k_{12}-A_2)(s+k_{12})]. \quad (12.11)$$

A similar process is applied to the second term on the right-hand side of Eq. (12.7) to yield a second expression like Eq. (12.11).
Therefore

$$\check{f}(s) = k_{12}A_1/[(k_{12}-A_2)(s+A_2)] - k_{12}A_1/[(k_{12}-A_2)(s+k_{12})] \\ + k_{12}A_3/[(k_{12}-A_4)(s+A_4)] - k_{12}A_3/[(k_{12}-A_4)(s+k_{12})]. \quad (12.12)$$

Reversing the Laplace transforms by means of Eqs. (12.3) and (12.5),

$$f(t) = a_2 = k_{12}A_1 e^{-A_2 t}/(k_{12}-A_2) - k_{12}A_1 e^{-k_{12}t}/(k_{12}-A_2) \\ + k_{12}A_3 e^{-A_4 t}/(k_{12}-A_4) - k_{12}A_3 e^{-k_{12}t}/(k_{12}-A_4) \\ = k_{12}A_1 e^{-A_2 t}/(k_{12}-A_2) + k_{12}A_3 e^{-A_4 t}/(k_{12}-A_4) \\ - k_{12}[A_1/(k_{12}-A_2) + A_3/(k_{12}-A_4)]e^{-k_{12}t}. \quad (12.13)$$

Thus we have converted the differential equation in terms of da_2/dt into an integrated expression in terms of a_2. A generalized form of this result, in which the forcing function may contain any number of exponential terms, is embodied in FUNCTN subprogram CA1 (Sect. 11.8). Eq. (12.13) is equivalent to equations (15) and (16) of Solomon (1960) and stated by him to be the solution to differential equations describing an identical compartmental system.

References

Aarons D, Reagan M (1977) SPSS subprogram SPECTRAL – spectral analysis of time series. Vogelback Computing Center, Northwestern University, Evanston, Ill.
Akbar AM, Nett TM, Niswender GD (1974) Metabolic clearance and secretion rates of gonadotropins at different stages of the estrous cycle in ewes. Endocrinology 94:1318–1324
Aleksandrov AD, Kolmogorov AN, Lavrent'ev MA (eds.) (1969) Mathematics: Its contents, methods, and meaning. MIT press, Cambridge, Mass London
Anderberg MR (1973) Cluster analysis for applications. Academic Press, New York London
Anscombe FJ (1960) Rejection of outliers. Technometrics 2:123–147
Aschoff J, Wever R (1976) Human circadian rhythms: a multioscillatory system. Fed Proc 35:2326–2332
Ashby WR (1956) An introduction to cybernetics. Wiley & Sons, New York London
Atkins GL (1969) Multicomponent models for biological systems. Methuen, London
Atkins GL (1977) Routines for calculating the first derivative of a function by numerical methods. Comput Biol Med 7:321–325
Atkinson AC (1978) Posterior probabilities for choosing a regression model. Biometrika 65:39–48
Atkinson AC, Hunter WG (1968) The design of experiments for estimation. Technometrics 10:271–289
Baird DT, Swanston I, Scaramuzzi RJ (1976) Pulsatile release of LH and secretion of ovarian steroids in sheep during the luteal phase of the estrous cycle. Endocrinology 98:1490–1496
Bard Y (1970) Comparison of gradient methods for the solution of nonlinear parameter estimation problems. SIAM J Numer Anal 7:157–186
Bard Y (1974) Nonlinear parameter estimation. Academic press, New York London
Basar E (1976) Biophysical and physiological systems analysis. Addison-Wesley, Reading, Mass London
Batschelet E (1974) Statistical rhythm evaluation. In: Ferin M, Halberg F, Richart RM, Vande Wiele RL (eds) Biorhythms and human reproduction. Wiley & Sons, New York London, pp 25–35
Baulieu EE, Raynaud J-P (1970) A "proportion graph" method for measuring binding systems. Eur J Biochem 13:293–304
Beck JV, Arnold KJ (1977) Parameter estimation in engineering and science. Wiley & Sons, New York London
Bellman R, Åström KJ (1970) On structural identifiability. Math Biosci 7:329–339
Benesch R, Benesch RE (1967) The effect of organic phosphate from the human erythrocyte on the allosteric properties of hemoglobin. Biochem Biophys Res Commun 26:162–167
Benham RD (1971) Interactive simulation language-8 (ISL-8). Simulation 16:116–129
Bergman RN, Bucolo RJ (1973) Nonlinear metabolic dynamics of the pancreas and liver. J Dyn Syst Meas Control 95:296–333
Berman M (1965) Compartmental analysis in kinetics. In: Stacy RW, Waxman BD (eds) Computers in biomedical research, vol II. Academic Press, New York London, pp 173–201
Berman M, Weiss MF (1977) Users manual for SAAM, 27th edn. Laboratory of Theoretical Biology, National Cancer Institute, National Institutes of Health, U.S. Dept. of Health, Education, and Welfare, Bethesda Md
Berson SA, Yalow RS, Bauman A, Rothschild MA, Newerly K (1956) Insulin-I^{131} metabolism in human subjects: demonstration of insulin bindig globulin in the circulation of insulin-treated subjects. J Clin Invest 35:170–190
von Bertalanffy L (1938) II. A quantitative theory of organic growth. Hum Biol 10:181–213
von Bertalanffy L (1973) General system theory. Penguin, London
Best EN (1975) Exploration of a menstrual cycle model. Simulation Today 25:117–120
Beveridge GSG, Schechter RS (1970) Optimization: theory and practice. McGraw-Hill, New York London
Beverton RJ, Holt SJ (1957) On the dynamics of exploited fish populations. Fish Invest Minist Agric Fish Food (GB) Ser. II Salmon Freshwater Fish 19:1–533

References

Bevington PR (1969) Data reduction and error analysis for the physical sciences. McGraw-Hill, New York London
Bogumil RJ (1974) Pulsatile variations in hormone levels. In: Ferin M, Halberg F, Richart RM, Vande Wiele RL (eds) Biorhythms and human reproduction. Wiley & Sons, New York London, pp 107–131
Bogumil RJ (1976) Computer simulation of endocrine control of the menstrual cycle. Excerpta Med Int Congr Ser 402:250–255
Bogumil RJ, Ferin M, Rootenberg J. Speroff L, Vande Wiele RL (1972 a) Mathematical studies of the human menstrual cycle. I. Formulation of a mathematical model. J Clin Endocrinol Metab 35:126–143
Bogumil RJ, Ferin M, Vande Wiele RL (1972 b) Mathematical studies of the human menstrual cycle. II. Simulation performance of a model of the human menstrual cycle. J Clin Endocrinol Metab 35:144–156
Box GEP, Draper NR (1969) Evolutionary operation. A statistical method for procress improvement. Wiley & Sons, New York London
Box GEP, Hill WJ (1967) Discrimination among mechanistic models. Technometrics 9:57–71
Box GEP, Lucas HL (1959) Design of experiments in non-linear situations. Biometrika 46:77–90
Box MJ, Davies D, Swann WH (1969) Non-linear optimization techniques. Mathematical and Statistical Techniques for Industry, Monograph No. 5. Oliver & Boyd, Edinburgh
Bradley DF (1968) Multilevel systems and biology – view of a subcellular biologist. In: Mesarovic MD (ed) Systems theory and biology. Springer, Berlin Heidelberg New York, pp 38–58
Bremermann H (1970) A method of unconstrained global optimization. Math Biosci 9:1–15
Brooks DE, McIntosh JEA (1975) Turnover of carnitine by rat tissues. Biochem J 148:439–445
Bross, I (1952) Sequential medical plans. Biometrics 8:188–205
Brown RF, Godfrey KR (1978) Problems of determinacy in compartmental modelling with application to bilirubin kinetics. Math Biosci 40:205–224
Builder SE, Segal IH (1978) Equilibrium ligand binding assays using labeled substrates: nature of the errors introduced by radiochemical impurities. Anal Biochem 85:413–424
Bush DS, Gann DS (1975) Hypothesis testing of time-variant features of adrenocortial control. In: Summer Computer Simulation Conference, LaJolla, Calif: Simulation Councils, pp 939–941
Chance B, Pye K, Higgins J (1967) Waveform generation by enzymatic oscillators. IEEE Spectrum 4(8):79–86
Chandler JP, Hill DE, Spivey HO (1972) A program for efficient integration of rate equations and least-squares fitting of chemical reaction data. Comput Biomed Res 5:515–534
Chatfield C (1975) The analysis of time series: theory and practice. Chapman & Hall, London
Cobelli C, Romanin-Jacur G (1976) On the structural identifiability of biological compartmental systems in a general input-output configuration, Math Biosci 30:139–151
Cobelli C, Polo A, Romanin-Jacur G (1977) A computer program for the analysis of controllability, observability and structural identifiability of biological compartmental systems. Comput Progs Biomed 7:21–36
Colquhoun D (1971) Lectures on biostatistics. An introduction to statistics with applications in biology and medicine. Clarendon, Oxford
Crick F (1966) Of molecules and men. University of Washington Press, Seattle, Wash London
Cronin J (1977) Some mathematics of biological oscillations. SIAM Rev 19:100–138
Dalziel K (1973) Kinetics of control enzymes. In: Rate control of biological processes: Symp. Soc. Exp. Biol. No. XXVII, University Press, Cambridge pp 21–48
Daniel C, Wood FS (1971) Fitting equations to data. Wiley & Sons, New York London
Danziger L, Elmergreen GL (1956) The thyroid-pituitary homeostatic mechanism. Bull Math Biophys 18:1–13
Danziger L, Elmergreen GL (1957) Mathematical models of endocrine systems. Bull Math Biophys 19:9–18
Daughaday WH (1956) Evidence for two corticosteroid binding systems in human plasma. J Lab Clin Med 48:799–800
Davies RG (1971) Computer programming in quantitative biology. Academic Press, London New York
DiStefano JJ (1976) Concepts, properties, measurement, and computation of clearance rates of hormones and other substances in biological systems. Ann Biomed Eng 4:302-319
DiStefano JJ, Wilson KC, Jang M, Mak PH (1975) Identification of the dynamics of thyroid hormone metabolism. Automatica 11:149–159

Dowd JE, Riggs DS (1965) A comparison of estimates of Michaelis-Menton kinetic constants from various linear transformations. J Biol Chem 240:863–869

Draper NR, Smith H (1966) Applied regression analysis. Wiley & Sons, New York London

Edmunds LN (1976) Models and mechanisms for endogenous timekeeping. In: Palmer JD An introduction to biological rhythms. Academic Press, New York London, pp 280–361

Ekins RP, Newman GB, O'Riordan JLH (1968) Theoretical aspects of "saturation" and radioimmunoassay. In: Hayes RL, Goswitz FA, Murphy BEP (eds.) Radioisotopes in medicine: in vitro studies U.S. Atomic Energy Commission, Oak Ridge Tenn, pp 59–100

Ekins RP, Newman GB, O'Riordan JLH: (1970) Saturation assays. In: McArthur JW, Colton T (eds) Statistics in endocrinology. MIT Press, Cambridge, Mass London, pp 345–392

Elliott JA, Stetson MH, Menaker M (1972) Regulation of testis function in golden hamsters: a circadian clock measures photoperiodic time. Science 178:771–773

Emmens CW (1948) Principles of biological assay. Chapman & Hall, London

Feldman HA (1977) A numerical method for fitting compartmental models directly to tracer data. Am J Physiol 233:R1–R7

Feldman H, Rodbard D, Levine D (1972) Mathematical theory of cross-reactive radioimmunoassay and ligand-binding systems at aquilibrium. Anal Biochem 45:530–556

Feldman K (1978) New devices for flow dialysis and ultrafiltration for the study of protein-ligand interactions. Anal Biochem 88:225–235

Feng L-J, Rodbard D, Rebar R, Ross GT (1977) Computer simulation of the human pituitary-ovarian cycle: studies of follicular phase estradiol infusions and the midcycle peak. J Clin Endocrinol Metab. 45:775–787

Finney DJ (1955) Experimental design and its statistical basis. Cambridge University Press, London

Finney DJ (1960) A introduction to the theory of experimental design. University of Chicago Press, Chicago London

Fisher RA (1952) Sequential experimentation. Biometrics 8:183–187

Fisher RA (1971) The design of experiments, 8th edn. Hafner, New York

Fletcher JE, Ashbrook JD (1973) Computer analysis of drug-protein binding data. Ann NY Acad Sci 226:69–81

Fletcher JE, Spector AA (1968) A procedure for computer analysis of data from macromolecule-ligand binding studies. Comput Biomed Res 2:164–175

Fletcher JE, Spector AA (1977) Alternative models for the analysis of drug-protein binding. Mol Pharmacol 13:387–399

Fletcher JE, Spector AA, Ashbrook JD (1970) Analysis of macromolecule-lingand binding by determination of stepwise equilibrium constants. Biochemistry 9:4580–4587

Fowler RE, Edwards RG, Walters DE, Chan STH, Steptoe PC (1978) Steroidogenesis in preovulatory follicles of patients given human menopausal and chorionic gonadotrophins as judged by the radioimmunoassay of steroids in follicular fluid. J Endocrinol 77:161–169

Gaddum JH (1945) Lognormal distributions. Nature 156:463–466

Gallagher TF, Yoshida K, Roffwarg HD, Fukashima DK, Weitzman ED, Hellman L (1973) ACTH and cortisol secretory patterns in man. J Clin Endocrinol Metab 36:1058–1068

Gann DS (1969) Parameters of the simulus initiating the adrenocortical response to hemorrhage. Ann NY Acad Sci 156:740–755

Gann DS, Cryer GL (1973) Feedback control of ACTH secretion by cortisol. In: Brodish A, Redgate ES (eds) Brain-pituitary-adrenal interrelationships. Karger, Basle London New York, pp 197–223

Gann DS, Cryer GL, Schoeffler JD (1973) Finite level models of biological systems. Ann Biomed Eng 1: 385–445

Gann DS, Ostrander LE, Schoeffler JD (1968) A continuous system of adrenocortical function. In: Mesarovic MD (ed) Systems theory in biology. Springer, Berlin Heidelberg New York, pp 185–200

Gann DS, Seif FJ, Schoeffler JD (1972) A quantized variable approach to description of biological and medical systems. In: Zeek RW, Showalter AE (eds) Applications of Walsh functions, 1972 Proceedings. National Technical Information Service, U.S. Dept. of Commerce, Doc. No. AD-744650, Springfield Va, pp 134–141

Garfinkel D, Garfinkel L, Moore WT (1977) Computer simulation as a means of physiological integration of biochemical systems. In: Solomon DL, Walter C (eds) Mathematical models in biological discovery. Springer, Berlin Heidelberg New York (Lecture notes in biomathematics, vol 13, pp 146–172)

Gear CW (1971) The automatic integration of ordinary differential equations. Commun ACM 14:176–179
Glass HI, de Garreta AC (1971) The quantitative limitations of exponential curve fitting. Phys Med Biol 16:119–130
Glandsdorff P, Prigogine I (1971) Thermodynamics of structure, stability and fluctuations. Wiley & Sons, New York London
Gold HJ (1977) Mathematical modelling of biological systems – an introductory guidebook. Wiley & Sons, New York London
Goodwin B (1970) Biological stability. In: Waddington CH (ed) Towards a theoretical biology, vol 3. University Press, Edinburgh, pp 1–17
Greep RO, Koblinski MA, Jaffe FS (eds) (1976) Reproduction and human welfare: a challenge to research. MIT Press Cambridge, Mass London, pp 81–164
Grizzle WE, Dallman MF, Schramm LP, Gann DS (1974) Inhibitory and facilitatory hypothalamic areas mediating ACTH release in the cat. Endocrinology 95:1450–1461
Gurpide E (1975) Tracer methods in hormone research. Springer, Berlin Heidelberg New York
Gurpide E, Mann J (1970) Interpretation of isotope data obtained from blood-borne compounds. J Clin Endocrinol Metab 30:707–718
Halberg F (1969) Chronobiology. Annu Rev Physiol 31:675–725
Hammersley JM, Handscomb DC (1964) Monte Carlo methods. Methuen, London
Hanks J (1972) Growth of the African elephant (*Loxodonta africana*). East Afr Wildl J. 10:251–272
Hanks J, McIntosh JEA (1973) Population dynamics of the African elephant (*Loxodonta africana*). J Zool 169:29–38
Hastings JW (1972) Timing mechanisms. In: Behnke JA (ed) Challenging biological problems. Directions toward their solution. Oxford University Press, New York, pp 148–167
Healey MJR (1972) Statistical analysis of radioimmunoassay data. Biochem J 130:207–210
Heineken FG, Tsuchiya HM, Aris R (1967) On the accuracy of determining rate constants in enzymatic reactions. Math Biosci 1:115–141
Heinmets F (1966) Analysis of normal and abnormal cell growth. Plenum, New York
Heinrich R, Rapoport SM, Rapoport TA (1977) Metabolic regulation and mathematical models. Prog Biophys Mol Biol 32:1–82
Higgins J (1967) The theory of oscillating reactions. Ind Eng Chem 59:18–62
Hill WJ, Hunter WG, Wichern DW (1968) A joint design criterion for the dual problem of model discrimination and parameter estimation. Technometrics 10:145–160
Himmelblau DM (1970) Procress analysis by statistical methods. Wiley & Sons, New York London
Holaday JW, Martinez HM, Natelson BH (1977) Synchronized ultradian cortisol rhythm in monkeys: persistence during corticotropin infusion. Science 198:56–58
Hollander M, Wolfe DA (1973) Nonparametric statistical methods. Wiley & Sons, New York London
Iberall A (1972) Toward a general science of viable systems. McGraw-Hill, New York London
Inoué S (1973) Regulatory mechanisms in the sex cycle. Theoretical and experimental studies in the rat. Adv Biophys 5:1–63
Inoué S, Nakamura T, Sekiguchi T (1970) A theoretical approach to the regulatory mechanism in the brain-hypophyseal-gonadal system with reference to its mathematical modeling and computer simulation. Endocrinol Jap 17:567–583
Jacquez JA (1972) Compartmental analysis in biology and medicine. Kinetics of distribution of tracer-labelled materials. Elsevier, Amsterdam London
Janson PO, Amato F, Weiss TJ, Ralph MM, Seamark RF (1978) On the isolated perfused ovary as a model for the study of ovarian function. Fertil Steril 30:230–236
Jenkins GM, Watts DG (1968) Spectral analysis and its applications. Holden-Day, San Francisco London
Jennrich RI, Sampson PF (1968) Application of stepwise regression to non-linear estimation. Technometrics 10:63–72
Johnson LE (1974) Computers, models, and optimization in physiological kinetics. CRC Crit Rev Bioeng 2:1–37
Johnson P, McIntosh RP (1976) Fluorescence depolarization in a model system: carbonic anhydrase-dansyl sulphonamide. Biochim Biophys Acta 453:521–532
Jones RW (1973) Principles of biological regulation. An introduction to feedback systems. Academic Press, New York London

Julius RS (1972) The sensitivity of exponentials and other curves to their parameters. Comput Biomed Res 5:473–478
Kalman RE (1962) Canonical structure of linear dynamical systems. Proc Nat Acad Sci USA 48:596–600
Kauffman S (1970) Bahaviour of randomly constructed genetic nets: binary element nets. In: Waddington CH (ed) Towards a theoretical biology, vol 3. University Press, Edinburgh, pp 18–37
Kauffman S (1977) Dynamic models of the mitotic cycle: evidence for a limit cycle oscillator. In: Solomon DL, Walter C (eds) Mathematical models in biological discovery. Springer, Berlin Heidelberg New York (Lecture notes in biomathematics, vol 13, pp 96–131)
Kauffman S, Wille JJ (1975) The mitotic oscillator in *Physarum polycephalum*. J Theor Biol 55:47–93
Keane PM, Walker WHC, Gauldie J, Abraham GE (1976) Thermodynamic aspects of some radioassays. Clin Chem 22:70–73
Kemp KW, Nix ABJ, Wilson DW, Griffiths K (1978) Internal quality control of radioimmunoassys. J Endocrinol 76:203–210
Ketelslegers J-M, Knott GD, Catt KJ (1975) Kinetics of gonadotrophin binding by receptors of the rat testis. Analysis by a non-linear curve-fitting method. Biochemistry 14:3075–3083
Klein DC (1978) The pineal gland: a model of neuroendocrine regulation. In: Richlin S, Baldessarini RJ, Martin JB (eds) The hypothalamus. Raven, New York, pp 303–327
Klein DC, Weller JL (1970) Indole metabolism in the pineal gland: a circadian rhythm in N-acetyltransferase. Science 169:1093–1095
Knobil E, Plant TM (1978) Neuroendocrine control of gonadotropin secretion in female rhesus monkeys. In: Ganong WF, Martini L (eds) Frontiers in neuroendocrinology, vol 5. Raven, New York, pp 249–264
Knott G (1977) MLAB: an online modelling laboratory, 7th edn. Division of Computer Research and Technology, National Institutes of Health, U.S. Departement of Health, Education, and Welfare, Bethesda, Md
Knudsen JF, Barraclough CA (1977) A longitudinal study of the changes in responsiveness of the hypothalamo-pituitary unit to medial preoptic area stimulation and to luteinizing hormone releasing hormone administration during diestrus-2 and proestrus in rats. Endocrinology 101:187–195
Kopell N, Howard LN (1973) Plane wave solutions to reaction-diffusion equations. Stud Appl Math 52:291–328
Krause RD, Lott JA (1974) Use of the simplex method to optimize analytical conditions in clinical chemistry. Clin Chem 20:775–782
Kropholler HW, Senior PR (1976) Successful use of Gear's method for solving a problem posed by Chandler et al. Comput Biomed Res 9:153–157
Lamport H (1940) Periodic changes in blood estrogen. Endocrinology 27:673–680
Laszlo E (1972) Introduction to systems philosophy. Gordon & Breach, New York London Paris
Laurence DJ, Wilkinson G (1974) Model for competitive binding assays – the shape and location of the inhibition curves. Anal Chem 46:1132–1135
Lawley DN, Maxwell AE (1963) Factor analysis as a statistical method. Butterworths, London
Lawton WH, Sylvestre EA, Maggio MS (1972) Self modeling nonlinear regression. Technometrics 14:513–532
Levenberg K (1944) A method for the solution of certain nonlinear problems in least squares. Appl Math 2:164–168
Levine HD, Rosen AL, DeWoskin R, Moss GS (1977) Application of self-modelling nonlinear regression to ventricular pressure data. Comput. Biomed Res 10:363–372
Levins R (1970) Complex systems. In: Waddington CH (ed) Towards a theoretical biology, vol 3. University Press, Edinburgh, pp 73–88
Licko V (1975) Simulation of responses of metabolic and endocrine systems to external stimuli. In: Summer Computer Simulation Conference, LaJolla, Calif: Simulation Councils, pp 931–934

Magar ME (1972) Data analysis in biochemistry and biophysics. Academic Press, New York London
Marquardt DW (1963) An algorithm for least-squares estimation of non-linear parameters. SIAM J 11:431–441
Matthews CME (1957) The theory of tracer experiments with 131I-labelled plasma proteins. Phys Med Biol 2:36–53
Matthews DE (ed) (1977) Mathematics and the life Sciences. Springer, Berlin Heidelberg New York (Lecture notes in biomathematics, vol 18)

May RM (1973) Stability and complexity in model ecosystems. University Press, Princeton NJ
May RM (1976) Simple mathematical models with very complicated dynamics. Nature 261:459–467
McArthur JW, Colton T (eds) (1970) Statistics in endocrinology. MIT Press, Cambridge, Mass London
McGuire RA, Berman M (1978) Maternal, fetal, and amniotic fluid transport of thyroxine, triiodothyronine, and iodide in sheep: a kinetic model. Endocrinology 103:567–576
McIntosh JEA, Lutwak-Mann C (1972a) Zinc transport in rabbit tissues. Some hormonal aspects of the turnover of zinc in female reproductive organs, liver and body fluids. Biochem J 126:869–876
McIntosh JEA, Lutwak-Mann C (1972b) Zinc in the luteal and interstial tissue of the rabbit ovary in early pregnancy. Nature [New Biol] 236:53–54
McIntosh JEA, Lutwak-Mann, C (1974) Calcium transport in the early conceptus and associated maternal tissues in the rabbit. Biochem J 138:97–105
McIntosh JEA, Moor RM, Allen WR (1974) Pregnant mare serum gonadotrophin: rate of clearance from the circulation of sheep. J Reprod Fertil 44:95–100
Mercier C, Alfsen A, Baulieu EE (1966) A testosterone binding globulin. Excerpta Med Int Congr Ser 101:212
Mesarovic MD (1968) Systems theory and biology – view of a theoretician. In: Mesarovic MD (ed) Systems theory and biology. Springer, Berlin Heidelberg New York, pp 59–87
Mishell DR, Nakamura RM, Crosignani PG, Stone S, Kharma K, Nagata Y, Thorncroft IH (1971) Serum gonadotrophin and steroid pattern during the normal menstrual cycle. Am J Obstet Gynecol 111:60–65
Mitchison JM (1971) The biology of the cell cycle. University Press, Cambridge
Moor RM, Hay MF, Dott HM, Cran DG (1978) Macroscopic identification and steroidogenic function of atretic follicles in sheep. J Endocrinol 77:309–318
Moor RM, Hay MF, McIntosh, JEA, Caldwell BV (1973) Effect of gonadotrophins on the production of steroids by sheep ovarian follicles cultured in vitro. J. Endocrinol 58:599–611
Mosley J, Bevan BR (1977) Spline function analysis applied to a human placental lactogen assay. Ann Clin Biochem 14:16–21
Myhill J (1968) Investigation of the effect of data error in the analysis of biological tracer data from three compartment systems. J Theor Biol 23:218–231
Naus AJ, Kuppens PS, Borst A (1977) Calculation of radioimmunoassay standard curves. Clin Chem 23:1624–1627
Nelder JA, Mead R (1965) A simplex method for function minimization. Comput J 7:308–313
Nicolis G, Auchmuty JFG (1974) Dissipative structures, catastrophes, and pattern formation: a bifurcation analysis. Proc Natl Acad Sci USA 71:2748–2751
Nie NH, Hull CH, Jenkins JG, Steinbrenner K, Bent DH (1975) SPSS: Statistical package for the social sciences, 2nd edn. McGraw-Hill, New York London
Njus D, Sulzman FM, Hastings JW (1974) Membrane model for the circadian clock. Nature 248:116–120
Olsen LF, Degn H (1977) Chaos in an enzyme reaction. Nature 267:177–178
Ostrander LE, Schoeffler JD, Gann DS (1968) Finite state models with Boolean variables. In: Enslein K (ed) Data acquisition and processing in biology and medicine, vol 5. Pergamon, Oxford New York
Overall JE, Klett CJ (1972) Applied multivariate analysis. McGraw-Hill, New York London
Papaikonomou E (1974) Biocybernetics, biosystems analysis, and the pituitary adrenal system. Nooy's Drukkerij, Purmerend
Palmer JD (1976) An introduction to biological rhythms. Academic Press, New York London
Pasteels JL (1977) Basic concepts in neuroendocrinology. In: Hubinont PO, L'Hermite M, Robyn C (eds) Clinical reproductive neuroendocrinology. Karger, Basel (Progress in reproductive biology, vol 2, pp 1–11)
Pattee HH (1970) The problem of biological hierarchy. In: Waddington CH (ed) Towards a theoretical biology, vol 3. University Press, Edinburgh, pp 117–136
Pavlidis T (1971) Mathematical models of circadian rhythms: their usefulness and their limitations. In: Menaker M (ed) Biochronometry. Symposium Proceedings, Friday Harbor, Washington, 1969. National Academy of Sciences, Washington DC, pp 110–116
Pavlidis T (1973) Biological oscillators: their mathematical analysis. Academic Press, New York London
Pittendrigh CS (1965) On the mechanism of the entrainment of a circadian rhythm by light cycles. In: Aschoff J (ed) Circadian clocks. Proceedings of the Feldafing Summer School, 1964. North-Holland, Amsterdam, pp 277–297

Prigogine I, Nicolis G (1971) Biological order, structure and instabilities. Q Rev Biophys 4:107–148
Prigogine I, Nicolis G, Babloyantz A (Nov. 1972) Thermodynamics of evolution. Phys Today 24:23–28
Provine WB (1977) The role of mathematical population geneticists in the evoutionary synthesis of the 1930's and 40's. In: Solomon DL, Walter C (eds) Mathematical models in biological discovery. Springer, Berlin Heidelberg New York (Lecture notes in biomathematics, vol 13, pp 2–30)
Rapoport A (1952) Periodicities of open linear systems with positive steady states. Bull Math Biophys 14:171–183
Rapp PE, Berridge MJ (1977) Oscillations in calcium-cyclic AMP control loops form the basis of pacemaker activity and other high frequency biological rhythms. J Theor Biol 66:497–525
Rassmussen H (1974) Organization and control of endocrine systems. In: William RH (ed) Textbook of edocrinology, 5th edn. Saunders, Philadelphia Pa, pp 1–30
Raynaud J-P (1973) A computer programm for the analysis of binding experiments. Comput Prog Biomed 3:63–78
Rebar R, Perlman D, Naftolin F, Yen SSC (1973) The estimation of pituitary luteinizing hormone secretion. J Clin Endocrinol Metab 37:917–927
Reiter RJ (1974) Circannual reproductive rhythms in mammals related to photoperiod and pineal function: a review. Chronobiologia 1:365–395
Rescigno A, Beck JS (1972) Compartments. In: Rosen R (ed) Foundations of mathematical biology, vol II. Academic Press, New York London, pp 255–322
Riggs DS (1963) The mathematical approach to physiological problems. Williams & Wilkins, Baltimore Md
Riggs DS (1970) Control theory and physiological feedback mechanisms. Williams & Wilkins, Baltimore Md
Riggs DS (1977) How models of feedback systems can help the practical biologist. In: Solomon DL, Walter C (eds) Mathematical models in biological discovery. Springer, Berlin Heidelberg New York (Lecture notes in biomathematics, vol 13 pp 175–205)
Roberts DV (1977) Enzyme kinetics. University Press, Cambridge
Roberts PJ, Coppola JC, Isaacs NW, Kennard O (1973) Crystal and molecular structure of cortisol (11β, 17α, 21-trihydroxy-pregn-4-ene-3,20-dione) methanol solvate. J. Chem Soc Perkin Trans II: 774–781
Robinson B (1977) SPSS subprogramm NONLINEAR – Nonlinear regression, Manual No. 433. Vogelback Computing Center, Northwestern University, Evanston, Ill
Rodbard D (1968) Mechanics of ovulation. J Clin Endocrinol 28:849–861
Rodbard D (1973) Mathematics of hormone-receptor interaction: I. Basic principles. In: O'Malley BW, Means AR (eds) Receptors for reproductive hormones. Plenum, New York London, pp 289–326
Rodbard D (1974) Apparent positive cooperative effects in cyclic AMP and corticosterone production by isolated adrenal cells in response to ACTH analogues. Endocrinology 94:1427–1437
Rodbard D (1977) "Specific" interference (parallel displacement) in radioligand assays by extraneous binding proteins. Endocrinology 101:1180–1183
Rodbard D (1978) Statistical estimation of the minimal detectable concentration ("sensitivity") for radioligand assays. Anal Biochem 90:1–12
Rodbard D, Catt K (1972) Mathematical theory of radioligand assays: the kinetics of separation of bound from free. J Steroid Biochem 3:255–273
Rodbard D, Feldman HA (1975) Theory of protein-ligand interaction. In: O'Malley BW, Hardman JG (eds) Methods in enzymology, vol 36. Academic Press, New York London, pp 3–16
Rodbard D, Hutt DM (1974) Statistical analysis of radioimmunoassays and immunoradiometric (labelled antibody) assays. In: Radioimmunoassays and related procedures in medicine, vol 1. International Atomic Energy Agency, Vienna, pp 165–192
Rodbard D, Lewald JE (1970) Computer analysis of radioligand assay and radioimmunoassay data. Acta Endocrinol [Suppl] (Kbh) 147:79–103
Rodbard D, Munson PJ (1978) Is there an osmotic threshold for vasopressin release? Editorial comment. Am J Physiol 234:E340–E342
Rodbard D, Tacey RL (1978) Radioimmunoassay dose interpolation based on the mass action law with antibody heterogeneity. Exact correction for variable mass of labelled ligand. Anal Biochem 90:13–21
Rodbard D, Bridson W, Rayford PL (1969) Rapid calculation of radioimmunoassy results. J Lab Clin Med 74:770–781

Rodbard D, Ruder HJ, Vaitukaitis J, Jacobs HS (1971) Mathematical analysis of kinetics of radioligand assays: improved sensitivity obtained by delayed addition of labelled ligand. J Clin Endocrinol Metab 33:343–355

Rodbard D, Munson PJ, De Lean A (1978) Improved curve-fitting, parallelism testing, characterization of sensitivity and specificity, validation, and optimization for radioligand assays. In: Radioimmunoassay and related procedures in medicine, vol 1. International Atomic Energy Agency, Vienna, pp 469–504

Rosen R (1970 Dynamical system theory in biology, vol 1: stability theory and its applications (Wiley & Sons, New York London

Rosen R (1977) The generation and recognition of patterns in biological systems. In: Matthews DE (ed) Mathematics and the life sciences. Springer, Berlin Heidelberg New York (Lecture notes in biomathematics, vol 18 pp 222–341)

Ross GJS (1972) Stochastic model fitting by evolutionary operation. In: Jeffers JNR (ed) Mathematical models in ecology. Blackwell, Oxford, pp 297–308

Routh MW, Swartz PA, Denton MB (1977) Performance of the super modified simplex. Anal Chem 49:1422–1428

Sandor T, Sridhar B, Hollenberg NK (1978) Multiexponential fit of data by using the maximum likelihood method on a minicomputer. Comput Biomed Res 11:35–40

Saunders DS (1976) The biological clock of insects. Sci Am 243:114–121

Scatchard G (1949) The attractions of proteins for small molecules and ions. Ann N Y Acad Sci 51:660–672

Schoeffler JD, Ostrander LE, Gann DS (1968) Identification of Boolean mathematical models. In: Mesarovic MD (ed) Systems theory and biology. Springer, Berlin Heidelberg New York, pp 201–221

Schwartz NB (1969) A model for the regulation of ovulation in the rat. Recent Prog Horm Res 25:1–55

Schwartz NB, Waltz P (1970) Role of ovulation in the regulation of the estrous cycle. Fed Proc 29:1907–1912

Schwartz NB, Dierschke DJ, McCormack CE, Waltz PW (1977) Feedback regulation of reproductive cycles in rats, sheep, monkeys, and humans, with particular attention to computer modeling. In: Greep RO, Koblinski MA (eds) Frontiers in reproduction and fertility control. MIT Press, Cambridge, Mass, pp 55–89

Seamark RF, Moor RM, McIntosh JEA (1974) Steroid hormone production by sheep ovarian follicles cultured in vitro. J Reprod Fertil 41:143–158

Seif FJ, Gann DS (1972) An orthogonal transform approach to the description of biological and medical systems. In: Zeek RW, Showalter AE (eds) Applications of Walsh functions, 1972 Proceedings. National Technical Information Service, US Dept of Commerce, Doc No AD-744 650, Springfield, Va, pp 128–133

Shack WJ, Tam PY, Lardner TJ (1971) A mathematical model of the human menstrual cycle. Biophys J 11:835–849

Sheppard CW (1962) Basic principles of the tracer method. Wiley & Sons, New York London

Sheps MC, Menken JA (1973) Mathematical models of conception and birth. University of Cicago Press, Chicago London

Shipley RA, Clark RE (1972) Tracer methods for in vivo kinetics. Academic Press, New York London

Siegel S (1956) Nonparametric statistics for the behavioural sciences. McGraw-Hill, New York London

Smith WR (in press) A mathematical model of the hypothalamic-pituitary-gonadal axis. II. Feedback control of gonadotrophin secretion. Bull Math Biol

Snedecor GW, Cochran WG (1967) Statistical methods, 6th edn. Iowa State University Press, Ames, Iowa

Sollberger A (1965) Biological rhythm research. Elsevier, Amsterdam London New York

Solomon AK (1960) Compartmental methods of kinetic analysis. In: Comar CL, Bronner F (eds) Mineral metabolism, vol 1A. Academic Press, New York London, pp 119–167

Solomon DL, Walter C (eds) (1977) Mathematical models in biological discovery. Springer, Berlin Heidelberg New York (Lecture notes in biomathematics, vol 13)

Spath H (1974) Spline algorithms for curves and surfaces. Utilitas Mathematica, Winnipeg

Spendley W, Hext GR, Himsworth FR (1962) Sequential application of simplex designs in optimisation and evolutionary operation. Technometrics 4:441–461

Speroff L, Vande Wiele RL (1971) Regulation of the human menstrual cycle. Am J Obstet Gynecol 109:234–247

Stear EB (1975) Application of control theory to endocrine regulation and control. Ann Biomed Eng 3:439–455
Stewart M, Stewart F (1977) Constant and variable regions in glycoprotein hormone beta subunit sequences: implications for receptor binding specificity. J Mol Biol 116:175–179
Sussmann HJ, Zahler RS (1977) Catastrophe theory: mathematics misused. The Sciences 17(6):20–23
Swann WH (1969) A survey of non-linear optimization techniques. FEBS Lett [Suppl 1] 2:S39–S55
Swartz J, Bremermann H (1975) Discussion of parameter estimation in biological modelling: algorithms for estimation and evaluation of the estimates. J Math Biol 1:241–257
Tait JF, Burstein S (1964) In vivo studies of steroid dynamics in man. In: Pincus G, Thimann KV, Astwood EB (eds) The hormones, vol V. Academic Press, New York London, pp 441–557
Tait JF, Little B, Tait SAS, Flood C (1962) The metabolic clearance rate of aldosterone in pregnant and non-pregnant subjects estimated by both single-injection and constant-infusion methods. J Clin Invest 41:2093–2100
Thom R (1975) Structural stability and morphogenesis. Benjamin, Reading, Mass
Thompson HE, Horgan JD, Delps E (1969) A simplified mathematical model and simulations of the hypophysis-ovarian endocrine control system. Biophys J 9:278–291
Treanor CE (1966) A method for the numerical integration of coupled first-order differential equations with greatly different time constants. Math Comput 20:39–45
Tuccy J (1977) SPSS subprogramm NPAR TESTS: Non-parametric statistical tests. Vogelback Computing Centre, Northwestern University, Evanston Ill
Turgeon JL, Barraclough CA (1977) Regulatory role of estradiol in pituitary responsiveness to luteinizing hormone-releasing hormone on proestrus in the rat. Endocrionology 101:548–554
Tyson J, Kauffman S (1975) Control of mitosis by a continuous biochemical oscillation: synchronization; spatially inhomogeneous oscillations. J Math Biol 1:289–310
Urquhart, J (1970) Blood-borne signals. The measuring and modeling of humoral communication and control. Physiologist 13:7–41
Urquhart J, Li CC (1968) Dynamics of adrenocortical secretion. Am J Physiol 214:73–85
Urquhart J, Li CC (1969) Dynamic testing and modeling of adrenocortical secretory function. Ann NY Acad Sci 156:756–778
Vagnucci AH, Wong AKC, Ciu TS (1974) Time series analysis of hormonal patterns in human plasma. Comput Biomed Res 7:513–532
Vande Wiele RL, Bogumil J, Dyrenfurth I, Ferin M, Jewelewicz R, Warren M, Rizkallah T, Mikhail G (1970) Mechanisms regulating the menstrual cycle in women. Recent Prog Horm Res 26:63–103
Waddington CH (1957) The strategy of the genes. Allen & Unwin, New York
Waddington CH (ed) (1968–1972) Towards a theoretical biology, vols 1–4. University Press, Edinburgh
Wagner RK (1978) Extracellular and intracellular steroid binding proteins. Properties, discrimination, assay and clinical applications. Acta Endocrinol [Suppl 218] (Kbh) 88:1–73
Wald A (1947) Sequential analysis. Wiley & Sons, New York
Wallen EP, Yochim JM (1974) Rhythmic function of pineal hydroxyindole-O-methyl transferase during the estrous cycle: an analysis. Biol Reprod 10:461–466
Walter C (1965) Steady-state applications in enzyme kinetics. Ronald, New York
Walter CF (1972) Kinetic and thermodynamic aspects of biological and biochemical control mechanisms. In: Kun E, Grisolia S (eds) Biochemical regulatory mechanisms in eukaryotic cells. Wiley & Sons, New York London, pp 355–489
Walter C (1974) Graphical procedures for the detection of deviations from the classical model of enzyme kinetics. J Biol Chem 249:699–703
Walter C (1977) Contributions of enzyme models. In: Solomon DL, Walter C (eds) Mathematical models in biological discovery. Springer, Berlin Heidelberg New York (Lecture notes in biomathematics, vol 13, pp 31–93)
Warme PK (1977) Space-filling molecular models constructed by computer. Comput Biomed Res 10:75–82
Weiss TJ (1978) Follicular development and gonadotrophins. Doctoral Dissertation, University of Adelaide, Adelaide, S. Aust.
Weiss TJ, Armstrong DT, McIntosh JEA, Seamark RF (1978) Maturational changes in sheep ovarian follicles: gonadotrophic stimulation of cyclic AMP production by isolated theca and granulosa cells. Acta Endocrinol (Kbh) 89:166–172
Weizenbaum J (1976) Computer power and human reason. From judgement to calculation. Freeman, San Francisco

Westphal U (1971) Steroid-protein interactions. Springer, Berlin Heidelberg New York
Whitby LG, Lutz W (eds) (1971) Principles and practice of medical computing. Churchill, Edinburgh London
Wilkinson GN (1961) Statistical estimations in enzyme kinetics. Biochem J 80:324–332
Wilkinson JH (1965) The algebraic eigenvalue problem. Clarendon, Oxford
Williams MB (1977) Needs for the future: radically different types of mathematical models. In: Solomon DL, Walter C (eds) Mathematical models in biological discovery. Springer, Berlin Heidelberg New York (Lecture notes in biomathematics, vol 13, pp 226–240)
Winfree AT (1970) Integrated view of resetting a circadian clock. J Theor Biol 28:327–374
Winfree AT (1974a) Rotary chemical reactions. Sci Am 230:82–95
Winfree AT (1974b) Patterns of phase compromise in biological cycles. J Math Biol 1:73–95
Winfree AT (1977) Some principles and paradoxes about the phase control of biological oscillations. J Interdiscip Cycle Res 8:1–14
Wold S (1974) Spline functions in data analysis. Technometrics 16:1–11
Worthing AG, Geffner J (1943) Treatment of experimental data. Wiley & Sons, New York London
Yanagishita M, Rodbard D (1978) Computerized optimization of radioimmunoassays for hCG and estradiol: an experimental evaluation. Anal Biochem 88:1–19
Yates FE (1974) Modeling periodicities in reproductive, adrenocortical, and metabolic systems. In: Ferin M, Halberg F, Richart RM, Vande Wiele RL (eds) Biorhythms and human reproduction. Wiley & Sons, New York London, pp 133–142
Yates FE, Brennan RD, Urquhart J, Dallman MF, Li CC, Halpern W (1968) A continuous system model of adrenocortical function. In: Mesarovic, MD (ed) Systems theory and biology. Springer, Berlin Heidelberg New York, pp 141–184
Yates FE, Russel SM, Maran JW (1971) Brain-adenohypophysial communication in mammals. Annu Rev Physiol 33:393–444
Yates FE, Marsh DJ, Iberall AS (1972) Integration of the whole organism – a foundation for a theoretical biology. In: Behnke JA (ed) Challenging biological problems. Directions toward their solution. Oxford University Press, New York, pp 110–132
Yen SSC (1977) Regulation of the hypothalamic-pituitary-ovarian axis in women. J Reprod Fertil 51:181–191
Zaroslinski JF, Keresztes-Nagy S, Mais RF, Oester YT (1974) Effect of temperature on the binding of salicylate by human serum albumin. Biochem Pharmacol 23:1767–1776
Zeeman EC (1972) Differential equations for the heartbeat and nerve impulse. In: Waddington CH (ed) Towards a theoretical biology, vol 4. University Press, Edinburgh, pp 8–67
Zeeman EC (1976) Catastrophe theory. Sci Am 234:65–83
Zeigler BP (1976) The theory of modelling and simulation. Wiley & Sons, New York London
Zilversmit DB, Entenman C, Fisher MC (1943) On the calculation of "turnover time" and "turnover rate" from experiments involving the use of labelling agents. J Gen Physiol 26:325–331

Subject Index

Definitions of terms appear on pages referred to in *italics*

Ablation
 of neural tissue 66
 of subsystems 40
Accuracy *69*
ACTH *see* Adrenocorticotrophic hormone
Adaptation
 of biological systems to step inputs 41
 of endocrine systems to stimuli 53
 to environment 45, 174, 189
 of organisms to stimuli 49, 207
Adrenal
 control, uncoupling of 52
 frequency analysis of response to ACTH 41
 gain in feedback to hypothalamus 50
 glands, rhythmic secretions in isolation 172
 models of action of 38
 non-linear response to ACTH 32
 in ovulatory cycle 203–204, 217, 221, 224
Adrenocortical system
 control, finite level modelling of 66
 cross-linking of, with ovarian system 190
 experimental problems in 69
 modelled using CSMP program 76
 models of, not inherently oscillatory 172
Adrenocorticoids, model for release of 175
Adrenocorticotrophic hormone (ACTH) 32, 38, 41
 secretion of 66, 68–69
 time-series analysis of 196
Aesthetic pleasure of modelling 24
Albumin
 equilibrium dialysis of ligands and 111, 145–150
 testosterone antibody production 157
 transport of 137–138
Aldosterone 200
Algorithm 28, 38, *77*, 80
Aliasing *196*, 200
Allosterism 32, *143*, 152–155
Amplitude *173*–174, 191, 290
 determination from discrete time data 179

 ever-increasing 49
 in frequency analysis 40
Amino acid sequences analysed 226
Anabolism 96, 98
Analytical
 experiments *103*
  design of 103–114
  importance of experimental frame in 103
  interpretation of parameters in 87
  physical meaning of parameters in 74
 models *see* Theoretical models
Androgens 203, 217–221 *see also* Testosterone
Angiotensin feedback loop 48
Anovular cycles 220–221, 223
Antibody
 antigen binding to 143, 155
 to testosterone, production of 157
Antidiuretic hormone 48, 54
Antigen-antibody binding 143, 155
Apples and the cosmos 4, 19
Approximation
 in applying mathematics to biology 26
 and computers in biological research 21
 of derivatives by central differences 257
 by linearization 10, 41, 44, 49–50, 52, 81–82, 91, 254
Association (equilibrium) constant *143–144*
 of CBG 149
 Michaelis-Menten equation *70*–72, 78
 precision of estimates of 149
 of SBG 149–150
 sequential binding model 152
 tracer and ligand differing in 156–159
Assumptions
 challenged 224
 in compartmental analysis 120
 in description of models 22
 different, give same result 224
 in measuring ligand binding 146
 in modelling
  enzyme kinetics 31
  ovulatory cycles 218
 of normality of distribution 73
 in parametric statistics 226

Assumptions
  reassessing 1
  require verifying 225
  testing sensitivity of model to 224
  in using mathematics to describe biology 26
Asymptotic mass 96, 98
Attractors 64
  orbits 43
  surfaces 64
Auto-correlation function *191*, 194–197
  coefficient *194*–195
  correlogram and *195*, 197
  cross-correlation *198*
  cross-covariance function 198
  lag *194*–195, 197–198, 200
  of menstrual cycle temperature variation 196–197
Automata theory 30, 65
Auto-regulation
  of blood flow 41
  of chemical reactions 62
Auto-regression *195*
AUX subprograms 133, 279, 281–282

Bartlett's test 248
Baseline of time-series *191*
von Bertalanffy equation of growth 96
Bias *69*, 72, 83
  linearization causing 91
  Lineweaver-Burke plot 70
  in parameter estimates 91, 93–94, 150
    competitive protein-binding assay 156, 165
    Monte Carlo simulation 72, 91–95, 135
    SIMUL program 92, 165, *260*–266
  systematic error causing 84, 150
  in testing models 24
Bicycle 45
Bifurcation *57*–58, 65
  in interacting rhythms 188
Binary
  nature of natural variables 68
  notation
    in finite level modelling 10, 68
    in model of
      gene behaviour 14–16
      ovulatory cycle 214
Binding sites *see* Ligand binding to macromolecules
Bio-assay 118
  logit-log plot in 162
  modelling of 162
Biological
  behaviour
    of models 5, 16, 43
    statistical mechanisms in studying 55
    synchronizing 186
  models 2
    scientists' responsibility 24–25

systems *see also* Complexity in biological systems
  assumed non-linear 32
  difficulties
    in frequency analysis with 41
    in studying feedback loops in 52
  dynamics described by compartmental analysis 31
  experimental uncertainty ill-defined in 97
  explaining stability and evolution in 54–55
  feedforward in 46
  functions of, not evident 53
  generalized descriptions of instabilities in 64–66
  homeostasis in 45, 52, 171, 174
  interacting feedback loops in 50
  linearity and non-linearity in 32–34, 40
  mathematics suitable for 26, 55
  models of feedback in 54
  nature of 26
  not neutrally stable 43
  open 42, 55
  periodic inputs advantageous in 41
  properties alter during tests 41
  response to environment 45
  structurally stable 42
  theoretical modelling superficial for 31
  and time 27, 69
  transport lags in 49
  variation 103 *see also* Individual variation
    in competitive protein-binding assays 169
    estimated from residuals 104
    non-normal nature of 73, 103
    uncontrolled 103
Biphasic secretion of LH 208
Birth 45, 226
Black box 34, 41
  approach to rhythms 176, 184
  appropriate to endocrinology 37
  methods applied to feedback systems 47
Blastocyst fluid 123
Block
  diagrams 9, *39*–40, 67
  of replicated samples 104, 230
Blood plasma
  binding proteins in 149
  clearance 116–119
    of PMSG from 89–95, 116–119, 139–142
    human pregnancy 146–150, 227–228
    mammillary compartmental model of 135–142
  reproductive hormones, levels in 221, 224
    during menstrual cycles 204
    steroid levels in 227

Subject Index

Blood plasma
  transport of albumin in 137–138
    calcium in 131
    carnitine in 131
    steroid hormones in 143, 146–150
    zinc in 123–130, 142
BMDX85 biomedical program 292
Bode diagrams 40–41, 49, 51
Boolean
  algebra 15, 68–69
  notation to describe finite level models 67
Bound-to-free, bound-to-total ratio see Ratio
Boundary conditions
  parameters to be optimized 282, 290
  of space influence dynamics 61–62
Bounds, parameter 83, 292 see also Constraints; Penalty functions
Butterfly effect 57

C, combined measure of discrimination 108–109, 111, 135, 276
CA1 FUNCTN subprogram 278–279, 281
  analytical integration of differential equations of 294–295
  exchange of zinc 125–128, 135
  forcing function and 125–129
  input format 126
CA2 FUNCTN subprogram 132, 279–281
CA2A FUNCTN subprogram 133–135, 281
CA3 FUNCTN subprogram 137–142, 282
Calcium
  and cAMP feedback loop 175
  feedback control of 52
  transport 131
cAMP see Cyclic 3′,5′-adenosine monophosphate
Carcinogenesis 31
Cardan's method 286
Cardinality 67
Carnitine 131
Catabolism 96, 98
Catalysts and steady state 43
Catastrophe theory 18, 64–65
Causality 3, 67
  in rhythms 202
Cause and effect 7
CBG see Corticosteroid binding globulin
Cells see also Granulosa, Theca cells
  diffusion between 66
  as open systems 42
  structural components and diffusion 30, 60
Central differences 257
Chaotic behaviour 11, 57–58
  from an enzyme 58, 63
Characteristic equation 43–44
Chemical reactions
  non-linear 32, 60
  producing

instabilities 61
limit cycles 62
rates of, and differential equations 28
Chi-square 231, 245–246, 257
  goodness of fit of model to data 85
  reduced 90, 257–258
  test of distribution using 246
CHISQR (R CHI SQUARE) 90, 92, 254, 260, 266 see also Reduced chi-square
Circadian
  changes in parameters 221
  disturbances to endocrine systems 53
  oscillator controlling pineal 180
  results of removing signals 172
  rhythms 55, 171, 175
    effects on models of ovulatory cycle 224
    entrained 182, 186
Classes, selecting
  of individuals to which models apply 12–13
  of systems for study 23
Classification
  cluster analysis 237–238
  discriminant analysis 238–240
  linear models 233–240
Clearance 116
  biological potency and 115
  contrast with exchange 119
  example, detailed, of model fitting 89–95
  half-time of 119, 121
  of hormones from blood plasma 38, 89–95, 116–119, 139–142
    determines hormone action 115, 180
    modelled as a transfer function 38, 39
    in ovulatory cycles 206–208, 210, 219, 221
    parameters assumed constant 206–207
    probably rhythmic 189, 224
  linearity 118
  mammillary compartmental model 137
  Monte Carlo simulation of 94–95
  parameter interaction common in models of 87
  physical model 118–119, 123–124
  of PMSG 38, 89–95, 116–119, 139–142
  potencies of gonadotrophins 118
  secretion rate 116
  Stewart-Hamilton equation 116–117, 119
Clinical trials 105
Clock see also Rhythms, inherent
  biological 173, 175–176, 184
  influencing pineal secretions 180
  inhibition of 188
  master, in central nervous system 172
  model of mitosis 184–185
  phase discontinuities in a biological 181–185
  in rat oestrous cycle 210–211
Closed systems 26 see also Isolated systems
  dynamic equilibrium 120

Closed systems
  influence of catalysts on   42–43
  unusual in biology   120
Cluster analysis   *237*–238
Coefficient of variation   92, 95, *243*
  in competitive protein-binding assay
    167–168
  reduction of   113
Coherency squared   199
Collaboration between biologists and mathematicians   5, 20
Communication
  between mathematicians and biologists   20
  channels   190
  endocrine   190
  of models   22
Comparative experiments   *103*   see also
    Controls, in comparative experiments
  design of   103–105
  statistical tests applied to   227
Compartments   *120*
  fusion of slime mould modelled using   187
  LH in the pituitary modelled using   218
Compartmental
  analysis   *120*–142
    inhomogeneity modelled by   31, 60
    simplification by   9
  models   *120*—142
    any number of compartments   135–142
    assumptions in   120
    FUNCTN subprograms   125–129, 132–135, 137–142, 278–282, 290
    combining experimental results   126
    computer routine   292
    definitions   120–122
    differential equations and   31, 122–123, 131–132
    dynamic systems analysed in terms of   115–142
    essentially empirical   120
    exchange   119–142
    forcing function   125–126, 131, 142, 294
    four-compartment model   137, 141–142
    identifiability analysis   122, 135
    inadequacies of linear models   121
    integration by Laplace transform   125, 128, 278, 294–295
    mammillary models   135–142
    non-linear dynamic models   88
    numerical integration   122, 131–142, 294–295
    one-compartment   122–123
    parameter interaction common in   87
    SAAM program   292
    simplifying assumptions   120
    stochastic elements   121
    terminology   120–122
    three compartment   123–124
    comparison of parallel and series   123–130, 132–135
    FUNCTN subprograms   127–130, 132–135, 278–281
    mean specific activity   279
    transients   120
    two compartment   123–124
      CA1 FUNCTN subprogram   125–128, 135, *278*–279, 281
      Zilversmit criterion   125
    uniqueness   121
    variable rate constants   121
    zinc transport   123–130
Competitive protein-binding assays
  155–170   see also   Ligand binding to macromolecules
  association constant of ligand   288
  association, dissociation rate constants   170
  characterization, importance of   170
  confidence intervals   169
  cross reaction   156–157
  empirical models   160–170
    advantages of   160–162
    Healey's model   *162*–165
    interpolation using   155–156, 160
    logit-log   162
    RIAH FUNCTN subprogram   162–165, *289*
    sigmoidal   162–165
    spline functions   165–167
  experimental conditions   157–160, 169
  maximization of response   169
  misclassification   156, 160
  non-specific binding   156, 160, 162–163, 168
  optimization   169–170
  parallelism   157
  precision   156, 169
  principles of   155
  sensitivity   156, *168*–169
  separation of free and bound fractions   146–147, 156, 170
  simulation of   164–165
  testosterone assay   157–160
  theoretical models   156–160
    difficulties in   156, 160–161
    MASSACT FUNCTN subprogram   156, 284–286
    optimization of assay   155–156, 160, 169–170
    RIA FUNCTN subprogram   157–160, 288
  thermodynamics of   170
  tracer and unlabelled ligand binding differently   156–157
  variance in   167–168
Complex
  behaviours of interacting oscillators   188
  frequency domain   33–*34*, 37   see also
    Spectral density function

Subject Index

Complex frequency domain
  analysis of biological systems 41
  response to addition of oestradiol in ovulatory cycle 223
  roots 44, 153–155
  spatial behaviour 61
  stimulus-response activities in endocrinology 53
  systems studied by finite level modelling 216
Complexity in biological systems 6–25
  affects feedback analysis 46
  computers and 20
  constrained by evolution 11
  controlling conditions of study 7
  depends on numbers of events observed 11
  from rhythm interactions 189
  hierarchies and 10–11
  individual variation and 12–13
  model of, leading to organized simplicity 14–16
  ovulatory cycle 203–204, 225
  and reductionism 4
Components of a system 6, 23, 53
  in ovulatory cycle model 203–204, 223–225
Computer
  advantages of 20–21
  analogue 31, 74–75, 77
  digital 75–77
  fallibility of 19
  hybrid 77
  and models 20–22
  limitations in using 6, 9, 21
  mystical powers attributed to 19
  programming languages 76 see also FORTRAN
  programs 75–77
    BMDX85 292
    CSMP 76
    biological 77
    DESIGN 109, 111, 134–135, 250, 253–254, 268–277
    fallacy-prone 22
    MIMIC 76
    MLAB 292
    are models 22
    MODFIT 89–102, 116–119, 250–260
    need description and verification 22
    NLIN 292
    NON-LIN 292
    ovulatory cycle models 211, 217, 223
    packages 76, 291–292
    SAAM 292
    SIMUL 59–60, 76, 85, 87, 89, 91, 93–94, 149–150, 156, 165, 186, 250, 258, 260–266
    splines 36
    SPSS 196–197, 227, 234, 236, 239, 292
  subprograms
    CA1 FUNCTN 125–129, 135, 278–279, 281
    CA2 FUNCTN 132, 279–281
    CA2A FUNCTN 133–135, 281
    CA3 FUNCTN 137–142, 282
    CUBIC 286, 288
    DISCRIMINANT 239
    D02AEF see STIFF
    EIGEN 250, 258, 260
    EXPCUBE FUNCTN 96, 266
    FACTOR 234–236
    FCHISQ 250, 257–260, 268
    FIT 250–258, 260, 268
    FOLL FUNCTN 100–101, 267–268
    GENBIND FUNCTN 153–155, 287
    GGNOF 260, 265
    LIMIT FUNCTN 59–60, 186, 290
    MASSACT FUNCTN 111–114, 146–150, 156, 159–160, 284–286
    NONLINEAR 292
    NPAR TESTS 227–228, 230
    POLYNOM FUNCTN 99–100, 254, 267
    RESERVR FUNCTN 89–95, 125, 253, 266, 278
    RIA FUNCTN 157–160, 288
    RIAH FUNCTN 162–165, 289
    SERDES 268, 276–277
    SIN FUNCTN 192–194, 290
    SPECTRAL 196–197
    STIFF 253, 279–282, 290
    TCALC 268, 275
  three-dimensional molecules drawn by 21
Conception and birth as probability processes 226
Concepts
  abstract explored 18
  aim of computing is to test 22
  of biological development 55
  clarifying 25
  of control theory 53
  deficiencies shown 201, 224–225
  of feedback 45–54
  inspired, needed 17, 23–24
  of model compatible with data 2
  necessary for mathematics 18
  unifying 19
Conclusions suspect 24
Condition number 87–88, 90, 92, 98, 258, 265
Confidence
  intervals 249
    in auto-correlation coefficient 195
    in competitive protein-binding assays 169
    in median (Nair's test) 228
    in new observations 249
    non-parametric 228, 249
    in parameter estimates 249
    in a ratio (Fieller's theorem) 243, 249
    t-test, use in calculating 249
  in model 108, 111, 135, 276
Constraints see also Penalty functions
  of evolution on biological systems 11, 19

Constraints
  fundamental to system function 25
  on model by solubility of equations 2
  on parameter values 67–68, 83, 292
  parameter values as 8
  shown by simulation 14
Continuous
  equations
    compared with finite level models 68–69, 213
    not suitable 66
  systems 26, *29*, 76
    CSMP computer program 76
    MIMIC computer program 76
    SIMUL 260–266
Contraception
  modelled by limit cycles 221–222
  by steroids, simulated 215–216, 220
Contrasts 231–232, 248
Control
  in biological systems 55, 61
    by dynamics 62, 188
    by rhythms 189–191
  chart 249
  hierarchies *11*
  network in endocrinology 189
  principles 4 *see also* Organization
    of feedback systems 189–190, 221
  systems modelled in compartmental terms 121
  theory 37–54
    in endocrinology 53–54
Controls, in comparative experiments 103
  independent sample tests 232
  managing biological variation 12, 103–104
  matched pairs 104
  related sample tests 229–231
Controllability 190–191 *see also* Identifiability analysis
Convolution integrals 38–39 *see also* Deconvolution integrals
  in modelling the ovulatory cycle 219–220
Co-operativity 32
  producing limit cycles 63
  in receptor response 54
  in sequential binding model *143*, 152–155
Coronary system, auto-regulation of blood flow 41
Corpus luteum
  in models of ovulatory cycles 212, 216–218, 224
  transport of zinc in 123, 127–130, 135, 142
Correlation 244
  auto-correlation 191, 194–195
  factor analysis *233*, 235–236
  multivariate analysis 233
  oblique rotation of axes, effect on 234–235
  orthogonality 233
  between parameters *87*, 90, 92, 98, 258, 265
  principle component analysis 233
  relationship to covariance 244
Correlogram *195,* 197
Corticosteroid binding globulin (CBG)
  properties of 110–114, 146–150
  simulation of 110–114
Corticosteroids, circadian rhythms 172
Corticosterone 38, 68, 200
Corticotrophin releasing factor 50, 68
Cortisol
  feedback models 48, 50, 67–69
  models based on synthesis of 38
  secretion studied by frequency analysis 41
  three-dimensional drawing of 21
Covariance 87, 235, *243*–244
  analysis 104
  auto-correlation 194
  time-series analysis 194
Creativity and modelling 6–7, 17, 24
Critical range tests *231*–232, 248
Cross-correlation *198*
Cross-covariance function 198
Cross-linking of endocrine systems 190
Cross-reaction 156–157
CSMP program 76
Cubic equation
  Cardan's method of solution 286
  CUBIC subprogram *286,* 288
  fitted to follicle growth data 99–101
  ligand binding to macromolecule 146, 284, 288
CUBIC subprogram *286,* 288
Cumulative
  frequency histogram, analysis of residuals 84
  sum control chart (CUSUM) *249*
Curvature matrix *88,* 257–258
  condition number *87–88*
  sensitivity coefficients 87
Curve fitting 34–36 *see also* Empirical models
Cusp model 65
CUSUM control chart *249*
Cycle, ovulatory *see* Oestrous cycle; Ovulatory cycle modelling
Cycles *see also* Oscillations; Rhythms
  associated with the ovulatory cycle 203
  biochemical, conditions for brevity and stability 16
  of responses 57
  of wave propagation 62
Cyclic
  3′,5′-adenosine monophosphate
    assay of 163
    and calcium feedback loop 175
    ovarian tissue production of 228–232
  data *see* Limit cycles; Oscillations; Rhythms; Time-series

Subject Index 313

Cyclic
   solutions of equations 202
   in modelling the ovulatory cycle 204–208, 210
   non-, model of rhythm 212
Cyclicity, events drive or are driven by 202, 216

$D0$, difference in response between models 107–109, 111–112, 135, 276
Damped non-linear feedback systems, magnification of 50
Damping of oscillations 42, 44, 56, 59–60, 174
Data *see* Experimental data
Decision functions 212–213, 217–219, 223 *see also* Thresholds
Deconvolution integrals 39 *see also* Convolution integrals
Degrees of freedom 83, 92, 96, 99, *242*, 254
   F-test and 248
   reduced chi-square and 246
   t-test and 247
Delta function *see* Impulse inputs
Dependence of parameters 87, 97, *257*–258, 265
Dependent variables 7–8, 18, 76, 254 *see also* Variables
   deterministic 29
   in differentials 26
   evolutionary operation (EVOP) 81
   maximization of 169
   more than one 77, 282, 290, 292
   optimization 80–88
   uncertainty in, measured by variance 82
Description
   mathematical, of biological models 26–73
   of models 22
Design of experiments *see* Experimental design
DESIGN program 109, 250, *268*—277
   comparison of parallel and series compartmental models 123–135
   examples of output 111, 135
   input format for 253–254, 275
   SERDES subprogram *276*
   simulation of binding of steroids to proteins 110–114
   TCALC subprogram 268, *275*
Deterministic
   behaviour *11*, 29
   equation producing stochastic outcome 57
   input, assumption challenged 224
   models
      contrasted with stochastic 226
      simplex search methods 81
   system 26, *29*, 67
      apparently random response from 58
Development in biology 5, 45, 54–66
   a model for 64
   not reversible 64
Diagrams 9
   analogue notation in 9

   block 9, 39–40, 67
   Bode *40*–41, 49, 51
   in describing models 22
   drawn by computer 21
   flow 9
   stereo-, of cortisol 21
   symbol and arrow 9
Dialysis, equilibrium
   advantages of 156, 160
   CBG 110–114, 146–150
   competitive protein-binding assays 170
   inability to distinguish between binding models using data from 154
   pregnancy plasma 146–150
   SBG 110–114, 146–150
Diapause in insects 176, 178
Difference equations *see* Equations, difference
Differential equation models *see also* Compartmental models; Dynamic systems; Integration; Stiff differential equations
   AUX subprograms 133, 279, 281–282
   ease of definition 122
   FUNCTN subprograms 132–135, 137–142, 279–282
   generalized mammillary compartmental model 135–142
   integrated before comparing with data 28–29, 88
   LIMIT FUNCTN subprogram 290
   MODFIT program 253
   SIMUL program 260
   writing mathematical descriptions of 28, 122–123, 131–132, 294–295
Differential equations 26–31 *see also* Compartmental models; Differential equation models; Integration; Partial derivatives; Stiff differential equations
   comparison with data 28–29
   in compartmental analysis 31, 120–142, 294–295
   conditions for use 27, 29–30
   with cyclic solutions in modelling the ovulatory cycle 204–207, 213
   defining 30
   to describe rhythms 176
   eliminated in ovulatory cycle model 213–216
   generalize algebraic equations 27
   instability in 56, 58–64, 88
   in modelling
      biological response 174
      the ovulatory cycle 205–206, 208, 210–212, 217, 219, 223
   order of 88
   ordinary, in catastrophe theory 64
   partial 30–32, 60, 64
   to produce limit cycles and chaotic behaviour 58, 290
   stability 43–44

Differential equations
  steady states from 30
  in theoretical models 31
  why used 27
Differentials 26–27
  defining attractor surfaces 64
  at equilibrium 42
  as operators 33
  at steady states 42–43
Differentiation, biological 53, 61
  metaphoric models of 64–66
Diffusion *see also* Transport
  and chaotic behaviour 58
  in compartmental analysis 31, 120, 122
  determines dynamic behaviour 61–62
  and differentiation 66
  near enzymes 30
  in feedback systems 49
  instantaneous 62, 290
  and limit cycles 63, 290
  of metabolites neglected 31
  in modelling
    interacting rhythms 187–188
    spatial inhomogeneity 60–61
  rates and differential equations 28
  in structural cell components 30
  and substrate inhibition producing instability 63
Dimensional analysis 8
Discontinuities *see also* Thresholds; Decision functions
  described continuously 212
  in phases of rhythms 181–182
  producing cyclicity 208–209
  in modelling the ovulatory cycle 205, 218
Discontinuous
  operator 207
  systems 65 *see also* Discrete systems
Discrete
  measurement of rhythms 179, 196
  systems 29—30, 76
    biological 26
    example of instability in 56–58
  time modelling in biology 69
Discriminant analysis 238–240
  classification of individuals by 238
  ovarian follicle steroid production 238–240
  training set 238
DISCRIMINANT, SPSS subprogram 239
Disposal, irreversible 118–119 *see also* Clearance
Distribution, statistical
  form unknown, suitable tests 232
  log-normal 73
  non-parametric tests, irrelevance of, in 228
  normal (Gaussian) 71, 73, 165, 227, 234, 242
  assumptions of 73
  calculation of parameter uncertainty requires 79
  and discriminant analysis 238
  experimental uncertainty 73
  and individuality 12
  measurement error 73
  method of least squares 79
  multivariate analysis 234
  tests for 227, 234, 246
  time-series analysis 192
  z-score 244
  skewed 73
Disturbances *see also* Perturbation; Stimuli
  from antagonistic hormones 52
  continual, in endocrine systems 53
  in homogeneous systems 61
  to limit cycles 181–188
  in ovarian function 190
Divergence *107 see also* Residuals
  between model and data 245–246
  between models 106–107, 110–114, 275
D02AEF subprogram *see* STIFF subprogram
Dose 122, *145,* 147, 162, 282
  minimum detectable (sensitivity) *168–169*
Drugs
  affecting auto-regulation of blood flow 41
  clearance of 115–116
  compartmental analysis 115, 120, 122, 135, 137
  effect on linear response 38
  opening feedback loops 51
  removal of subsystems by 40
  responses of circadian rhythms to 172
Dynamic *see also* Compartmental models; Differential equation models; Integration; Stiff differential equations
  behaviour of catastrophe model 65
  control in biology 62
  descriptions related to observable parts 66
  models 28
    behaviour of non-linear 61
    of clearance 115–119
    of discrete time data 69
    linear 33
    tests for stability in linear 43
    writing differential equations of 122–123, 131–132
  pools of LH in the pituitary 208
  stability in endocrinology 53
  systems 28, 30
    tracers in *120*

EIGEN subprogram 250, *258,* 260
Eigenvalues
  calculated by EIGEN subprogram *258*
  condition number and 87–88
  and stability 43–44
  in feedback 49

Subject Index 315

Elephants
  empirical growth model of 95–99, 266
  population dynamics of 76
Emergent behaviour of models 4
Empirical
  devices used in ovulatory cycle model 223
  equations 26, 34
    choice of 35
    converting data for comparison with differential models 28
    to describe pools 9
    in describing models 22
    in determining transfer functions 37
    in finite level models 67
    in ovulatory cycle models 202, 212–213, 219
    too restrictive 35
    in self-modelling 36
    splines 35–36, 165–167
    simple, from complex interactions 35
  modelling 34–41, 224
    of feedback systems 47
    of instability and development 56
    using thresholds 208
  models *3,* 23, 25, 74, 103, 155
    clearance from the blood stream as 89–95, 115
    competitive protein-binding assays 143, 160–170
    disadvantages of 3, 8, 35, 74
    equations of, are non-unique 74
    exponentials, sum of, in 89–90, 125
    frequency domain analysis in biology 196
    growth of elephants 95–99
    Healey's, of competitive protein-binding 162–165
    often over-parameterized 100
    ovarian follicular wall growth 99–102
    parameters may have no physical meaning 74, 125
    of rat oestrous cycle 212
    results, explaining 61, 184
Endocrine systems (generalized discussions of)
  behaviour described by transfer functions 37
  controllability and observability in 190
  convolution integrals in 39
  empirical modelling of 34
  involved in homeostasis, development 45
  measurement of steady states in 53
  modelled by feedback 46, 52–54
  respond to environment 45
  rhythms in 189–191
  suited to finite level modelling 66
  theoretical modelling of 31
  usefulness of modelling 6
Endometrium 123–126, 130, 278
Energy
  exchange with environment 42, 55
  metabolism and hormone action 54
  for response to hormone signals 190
Entropy in isolated and open systems 54–55
Entrainment
  of a limit cycle 185–186
  of nerves to noise frequency 186
  of rhythms 59, *174*
    biological to geophysical 172, 175–176, 178, 181
    phase changing by 181–185
Enzyme
  chains and limit cycles 63
  kinetics
    assumptions in theoretical models of 31
    Lineweaver-Burke plot 70–72, 243
    Michaelis-Menten equation *70–72,* 78
    simulation of 31, 77
    substrate binding 143
Enzymes
  circadian rhythms in activity of 171
  determine steady states in cells 43
  dynamic instability in 61–63
  and rhythm control 175–176
Epidemiology, difference equations used in 56
Epigenetic landscape 64
Episodic hormone release *see* Pulsatile hormone release
Equations *see also* Differential, Empirical equations
  aim of modelling 26
  algebraic 26–28, 30, 217
    in theoretical modelling 31
    used with rapid reactions 220
  changed at fixed times in modelling rhythms 212
  constraint of model to soluble 2, 20
  defining model 30–31
  describe how interpreted by computer 22
  describing
    models 7, 22
    rhythms 173
  difference 30, 56, 58, 211–212
  minimum number 31
  multiple in ovulatory cycle model 218
  nature of 18
  not used in some modelling 2
  partial differential 30–31, 60, 64
  redundant 31
  simplified by linear approximations 10, 41, 49–50, 52, 81–82, 91
  solved 31
  state *31*
  variety of, capable of simulating data 224
Equifinality in linear systems 43
Equilibrium 26, *42,* 54–55, 120
  constant *see* Association constant
  effect of catalysts on 43
  of fast processes 65
  importance of distance from 61

Error 69, *243 see also* Coefficient of variation; Confidence intervals; Standard deviation; Uncertainty; Variance
  actuating, in feedback 47
  bar 78
  prevents estimation of "true" parameter values 74
  systematic *see* Bias
  Type I, Type II *245*
Erythrocytes, zinc transport in 130
Evolution
  and dependence of biological systems on time 26
  ease of selecting organized simplicity in 16
  explaining, by physical laws 54
  history of mathematical modelling of 6
  principles of, derived from reductionism? 5
  providing constraints on kinds of development 11
  theory of, and choice of biological models 19
  through random fluctuations 55
Evolutionary operation (EVOP) 81, 169
Evolving organization in biology 54
EXPCUBE FUNCTN subprogram 96, *266*
  growth of elephants 95–99
Experimental
  basis of ideas 1, 19
  data 13
    amount required 13–14, 83
    analyzing rhythmic 173, 191–200
    are based on models 1
    comparison with
      models 1–2, 5, 19, 30–31, 74–102
      differential equations *see* Integration
    deficient 201, 221–225
    described empirically 34–35
    in describing models 22
    determines quality of support for model 13
    different kinds of 13
    ignoring variance in biological 213
    objective comparison with models 17
    quantized 213–214
    related to state variables 31
    summarized by interpolation 34
    to support assumptions 22
    used in modelling the ovulatory cycle 203–204, 213–214
  design 1, 5, 20, 73, 103–114
    efficient 25, 103–114
    factorial 105, 169
    importance of experimental frame in 103
    parameter interaction 86
    sequential methods *105*–114, 170, 268–276
  frame *7*, 23, 97–98, 108
    and cross reactants 156–157
    defined by physical constraints 106
    in description of models 22
    and general statements 7
    importance to experimental design 103
    influences condition number 88, 90
    and ligand-macromolecule interaction 145, 149
    in models of ovulatory cycle 204, 223–224
    and physiological conditions 7, 23, 224
    predictions outside 7
    restricted
      in analytical experiments 105
      leads to parameter interaction 86
      rigid in empirical modelling 35, 88
      selection of 23
      simplifications by restricting 9
    SIMUL program 92
    widened in comparative experiments 105
  measurement of feedback 52
  observables related to dynamic descriptions 31, 66
  observations *see also* Experimental data
    on response of rhythms to stimuli 176
  techniques, invention of 23, 201
  uncertainty *see* Uncertainty, experimental; Variance
Experiments
  biological, at steady states 30
  framework for, from control theory 53
  limits of feedback control measured by 49
  need for interplay of model and 1, 12–13, 17–19, 23
  needed in ovulatory cycle 221, 223–224
  new suggested 14, 17–18, 25, 61
  role of, in studying biological rhythms 173
  suggested from finite level models 67
  for testing model of rhythms 173
Explanation
  of biological functioning 23
  from models 3, 5, 7
  of observations 6, 25
Exponential decay
  clearance
    of PMSG from blood 38, 89–95, 116–119
    of ^{65}Zn from the blood plasma of rabbits 125
  difficulty of fitting models of, to data 87
  empirical model of 89, 116–118
  example of model fitting to 89–95, 116
  mammillary compartmental model of 135–142
  multiexponential model, examples 116–119, 125, 135–142
  non-linear dynamic models, of, special problems 88
  parameter interaction likely in models of 87
  RESERVR subprogram 125, *266*
Exponentials *see also* Exponential decay
  in curve fitting 35, 87, 89–95, 116, 125, 135–142, 266
  describing growth 95–99, 266

Exponentials
   in model of ovulatory cycles   219
   and non-linear responses   32–33
Extrapolation *see also* Predictions from models
   none from empirical modelling   35
   outside experimental frames   7

F-test   105, 227, *248*
   must preceed a *t*-test   247
$f(x)$, function of x 8
FACTOR, SPSS subprogram   234, 236
Factor analysis   *233–237*
   "explaining" correlation   233
   rotation of axes   234
   steroid production of ovarian follicles   234–237
Factorial experiments   105, 169
Factors (independent variables)   *105*
   advantages of varying several simultaneously   105
   classification   234
   clustering   110
   graph   234–235
   interaction of (non-linearity)   105
   summary variables   233
"Facts", dependence on models   1
Falsification of models   19
FCHISQ subprogram   250, *257–260*, 268
Feedback
   activating stimuli for   53
   concepts of   45–54
   control   46–48
      in endocrinology   54
   effectiveness of   48, 50–52
      examples of models of endocrine systems showing   54
   gain and magnification of   50–52
   homeostatic in biology   28
   loop   8, 190
      generalized   50
      opening   51
   loops
      interacting   50, 52
      with unidentified components   51
   in models of the ovulatory cycle   201–225
   negative   *46–47*
      behaviour of models containing   48
      biological   47, 171, 174
      calcium/cAMP   175
      characteristics of   47–48
      inadequate concept for endocrine control   191
      loop   50
         mechanisms for, in endocrinology   52–54
         in modelling ovulatory cycles   201–225
   positive   *46*, 55 *see also* Instability
      in Raschevsky-Turing metaphor   65
   prediction from   202
   producing limit cycles   63
   system
      bicyclist as   45
      energy supply for   45
      very sensitive control in   221
Feedforward   *46*, 52
Fieller's theorem   146, 243, 249
Finite level modelling   30, 65, 66–69
   applicable to qualitative results   13
   experimental error and   10
   and individual variation   12
   of ovulatory cycle   213–216
   symplifying data by   10
Fish, growth of   96
FIT subprogram   *250–258*, 260, 268
Fitted y value   78, 90–93
Fitting function, linearization of
   Gauss-Newton method   81
   Marquardt-Levenberg algorithm   82, 254–257, 292
FL (LAMBDA)   92, 112, 136, *254–257*
Flux   *121*
   calcium in rabbit   131
   carnitine in rat   131
   compartmental models   123
   corpus luteum zinc   128–130
   endometrial zinc   126
   zinc in rabbit   126, 128–130
Fly, flesh
   annual rhythm in diapause   176
   circadian rhythm in eclosion of   182–183
Foetus, transport of zinc to   123
FOLL FUNCTN subprogram 100–101, *267–268*
Follicle, ovarian
   atresia of, characterized by steroid output   234–238
   cAMP production   228, 230–231
   cultured   234–238
   FOLL FUNCTN subprogram   100–101, *267–268*
   gonadotrophins influencing   228–231
   human 238
   idealized   100–102
   mass of wall   99–102, 267–268
   models of ovulatory cycles concerning   203–204, 208–209, 211–213, 217–220, 223–224
   morphology   236
   ovulatory, preovulatory distinguished   238
   PMSG influencing   116–117
   POLYNOM FUNCTN subprogram   99–100
   sheep   234–238
   steroid production characterized by
      discriminant analysis   238–240
      factor analysis   240
   thickness of wall of   99–102
Follicle stimulating hormone *see also* Gonadotrophins
   assay of   163
   in a negative feedback loop   205, 208–209, 211–214, 216–220, 222–224
   in ovulatory cycle models   203–205, 209–210, 212

Follicle stimulating hormone
  plasma clearance rate in sheep 118
Follicular phase 203, 217, 222
Forcing functions *30*
  advantages and disadvantages of 125, 131, 142
  FUNCTN subprograms using 125–126, 186, 278–281, 294
  clearance from the blood stream modelled as a 125
  in "natural" responses 43
  periodic 40, 185–186
FORTRAN 76–77, 89, 250–253, 260, 268
Fourier
  analysis *see* Spectral density function
  transform *196, 199*
Fraction of dose administered 122, 282
Free-to-bound ratio *see* Ratio
Frequency *173*
  altered by rhythmic stimuli *see* Entrainment
  characteristics of biological systems 40
    compared 41
    difficulties in measuring 41
    from step or impulse inputs 41
  distributions *see* Distribution
  domain, analysis in the 40–41, 191, 195–197
    of feedback systems 41, 47, 49
    gain in 40, 51
    menstrual cycle temperature variation example 197
    resonant 49
    of time-series 191–192
Friedman test 230–231
FSH *see* Follicle stimulating hormone
Functionality 67–68

Gain
  of feedback loop 48–52 *see also* Open loop gain
  in frequency analysis 40
  high, in biological systems 52
  spectrum *199*
Gamma-globulin 157
Gaussian distribution *see* Distribution, normal
GENBIND FUNCTN subprogram 153–155, *287*
General statements
  from mathematics 12, 18–19
  from modelling 7
  not made by computers 21
Generalized mathematical descriptions
  of dynamics 66 *see also* Metaphoric modelling
  of endocrine systems using control theory 54
  of instabilities in biology 64–66
  of linear system behaviour 40
  not global for non-linear instability 61
  of system behaviour in frequency analysis 40
Genes
  behaviour of 65
  a model of 14–16
  and circadian rhythms 176
  and differentiation 64, 66
  directing development 45
  information from, controlling feedback response 52
  repression of, and limit cycles 63
Genetics, difference equations used in 56
GGNOF subprogram 260, 265
GH (growth hormone) 200
Glycolysis
  oscillations in 62
  theoretical modelling of 31
GnRH *see* following entry
Gonadotrophin releasing hormone
  assay of 163
  feedback 206–208, 223
  in models of the ovulatory cycle 203–204, 211, 217, 222–223
Gonadotrophins *see also* Follicle stimulating hormone; Human chorionic gonadotrophin; Luteinizing hormone; Pregnant mare serum gonadotrophin
  analyzing effect on ovarian tissue 228–232
  beta-subunit sequences analyzed 226
  influence on
    ovarian follicular development 99
    zinc transport 123–130
  in modelling ovulatory cycle 203–204, 212, 218–219, 221–224
  plasma clearance rates 115–119
  rhythmic secretion of 190
Granulosa cells
  mass of 99
  production of cAMP analyzed 228, 230–231
Graphic display
  by computer 21, 75
  CSMP program 76
  light-pen 76
  MLAB program 292
  three-dimensional drawing of cortisol 21
Growth 32, 53
  of elephants, empirical model 95–99
  EXPCUBE FUNCTN subprogram 96, *266*
  hormone 200
  of ovarian follicle 99–102

Haemoglobin interaction with oxygen 23, 143
Half-time (half-life) *see also* Clearance
  of disposal *119*
  inappropriate term in compartmental models 121
Hamster testes 176–178
Hand calculations
  elephant growth 99
  of integration 29
  non-parametric tests 227
Harmonic analysis *see* Spectral density function
hCG *see* Human chorionic gonadotrophin

Subject Index

Healey's empirical model *162*–165
  RIAH FUNCTN subprogram *289*–290
  testosterone assay 163–165
Heat shock, models of effects on mitosis 184–185
Hierarchical levels *10*–11
  change between forms of stability 55
  collaboration when working at different 5
  and evolution 11
  and lumping 10
  and reproduction 45
  and stochastic and deterministic behaviour 11
High-affinity binding *see* Specific binding
Hill coefficient 162, 289
HIOMT (Hydroxyindole-O-methyltransferase) 178–180
Historical fate of models 17
History
  determines future organization 64
  effects of previous 12
  of mathematical modelling in evolution 6
  of mathematics 18
  well-tried paths of 1
Hologram, biological 189
Homeostasis 45, 174
  biological feedback systems producing 45, 52, 171
  and biological rhythms 171
  model of complexity producing responses like 16
  and reproductive function 45
Homogeneous
  concentrations assumed, in enzyme kinetic modelling 31
  systems
    becoming organized 55
    oscillations in 61
  variables in differential equations 29–30
Homogenizing a car 23–24
Homology of protein structures 226
Hormones *see also* Gonadotrophins; Steroid hormones
  antagonistic 52
  assay of 155
  binding of protein 224
  circadian rhythms in 171
  clearance 115
  and differentiation of tissues 66
  communication by 190
  energy for response to 190
  episodic release of and implications 39, 189–190, 200, 213, 221
  generally spatially inhomogeneous 60
  influence on calcium and zinc transport 123–131
  insect 176
  interaction with receptors 54, 144–146, 190, 221, 223
  involved in response, homeostasis, development 45
  levels of
    averaged, inappropriate 12, 213
    in blood plasma, of reproductive 204
    determination of pulsatile secretion of 39
    effect of, over time 39
    model of mechanism determines measurements of 2
  menstrual cycle temperature variation 193
  production modelled by finite levels 67, 213–216
  relative potencies of 118
  rhythms and their interactions 171, 176, 189
  secretion inhibition in feedback 48
  stimulation, influenced by membrane rhythms 175
HPL (human placental lactogen) 167
Human chorionic gonadotrophin (hCG) 228–229
Human placental lactogen (HPL) 167
Hydroxyindole-O-methyltransferase (HIOMT) 178–180
Hypothalamus
  feedback on 48, 50, 52, 206–207
  in ovulatory cycle 203, 211, 217, 221, 223
Hypotheses
  of causality in ovulatory cycle models 202, 213–214, 216–217
  confirming by reductionism 5
  in model discrimination 108
  in multivariate analysis 233, 235
  null 226–228, *245*
  testing 25, 72–73, 245
    of, that model describes data 19
    too many 19, 66, 212
  working, from comparing frequency characteristics 41

Identifiability analysis *122*, 135
Identification of variables 67
Identifying differences between samples *see* Critical range tests
Ill-conditioning of matrix 258
Imagination in modelling 1, 7, 17, 24
Impulse inputs *37*–38
  and the characteristic equation 43
  clearance rate of 116
  convolution integral as sum of 39
  frequency characteristics from 41
  as stimuli to inherent rhythms 181–185
Independent
  samples
    more than two, compared 232
    two, compared 228–229
  variables *7*–8, 105 *see also* Factors
    assumed to be free of uncertainty 82
    choice of effective values of 13
    effect reduced by feedback 48
    equation using single, not helpful in physiology 35

Independent variables
  multivariate analysis 232, 234
    restrictions of range 9, 105
      lead to parameter interaction 86
    several 77, 232, 234, 292
    time as 26, 35 see also Clearance; Compartmental models; Exponential decay
Indeterminate see Stochastic
Individual
  mortality, price of adaption 45
  variation 12–13, 26, 103 see also Biological variation
    basis of data for generalized models 12
    and experimental error 12
    and finite level modelling 12, 69
    ignoring 213
    and normal distributions 12
    and use of control samples 12
Individuals
  blood plasma hormone levels from 205
  classification of 12–13
  measurements on, to detect rhythms 12, 189
  self-modelling for data from 12, 36–37
Information
  for discrimination *107*
  relationship to precision 106
  in rhythmic secretion of hormones 189–190
Infusion
  into Ca^{2+} control feedback loop 52
  causing cessation of pulsed hormone release 207
  clearance of hormones during any schedule of 38
  of corticosterone studied 38
  response to, of oestradiol and GnRH modelled 221–222
  short, as impulse input 38
Inhibitory reactions in feedback 50 see also Sign reversal
Inhibition of hormone secretion 48, 54
Inhomogeneity
  with positive feedback 65
  spatial, and stability behaviour 60–61, 63
Inhomogeneous systems 26, 30
  modelled by compartmental analysis 31
Initial
  conditions
    determine dynamic behaviour 61, 188
    difficulties in obtaining 41
    and equifinality 43
    homogeneous, produce inhomogeneity 61
    in Laplace transformation 34, 37, 294
    in model of oestrous cycle 211, 213
    need for, in dynamic models 88
    and non-linearity 33, 43
    as parameters to be optimized 88, 137, 140, 282, 290
    similar, leading to divergent outcomes 57, 181–185
  parameter estimates
    importance in gradient search 81–82
    required as input to programs 91, 109, 253–254
  volume of distribution 119
Injection
  described by impulse input 38
  of hormones 38
  volume 119
Input see also Disturbances; Factors; Impulse inputs; Perturbation; Stimuli
  analysis of response to rhythmic 40–41
  calculated by convolution integrals 39
  critical value of, for change of behaviour 55
  to feedback loops 49–52
  in finite level modelling 67, 69
  format for
    compartmental analysis FUNCTN subprograms 278
    DESIGN program 253–254, 275
    MODFIT program 253–254, 278, 282
    SIMUL program 253–254, 265, 278
  frequency characteristics from step or impulse 41
  functions 37–40
  and output 7, 39
  in ovulatory cycle model 204
  parameters as 8
  random, in endocrine systems 53
  small, for linear approximations 41
  step versus periodic in biology 41
  stochastic, tests ability 45
Insects
  breeding, number of 56
  hormonal diapause 176, 178
  larvae growth 23
Instability see also Unstable
  critical state for 55
  example of 56–58
    non-linear equations showing 61–64
  evolving through 55
  in feedback systems 46, 49, 65
  generalized descriptions of, in biology 64–66
  mathematics beyond 54–66
  structural 64
  at thresholds 208–209
Insulin
  feedback model concerning 54
  feedforward in release of 47
  model of secretion 175
  sign reversal in feedback loop producing 48
Integer parameters, optimization of 151
Integral, form of, in stable linear models 43
Integrated equation dynamic models see also Differential equation models
  CA1 FUNCTN subprogram 125–129, 278–279, 294–295
Integration 28–29, 31, 88, 122, 131 see also Stiff differential equations
  analytical 28, 117, 122, 294–295

Subject Index

Integration
  analytical
    compartmental model, Laplace transforms 294–295
    general solution of compartmental model 137
    by Laplace transforms 28, 34, 125, 294–295
    restrictions on 115
  approximate 117
  constants 27–28, 30, 34
  numerical
    AUX subprograms define models for 279, 281–282, 290
    computer removes restrictions on 20, 29, 115, 122, 131
    at discrete intervals 29
    generalized mammillary model 135–142
    MODFIT program, differential equation models 253
    speed of 77
    three-compartment models 132, 135
    two-compartment models 131–132
  range (step length) 281
  Stewart-Hamilton equation 117
Interference, technological 24
Interpolation 34
  competitive protein-binding assays 143, 156, 160, 169
  mass of ovarian wall tissue 102
  in self-modelling 36
Iodide transport 292
Iodine
  albumin, labelled with 137–138
  radioactive tracer 137–138, 156, 158
Irreversible loss 118–119 see Clearance
ISEED 91, 265
Isochron 181, 183–187
Isolated systems 42, 54, 120
Iterations in search algorithm 80

KEY 91, 165, 265–266
Kidney
  auto-regulation of blood flow in 41
  transformation of steroids in 54
Knots 36, 167
Kolmogorov-Smirnov test 227, 234, 246
Kruskal-Wallis test 232

Label, radioactive see Tracers
Lag 194–195, 197, 200
  in linear system analysis 198
  transport, in feedback loops 49
Laplace transforms
  in clearance of hormones 38
  conditions for use of 34
  and impulse input 37
  of input to block diagrams 40
  integration by 28, 34
    of compartmental model 120, 125, 128, 278, 294–295

linear operator 33
  starting conditions in 37
  in transfer functions 37–38
Latent roots 87–88
Laws, physical
  applied to biology 4–5
  of conservation 30
  described by differential equations 27
  empirical modelling and 3
  explaining evolution 54
  first order rate 122
  growth models and 96
  of mass action 28, 30, 61
  theoretical modelling and 3
Least squares, method of 35, 78–80
LH see Luteinizing hormone
Ligand binding to macromolecules see also Competitive protein-binding assay
  allosterism in 143, 152–155
  association constant 143–146
  assumptions in measuring 146
  choosing between models of 154–155
  classes of sites 143, 145
  comparison of models 149
  confidence intervals 169
  co-operativity 143, 152–155
  corticosteroid binding globulin 110–114, 146–150
  dose 145
  equilibrium constant 143–146
  experimental technique 146–147
  GENBIND FUNCTN subprogram 153–155, 287
  general model 151, 153–155
    compound, factor terms 287
  independent classes of sites 143, 284–285
  infinite dose 162, 289
  integer number of sites 145, 151, 287
  interactive sites 152–155
  low-affinity 110–114, 145, 284–285
  MASSACT FUNCT subprogram 111–114, 147–150, 156, 158–160, 284–286
  mathematical identity of independent site and sequential binding models 153
  models of
    empirical 162–165, 289–290
    theoretical 111–114, 143, 147–150, 156, 157–160, 168, 284–286, 288
  molar ratio 151, 153
  non-interactive 143, 184–285
  non-specific 110–114, 145–146, 147–151, 158, 168, 284–285
  precision 156, 169
  pregnancy plasma binding 146–150
  simulated 110–114
  reversible association 143–146
  RIA FUNCTN subprogram 157–160, 168, 288
  RIAH FUNCTN subprogram 162–165, 289

Ligand binding to macromolecules
  saturable   285
  Scatchard plot   144
  sequence on interaction   143
  sequential   152–155
  sensitivity   156, 168–169
  sex steroid binding globulin (SBG)   110–114, 146, 150
  simulation using DESIGN program   110–114
  single class of sites   110, 159–160, 288
  specific sites   110, *145*, 147–150, 284–286
  statistical considerations   150
  stochiometric binding constants   154
  testosterone   110, 146–150, 157–160, 167–168
  tracer binding differently from ligand   156–157
  zero dose   162, 289
Light, effect on biological rhythms   171–172, 174, 176–178, 180–183, 190, 204, 211
Light-pen   76
Likelihood   107–*108*, 275–276
  confidence   108
  divergence and   107
  ratio   *108*, 276
    examples   113, 135
  test   107–108
Limit cycles   *58*–60, 62, 181 see also Rhythms, inherent
  behaviour from chemical reactions   63
  biological control from   171
  in biology   59, 61, 174
  and catastrophes   65
  coupling   174, 186–188
  disturbances in models involving   181–188
  entrainment   185–186
  examples illustrating   61–64
  in feedback loops   49, 63
  interpretation of phase changes   182–185
  LIMIT FUNCTN subprogram   *290*
  models using   175
    for biological rhythms   171
    of hormone release   207
    of the timing of mitosis   182–185
  type of model for ovulatory cycle   212, 221–222
LIMIT FUNCTN subprogram   59–60, 186, *290*
Linear
  analysis of non-linear systems   38
  approximations   10, 44, 49, 81
  components, order of acting   33
  equations   32
    integration of   34
  feedback system analysis   46–47, 49–52
  models
    compartmental analysis   *120*–142
    multivariate analysis   232–240
    parameter estimation in   85
    in parameters   *78*
    of response   174
    stepwise regression   87
  sensitivity coefficients   78
  tests for stability of   43–44
  operator   32–33
  systems   26, *32*
    analysis in the frequency domain   40–41
    controllability and observability in   190
    dynamics of   33
    and equifinality   43
    represented by block diagrams   40
    response to sinusoidal stimuli   33
    studied by
      convolution integrals   38–39
      transfer functions   37–38
    techniques of analysis   32
Linearity   *32*–34
  in compartmental analysis   120
  effects of drugs and manipulation on   38
  limits on   38
  in physiological systems   32
  tests of   32–33, 38
Linearization of fitting function   81–82, 91–92, 254
Lineweaver-Burke plot   70–72, 244
Liver   54, 123, 130
Loadings see Multivariate analysis, parameters
Logic
  biological   19
  in mathematics   18–19
Logit-log transformation   162 see also Transformation of data
Low-affinity binding see Non-specific binding
Lumping   9
  in block diagrams   40
  in clearance of PMSG from blood plasma   140
  comments on, in model description   22
  and hierarchical levels   10
  simplification by   9–10, 60, 217
Luteal
  phase   203–204, 219–220
  tissue see Corpus luteum
Luteinizing hormone see also Gonadotrophins
  assay of   163
  biphasic secretion of   208
  feedback loop   206–210
  in models of ovulatory cycles   203–206, 208–224
  multiple frequencies in levels   172
  pituitary pools of   208, 217–218
  plasma clearance of, in sheep   118
Lyapunov functions   44

Magnification of feedback   48, *50*—51
Mammillary compartmental models
  FUNCTN subprograms   125–128, 132, 137–142, 278–282
  clearance of PMSG   139–142
  difficulties   135
  extensions   141–142
  transport of albumin   137–138

Subject Index

Man, the nature of   24
Mann-Whitney test *see* Wilcoxon two-sample randomization test
Markov chains and processes   30, *195*
Marquardt-Levenberg algorithm   82, 254–257, 292
Mass
  action law *see* Laws, physical
  of elephants   95–99
  of ovarian follicle wall   99–102
MASSACT FUNCTN subprogram   146, *284–286*
  competitive protein-binding assays   156, 159–160
  testosterone binding   111–114, 147–150
Matched pairs   104 *see also* Paired tests
Mathematical
  descriptions of biological models   26–73
  metaphor, a   64
  modelling
    of biological response to stimuli   174–175
    of biological rhythms   171–200
    in endocrinology   6
    generalizations from   12–13
    historical usefulness   6
    processes of, and aspects on which it depends   2, 201
Mathematics
  advantages and limitations in biological modelling   13, 18–20, 24–26, 61, 181, 201, 225
  aims of   18
  beyond instability   54–66
  biological relevance required   19
  challenged by biological problems   19, 61
  compliantly complicated   24
  communication difficulties in, to biologists   20
  contribution to studying biological rhythms   173, 181
  stability   45
  development of   18
  different approaches needed   13
  and explanation of
    biological development   55
    observations   6, 18
  general statements from   19
  interpretation needed in biology   18
  of limit cycles   59
  limitations of, in explaining biology   19
  logic in, use of   18–19
  in modelling in biology   18–20, 25
  modifying, of a model to improve fit   19
  nature of systems dealt with readily   26
  peculiar to biology   26
  responsibility for appropriateness of   20
  results non-intuitive   61
  techniques, inadequate   26, 201, 225
  unexpected predictions from   181

Maximum
  likelihood, method of   78
  local, in model discrimination   108
MCR   116 *see also* Clearance
Mean
  MODFIT program, input of   253–254, 278
  as a parameter of a model   1, 227
  precision of   83
  response of a time-series   290
  rhythm characterization   *174*, 191
  specific radioactivity of combined compartments   124, 132, 279, 281
  weighted   267
Measurements, need for models when making   2
Mechanisms
  not available in empirical modelling   34–35
  of biological rhythms   175–176
  control, using dynamics   188
  of feedback loops   48, 52
    in endocrinology   52–54
    in ovulatory cycle required   223
  modelling of unknown internal   69
  proposed, frequency characteristics of   41
  of response of biological systems to environment   45, 174
  stabilizing, range of effectiveness   50
  of target cell response   53, 223
Mechanistic models *see* Theoretical models
Median, confidence limits on   228
Melatonin   53, 163, 180
Membranes
  in biological rhythms   175–176
  diffusion through   28, 60
  immobilized enzyme behaviour on   63
  spatial inhomogeneity from   60
Menopause   204, 220
Menstruation   203–204, 213–216
Menstrual cycle *see also* Ovulatory cycle modelling
  cycles related to   203
  modelled as a dynamic, discrete time system   69
  models of the   201–225
  multiple frequencies related to   172
  structural stability tested   45
  temperature variation in   192–197
Metabolic
  clearance rate (MCR)   *116 see also* Clearance
  pathways, modelling of   31
Metabolism
  circadian rhythms in   171
  peripheral, of hormones   54
Metaphor
  Raschevsky-Turing   65–66
  Waddington's   64
Metaphoric
  basis of equations   26
  interpretation of data from rhythms   184

Metaphoric
  modelling *4*, 64
    and behaviour of individuals 13
    conflict with theoretical modelling 5, 66
    cyclic release of LH 206–207
    of feedback 47
    of gene behaviour 14–16
    of mitosis 62, 184–185, 187
    of rhythms 180
Metaphysical reality, models as 24
Michaelis-Menten equation 70, 78
  in modelling response to hormones 54
  weighting data 70–72
MIMIC program 76
Mini-computer 21, 76–77, 163
Minimization of fitting function 78–82
Minimum, local
  identifying *80*
  sine wave model 192, 194
Mitosis, models of 14, 53, 62, 175, 184–185, 187–188
MLAB program 292
MODE 92, 94, 165, *253*–254, 258, 265–267, 275
MODFIT program *250*–254
  advantages of 89
  differential equation models 115, 123, 131–142, 253
  input format for 253–254, 278, 282
  output, detailed description of 90, 92
  scope of 89
Monte Carlo simulation
  comparing parallel and series compartmental models 135
  examples of 72, 91–95, 135
  experimental error and parameter uncertainty 95, 104
  exponential decay models 87, 91–95
  principle *72*, 91, 95
  sequential ligand-macromolecule interaction 153
  SIMUL program 89, 91–95, 250, *260*—266
  testosterone assay 164–165
  validation of sequential design 110–114
Multiple regression analysis 232
Multivariate analysis 232–240
  biological aspects of 233–240
  cluster analysis 235, *237*–238
  correlation analysis 233
  discriminant analysis *238*–240
  factor analysis *233*–237
  multiple regression analysis 232
  non-metrical multidimensional scaling *237*
  normal distribution in 234
  parameters (loadings) 232–234, 239
  principal component analysis *233*, 237

N-acetyl transferase 180
Nair's test 228

Neurosecretions modifying rhythms 189, 211, 220, 223
NLIN program 292
Noise in feedback loops 49
NON-LIN program 292
Non-linear
  behaviour in finite level modelling 66–67, 69
  equations
    for chemical reactions 60
    with cyclic solutions 56–64, 206
    showing instabilities 61–64
  frequency characteristics in blood flow 41
  memory properties of tissues 172
  models 64
    computer programs 250–260, 291–292
    difficulty of fitting to data 78
    effects investigated by replication and simulation 165–167
    of feedback 47, 49
    location of minimum of objective function 79, 82
    Michaelis-Menton equation 70–71
    modelled by analogue computer 75
    MODFIT program *250*–260
    parameter search 80–82
    in parameters 78
    practical details 82–88
    sensitivity coefficients 78, 81, 87, 257, 275
    tests of stability 44–45, 49
  systems
    approximated as linear 32
    in biology 26
    combining subsystems in 40
    feedback 49–51
    frequency analysis of 41
    responses of 33
    stable behaviours of 172
    steady states 43
    transfer functions 37
NONLINEAR, SPSS subprogram 292
Non-linearities *32*–34
  affect feedback 46, 48
  consequences of 61
  described in endocrinology 53
  effect of, in ovulatory cycle model 220–221, 224
  hypotheses about, removed 213
  and instability 56
  modelling of, in glycolysis 172
  need identifying 223
  in physiological systems 32
  of receptor response 54
Non-metrical multidimensional scaling *237*
Non-parametric statistics and tests 71, 73, 226–232, 242
  as alternatives to *t*-test 247

Non-parametric statistics and tests
  basis of randomization tests 228
  chi-square test *245*
  confidence limits 228
  examples of 228–232
  Friedman test 230–231
  Kolmogorov-Smirnov test 227, 246
  Kruskal-Wallis test 232
  Mann-Whitney test 228
  many independent samples 232
  median 228
  Nair's test 228
  and qualitative data 13
  runs test 96, 147, 149, *245*
  suitable for individual variation 12
  two independent samples compared 229
  Wilcoxon tests 228–229
Non-specific binding *145*–146, 162
  by albumin 110–114
  estimated by
    MASSACT FUNCTN subprogram 147–150, *284*–286
    RIAH FUNCTN subprogram 162–165, *289*–290
  RIA FUNCTN subprogram makes no allowance for 158, 168
Normal distribution *see* Distribution, normal
Normalization *see* z-Score
NPAR TESTS, SPSS subprogram 227
  FRIEDMAN procedure 230
  M-W (Wilcoxon/Mann-Whitney test) procedure 228
  K-S (Kolmogorov-Smirnov test) procedure 227
NSETS 91, *265*
NTERMS 92, *250*, 254
Null hypothesis 19, 226–228, *245*
Nyquist plot 49

Objective
  comparison of model with data 17
  function
    geometric representation of 80
    method of least squares *78*
    minimization by parameter adjustment 78–82
    non-linearity of 81
    penalty function influence on 83
    problems with non-linear dynamic systems 88
    stability of behaviour goes with low parameter interaction 86
Observability in endocrine systems 190–191
Obsolescence in models 5, 24
Oestradiol
  exogenous, modelled 211, 221–224
  ovarian follicle, production of 234–240
  in ovulatory cycles 203–205, 209–210
    in feedback loops 204–224
    pituitary desensitized to 135
    as stimulus 53
Oestrous cycle
  models of 201–225
  rat 209–212
    and HIOMT rhythms 178–180
    modelled by CSMP computer program 76
  of sheep 221
Open
  feedback loop 48, 50
  loop gain *50*–51
  systems 45, 61
    in biology 26, 45, 55
    and equifinality 43
    and equilibrium 42
    physical models of 123–124, 137
    steady state 120, 123
    structure development in 55
Operating point of feedback loop *51*–52
Operators *32*–33
Optimization
  parameter *78*–85
    competitive protein-binding assays 157, 169–170
    difficulties of 86–87
    integer parameters 151
    progress of 90, 92
    techniques 292
    validated by Monte Carlo simulation 91–95
  of performance of models in biology 19
  of resources 25
Order of differential equations 88
Organization
  by dynamics 189
  general principles of, in biology 4–5
  of genotype maintained 45
  increasing 54–55
  through instability 55
  principles of, in common 4, 19 *see also* Metaphoric modelling
  of processes from random elements 11
  product of history 64
  self-, in biology 4–5, 45, 54
  structural, modelled 66
  of whole more than sum of parts 4
Orthogonality in multivariate analysis 233–234
Oscillations *see also* Cycles; Limit cycles; Rhythms; Time-series
  amplifying near steady states 42
  in biological systems 26
  from constant inputs 33
  from complex eigenvalues 44
  damped, near steady state 42, 44, 56, 60, 174
  explaining the design principles of life 172
  in feedback 48–49

Oscillations
  in NADH in cell-free yeast extracts 62, 172
  from peroxidase 63
  in plasma hormone levels, modelled 207
  short-term random, modelled in ovulatory cycle 220–221
  spontaneous 41
  stable 57–58, 63 *see also* Limit cycles
Oscillators
  networks of, in biology 189
  relaxation, entrainment of 185, 187
Outliers 84
  biological variation and 97, 99
Output 7, 39, 43, 67, 69, 204 *see also* Response
  in block diagrams 40
  of DESIGN program 111, 135
  of MODFIT program 90, 92
  of SIMUL program 91, 93–94
  of stable models 43
Ovariectomy modelled 204, 211, 220
Ovary 203, 217, 224 *see also* Follicle, ovarian
  ascorbate depletion bioassay 118
  interstitial tissue, zinc transport 123
  rhythmic secretion of steroids by 190
  cross-linked with adrenal 190
Overdose conditions uninformative 23
Over-parameterization of a model
  competitive protein-binding assay 162
  condition number and 87–88, 90, 92, 98, 100, 258
Ovulation modelled 204, 209–217, 219, 223–224
  delayed 221–222
  feedback and 54
Ovulatory cycle modelling 191, 201–225
  conclusions 223–225
  description 203–204
  in detail 217–223
  by discontinuities 204–209
  empirically of 212
  by finite levels 213–216
  as limit cycle 221–222
  metaphorically 204–205
  species differences in 204
  stochastically 220, 222
Oxygen-haemoglobin interaction 143

Paired tests *see also* Matched pairs
  Friedman two-way analysis of variance 230–231
  Wilcoxon matched-pairs signed-ranks test 229
Parable of biochemist and car 23–24
Parallel exchange between compartments 125–129, 132, 135, 137–142, 278–279, 281
Parameters 7–8
  and bifurcation 65, 188

Parameters
  bounds 292
  in catastrophes 64–65
  causes of changes in, in endocrinology 53
  comparison of any number of
    control chart 249
    critical range test 248
    null hypothesis 226–228, 245
  comparison of two
    example 227
    t-test 92, 98, 160, 168–169, 191, 195, 227, 246–248
  as constraints on model behaviour 8
  constraints on values of 30
    found by simulation 14
  correlation in non-linear models 86
  in curve-fitting 35
  cyclical changes in 41, 172
  define trajectories 42
  in description of models 22
  determine feedback effectiveness 48
  different, give same results 224
  effect on model behaviour 61, 75
  empirical 98
  estimates 31, 74–102, 90, 92
    from additional experiments 30
    approximate 74–76
    difficulties in making 86–88
    in finite level modelling 67, 69
    importance in fitting model to data 74
    initial 90, 92, 253–254
    integer 151
    interpolation of 85
    linearity and non-linearity 77–78, 81
    precision of 69–71, 85, 106
      estimated by Monte Carlo simulation 72, 85, 91, 95
      influenced by experimental design 106, 268–276
    rapid 74–76
    statistical basis of 69–70
    well-determined 97
  excess of 19, 66, 86, 212
  for hormone rates, assumed constant 206
  integer, optimization of 151
  integration constants as unknowns 30
  interaction between 86–88, 97
    competitive protein-binding assays 161
    condition number 88, 90, 92, 98
    correlation 87, 90, 92, 98
    dependence 87, 90, 92, 97, 257–258, 265
    experimental frame restricted 86–87
    exponential decay models 87, 90
    measures of 90–92
    minimization 87
    parameter precision in models with 85, 90
    redundant parameters 86–87
  interpretation in theoretical models 8, 31
  loading 233

Subject Index

Parameters
  of model allow simulation of puberty 207
  multivariate analysis 232–234
  non-linearity of, in model 78
  not constant in feedback 46
  "nuisance" 80, 142
  optimization 78
  of ovulation model 224
  in ovulatory cycle models 202, 210, 212–213, 219
  poorly determined 86
  random variations in, in ovulatory cycle model 221, 224
  redundancy
    signalled by condition number 87, 98
    sometimes necessary 88
  require experimental manipulation 224
  in rhythms 189
  search methods 78, 80–82
  in self-modelling 36
  semi-redundancy in exponential decay models 87
  significance to model behaviour required 22
  space, geometric representation of 80
  in splines 36
  none suitable found 31
  termination of optimization 84
  unidentified in modelling instabilities 64
  values
    must be feasible 31
    physiological significance 219, 225
    response mapped over a range of 44
    stability depends on 43–44, 50, 56–59
  well-determined 97
Parametric statistics and tests 71, 73, 226, 232–240, 242, 246
  analysis of variance 247–248
  apply to defined classes 12
  comparing
    any number of samples 248
    two samples, example of 227
  multivariate analysis 232–240
  Scheffé's test 248
  t-test 92, 98, 160, 168–169, 191, 195, 227, 246–248
Parathyroid hormone 52, 54
Parsimony, principle of 19
Partial derivatives 30–32, 60, 65, 75
  sensitivity coefficients 78, 81, 86–87, 257, 275
Pathological states in testing normal function 224
Pattern matrix (factor analysis) 235, 237
Penalty functions 83, 86, 88, 254, 257, 275, 292
  see also Constraints
Peptide hormone amino acid sequence analysed 226

Percent coefficient of variation 243
  competitive protein-binding assays 167–167
  in parameters 90–91, 258
Perception in modelling 1, 17
Periods of time-series 173–174, 192, 290
  in biological rhythms 191, 194
  determination from discrete data 179
  interplay of similar 179
  SIN FUNCTN subprogram 192–194, 290
Peroxidase, oscillations and chaotic behaviour of 58, 63
Peripheral compartments
  any number of, modelled 137–142, 282
  FUNCTN subprograms 125–135, 137–142, 278–282, 294–295
  mean specific radioactivity in 279, 281
Peritoneal fluid, transport of zinc in 116
Perspective, modelling in 23–25
Perspectives, different, in modelling 17
Perturbation
  amplified 42
  of biological systems 52
  in catastrophe theory 65
  and development 64
  effects in non-linear models 44
  of feedback loops 48
  from the steady state 61
  with positive feedback 65
  small in linear approximations 44, 49–50
  stability to, in a model of gene action 16
  test stability to 42–43, 224
Phase 173–174 see also Follicular, Luteal
  phase changes
    causing discontinuities in responses 181–185
    by entrainment 185–186
    by interactive rhythm coupling 186–188
  in, signals in feedback loops 49
  lag in feedback 49
  latent see Isochron 181, 183–186
  mixing in rat oestrous cycle 212
  space 43, 58–59
  of time-series 191, 290
Phases
  of ovulatory cycle 203–204, 221–222
  sensitive to stimulation 174, 176–180
Phosphofructokinase producing oscillations 62
Phospholipid 125
Physiological
  behaviour, modelling 35, 224
  components, identification in compartmental analysis 31
  conditions 7, 23
    testing models outside 23, 50
  response 32, 50
  systems
    and the butterfly effect 57

Physiological systems
  linearity and non-linearity in 32
  potentially chaotic 58
Pineal gland
  as master clock 172
  rhythms in activity 177–180
Pituitary
  in cortisol feedback 68
  desensitized to oestradiol 135
  in feedback loop 48
  in ovulatory cycle 203, 207–209, 211, 217–219, 221, 223
  pulsed release of hormones from 39, 175, 190
Placenta, transport of zinc in 123, 130
Plasma clearance rate *116*–119 see Clearance
PMSG see Pregnant mare serum gonadotrophin
Polyethylene glycol 157
POLYNOM FUNCTN subprogram 99–100, *254*
Polynomials
  competitive protein-binding assays 165
  in curve-fitting *35*–36
  ovarian follicle wall thickness 99–102
  POLYNOM FUNCTN subprogram 267
  sequential binding model 153
Pooled data, information loss 12
Pools 9 see also Compartmental analysis
  dynamic, in model of LH in the pituitary 208
Population (statistical) 98, 228, *242*, 244
Precision 69 see also Standard deviation; Uncertainty
  competitive protein-binding assay 156, 169
  estimated
    before experimentation 104
    by pooling values 169
    by replication 72, 104
  improvement by replication 104
  standard deviation 83
  weighting 70–71
Precursor cells or hormones 48, 53
Predictions from models 3–4, 22, 202
  finite level 67
  hindered 223
  impossible sometimes 57
  improving comparison of, with data 19
  non-intuitive 17, 20, 25
  outside experimental frame 7
  on range of application 23
  by simulation 13–14
  testing by experiment 17, 24
Pregnancy
  comparison of samples in 227
  effect on endometrial zinc transport 130
  occurrence discrete or continuous 29
  plasma 110–111, 146–150
  rabbits, zinc transport in 123–130
  sex steroid binding globulin 110–114, 146–150

testosterone 110
Pregnant mare serum gonadotrophin
  clearance from blood of sheep 38, 89–95, 116–119, 139–142
    Monte Carlo simulation of 94–95
  ovarian follicles 116–117
  relative potency 118
Principal component analysis 36, *233*, 237
Principle of superposition 33
Probability
  calculation of, as basis of randomization tests 228
  functions 9, 11
  hypothesis testing and 227, 245
  level of, in stastitical tests 249
  misclassification, discriminant analysis 238, 240
  models based on 29, 226
  stochastic process, outcome governed by 226
Probit plot 246
Progesterone
  in models of ovulatory cycles 203–205, 211–214, 217–223
  ovarian follicle, production of 234–239
Programs see Computer programs
Prolactin in ovulatory cycle models 203, 211, 223
Prostaglandins 53, 163
Puberty 207, 223
Pulsatile hormone release
  biological function of 189–190
  of cortisol 200
  determination of 39
  difficulties of modelling 200
  model of 206–207
  in ovulatory cycle 220–223

Quadratic equation
  ovarian follicle growth 99
  POLYNOM FUNCTN subprogram 99, *267*
  solution 286
Quantized variables 66–67
  in menstrual cycle model 213–214

R CHI SQUARE see CHISQR
Rabbit
  calcium transport in 131
  zinc transport in, hormonal influence on 123–130
Radio-immunoassay (RIA) of hormones 155–170, 201
  see also Competitive protein-binding assay; Ligand binding to macromolecules
Radio-immunometric assay 155, 162, 167
  see also Competitive protein-binding assay
Radioisotope dilution method 155
Random
  numbers 104, 165, 260, 265

Subject Index

Random
  oscillations in hormones 220–221
  selection of samples 103–104, 150, 227–229
  time-series 192
  variation 69, 104
Randomization *103 see also* Non-parametric statistics and tests
  managing biological variation by 103–104
  tests on ranks 227–232
Randomized block design *104*
Rankit plot 246
Ranks *227–232 see also* Non-parametric statistics and tests
  Friedman test 230–231
  Kruskal-Wallis test 232
  non-metrical multidimensional scaling *237*
  Wilcoxon tests 228–229
Rao's V 239
Raschevsky-Turing metaphor 65
Rat
  oestrous cycle models 179, 209–212
  prostate augmentation bioassay 118
  transport of carnitine in tissues of 131
Rate constants *121*
  of chemical reactions and diffusion 28
  in competitive protein-binding assay 170
  determine dynamic behaviour 61
  of exchange 118–119, 282
  in feedback 48–49
  in frequency domain 34, 40
  of irreversible loss 118–119, 122–123, 282
  in ovulatory cycle 205–206, 210
  reciprocal of turnover time 121
  and steady states 43
Ratio
  bound-to-free ligand *144*, 146, 168
  bound-to-total ligand *145*–146, 156, 159–160, 162
    MASSACT FUNCTN subprogram 111–114, 147–150, 156, 158–160, *284*–286
    RIAH FUNCTN subprogram 162–165, *289*
  free-to-bound ligand 146, 156–160, *288*
    RIA FUNCTN subprogram 158–168, *288*
  rate constants 144
  molar in ligand-macromolecule interaction 151
Receptors
  aspects of hormone signals distinguished by 221, 223
  assays using 155, 162–163
  and communication by hormones 190
  coupling stimulus to energy source for response 190
  in homeostastic feedback 52
  hormone interaction with 54
  identification of likely amino acids in 226
  interactions between ligands and 143
  responses
    assumed constant 206–207
    non-linear 54
    and rhythm coupling 176
  sensitivity, rhythmic 189
Reduced chi-square 90, 92, 99, 101, 109, *246*, 258, 266
  see also CHISQR (R CHI SQUARE)
  absolute measure of model's suitability 108
  testing goodness of fit 85, 96, 99
Reductionism in biology 4–5, 244
Related sample tests 229–231
  critical range tests 231, 248
Relaxation oscillator, entrainment of 185–187
Relaxin 53, 224
Reliability 74, 243 *see also* Coefficient of variation; Confidence intervals; Standard deviation
Renin 68, 200
Replication *104*, 113, 228
  experimental precision estimated by 82–83, 104, 109, 147
  parameter uncertainties checked by 164–165
  reduced chi-square test 85
  SIMUL computer program 91, 93–94
  within-group variation determined by 104
Reproduction
  and homeostasis 45
  and the physical laws 5
RES VARIANCE 90, 92, 94, 111, *254*, 258
  see also CHISQR (R CHI SQUARE); Residual sum of squares; Variance, residual
Research, problems identified in 14, 17–18, 25, 223–225
Reservoir compartment *see also* Forcing functions
  peripheral compartments fitted simultaneously 137
  physical model 123, 124
  RESERVR FUNCTN subprogram 266
  sampling only from 135–142
RESERVR FUNCTN subprogram 266
  CAI FUNCTN subprogram and 125–126, 278
  example of use with MODFIT program 89–95
  exponential decay 90–95, 125
  input format for 253
Residual sum of squares 78, 92, 258 *see also* Root mean square
Residuals *78*–79, 90, 92, 258
  estimated from replication 104
  examining 84
  graph of 116
  as measure of experimental uncertainty 83
  minimized by method of least squares 78
  outliers 84
  runs test on *245*
  testing 245

Residuals, trends shown by 116
Resonance in feedback 49
Response *see also* Dependent variables; Output
 of adrenals 32, 41
 of biological systems to environment 45
 calculated from convolution integrals 38–39
 controlled in negative feedback 46–47
 to hormones 48, 53–54 *see also* Receptors
 linear and non-linear 32, 40, 44
 mathematical models of biological 54, 174–175
 multiphased 53
 non-linearity in physiological systems 32
 physiological compared with model 50
 predicted from transfer functions 37
 to rhythmic input, analysis of 33, 40–41
 of rhythms to stimuli 176–188
 similar to natural variation 45, 220
 to stimuli described empirically 34
 stimulus and 7
 unforced 43, 49
Responsibility in modelling 24–25
Resting value *191*
Reversible
 interactions in block diagrams 40
 reactions 8
  do not undergo catastrophes 65
Rewards of modelling 4–6
Rhythms *see also* Circadian rhythms; Cycles; Oscillations; Time-series
 annual 176
 and biological control 189–191
 causality in 202
 contact inhibition of 188
 contribution of mathematics to 173
 coupling 172, 175–188
 detected in individuals 12, 191
 empirical description of 35, 191–200
 and endocrinology 189–191
 and environment 172–173
 experimental evidence 171–172
 inherent 172, 174–175, 178, 180
  see also Limit cycles; Clock
 in isolated tissue 172
 modelling 171–200
 models behaving like biological 50
 physiological implications of detected 180
 representation of 173–174
 response to stimuli 175–188
 stable *see* Limit cycles
Rhythmic
 data *see* Time-series
 input and output analysis 40–41
 inputs to endocrine systems 53
 release of hormones
  cessation of 207
  function for 189–190

 systems, magnification in 50
RIA FUNCTN subprogram 158, 168, *288*
RIAH FUNCTN subprogram *289*
 testosterone assay 163–165
 uncertainties checked by simulation 164–165
Root mean square (RMS) *83,* 90, 93 *see also* Residual sum of squares
Roots
 complex 44, 286
 cubic equation solved by Cardan's method 286
 real 286, 288
Rotation of factors (axes) 234–235
Routh-Hurwitz test of stability 44
Run *245*
Runs test 96, 147, 149, *245*
 outliers analysed 84, 90
 time-series analysis 192

s see Complex frequency domain
SAAM program 292
Salicylate, binding to albumin 153–155
Sample from a population 97, *242*
Samples, comparison of
 any number of
  analysis of variance 230–232, 247–248
  Bartlett's test 248
  coefficient of variation *243*
  critical range tests 231, 248
  distributions 227, 246
  F-test 105, 227, 248
  Friedman test 230–231
  Kruskal-Wallis test 232
  multivariate analysis 232–240
  non-parametric tests, examples 230–232
  null hypotheses 226–228, *245*
  Scheffé's test 248
 two
  non-parametric tests, examples 228–229
  parametric tests, example 227
  t-test 92, 98, 160, 168–169, 191, 195, 227, 246–248
  Wilcoxon (Mann-Whitney) test 228
Sampling
 data at discrete intervals 29
 errors and biological variation 12–13, 97
Saturation
 analysis *see* Competitive protein-binding assay
 of feedback 48
 of linear systems 32, 118
SBG *see* Sex steroid binding globulin
Scaling
 causes difficulty in parameter optimization 86
 non-metrical multidimensional *237*
Scatchard plot 144, 153
Scheffé's test 248
Score see z-Score

Subject Index

SDEV 91, 95, *265*
Search
 direct *80*–81, 88
 direction 79
 gradient 80–82
Secretion
 of hormones, calculated using deconvolution 39
 rate *116*
Selection of
 classes see Classes, selecting
 suitable or best models 9, 14, 19, 106–114
Self-modelling
 and individual variation 13
 non-linear regression 36–37
Sensitivity
 coefficients *78*, 81, 87, 257, 275
  experimental design 106
  graphs of 87
  parameter interaction and 86–87
 of competitive protein-binding assay 156, *168*–170
  improved by optimization 169
 of model to assumptions 224
Sequential
 experimental design *105*–114
  advantages of 105, 110–114
  comparison of parallel and series compartmental models 134–135
  DESIGN program 108–109, *268*–277
  determining SBG in early pregnancy blood plasma 110–114
  doubts concerning application in biology 106
  implementation 108–109
  integer parameter models, choosing between 151
  joint design criterion *107*
  kinetic experiments 107
  models differentiated between by 106–114, 155
  parameter precision increased by 106–107, 113–114, 276
  results compared with factorial design by simulation 113–114
  simulation gives evidence of advantages of 110–114
  termination criteria 107–108
  useful even when condition variable 114
 search of parameter space 80
SERDES subprogram 268, *276*–277
Serial exchange between peripheral compartments 123–124, 133
 AUX subprogram 281
 CA2A FUNCTN subprogram 133–135, 281
Series configuration see Compartmental models
Serum volume estimation 119

Sex steroid binding globulin (SBG)
 determined in presence of excess CBG 113
 properties of 110–114, 146–150
 simulation of testosterone binding to 110–114
Sheep
 clearance of PMSG from the blood of 38, 89–95, 116–119
 ovarian follicles of 116–117
  in culture 234–238
 ovary responds to individual LH pulses 221
Sialic acid 118
SIGMAY 90, 92, 135, 165, *260,* 265
Sigmoidal
 data, empirical description 35
 models
  competitive protein-binding assays 162, 165
  growth of elephants 95–99, 266
  radio-immunoassays 162–168, 288–290
Sign reversal in feedback loops 47–49
Significance
 comparative experiments, tests of 227–232
 level of *245*
 tests of 227–232, 242, 245–248
Simplex *80*–88
 competitive protein-binding assay 169
 direct maximization of response 81
 evolutionary operation (EVOP) 81
 minimization of objective function 80–81
Simplifications
 appropriate in endocrinology 53
 computer programs are 22
 of data by finite level models 10
 in diagrams 9
 different, give same result 224
 by experimental frames 7
 by lumping 9–10
 meaningful 23
 in modelling ovulatory cycles 202
 models necessarily limited by 5
 of models using simulation results 14
 by piecewise equations 213
 valid 20
 verifying 225
SIMUL program 59–60, 76, 85, 87, 89, 186, *258, 260*–266
 competitive protein-binding assays 156, 165
 examples 91, 93–94, 165
 input format 253–254, 265, 278
 ligand-macromolecule interaction 149–150
 linearization of model tested using 92
 Monte-Carlo simulation 72, 91, 93–94
 output interpreted 91, 93–94
 testosterone-SBG interaction 149–150
Simulation 13–14, 22, *72* see also Monte Carlo simulation
 analogue 74

Simulation
  analogue
    blood clearance   75
    computer   74–75
    non-linear models   75
    scaling problems   75
    subjectivity in parameter estimation   75–76
  competitive protein-binding assays   156, 164–165, 170
  showing constraints on variables and parameters   14, 25
  CSMP program   76
  of data inadequate   202, 220
  determining amount of data required   14
  of effects of contraceptive steroids   214, 216
  showing effects of experimental uncertainty   14
  enzyme kinetics   77
  experimental design   104, 110
  finding stability of model   14
  impractical   212
  of infusions of reproductive hormones   221–222
  interaction of steroids with pregnancy plasma   110–114
  ligand-macromolecule interaction   149–150
  MIMIC program   76
  in models of ovulatory cycles   211, 216, 219, 222–224
  of precision of parameter estimate   164–165
  predictions from   13–14
  program packages   76, 292
  of rhythms   202
  simplification using   14
  SIMUL program   89, 91, 93–94, 149–150, 260–266
  testosterone-SBG interaction   149–150
SIN FUNCTN subprogram   290
  menstrual cycle temperature analysis   192–194
Singularity
  biological significance   183
  in limit cycles   59–60, 181, 183, 186
  locus of, in interactive rhythm coupling   187
Sine function   173–174, *191–194*
  amplitude   191, 290
  as empirical description   35
  as input forcing function   185
  local minimum   192, 194
  menstrual cycle temperature variation   192–194
  parameter stability   193–194
  period   173, 191, 290
  phase   173, 191, 290
  SIN FUNCTN subprogram   *290*
Sinusoidal stimuli and transients   33
Sipps coefficient   162
Slide rule   74
Specific
  activity   *122*

binding between ligand and macromolecule   *145 see also*
  Ligand binding to macromolecules
  MASSACT FUNCTN subprogram   284–286
  simulated   110
  single class of sites   149
  two independent classes of sites   145, 147–150
radioactivity
  calculation of   123, 131
  FUNCTN subprograms   278–282
  mean   124, 132, 279, 281
Spectral density function   191, *196*
  constraints on experimental application   200
  cross-spectra   *199*
  properties of linear systems   198
  SPECTRAL, SPSS subprogram   196–197
Spline function   *35–36*
  competitive protein-binding assay   165–167
  quadratic   167
  in self-modelling   36
SPSS (program package)   227
  DISCRIMINANT   239
  FACTOR   234, 236
  NONLINEAR   292
  NPAR TESTS   227
    FRIEDMAN procedure   230
    M-W (Mann-Whitney/Wilcoxon test) procedure   228
    K-S (Kolmogorov-Smirnov test) procedure   230
  SPECTRAL   196–197
Stability
  of biological systems   45, 54, 64, 172
  concept of   42
  in endocrinology   53
  from energy relationships   45
  of feedback loops   48–50, 63
    in biology   45, 52
  global   44
  and homeostasis   45
  from instability   55
  mathematics and biological   45
  of model behaviour
    tested by simulation   14
    tests for, in linear models   43–44
    in very complex systems   14–16
    when noise introduced   16
  neutral   42
  of non-linear
    models   44–45, 220–221
    systems   43, 88
      analogy for   44
  parameter-dependant changes in   56–58
  point   *42–43*, 49–50, 61
  and spatial inhomogeneity   60–61
  structural   42, 45, 64, 220–221

Subject Index

Stability, topology of, in biology 42
Stable steady state 42, 56, 58, 207
  analogy for 42
  tested in linear model 43
  unstable steady state 57 *see* Singularity
Standard
  deviation 1, *242*–243
    estimated from replicates 72, 82–83
    normalization of residuals 84
    SIMUL program 92, 165
    simulated competitive protein-binding assay 167
    weighting by inverse of variance 83
    z-score *244*
  error of the mean *242*
  partial regression coefficient *232*
Standardized measure *see z*-Score
State *see* Steady states; Equations, Variables, state
Statistical mechanics 30, 54–55
Statistics 11, 69–73
  in comparing model with data 19
  experimental design 73
  formulae *242–249*
  mathematical models *see* Stochastic models
  methods, dependence on randomization 104
  non-parametric 71, *242*
  parameter estimation 69–70
  parametric 71, *242*
  tests, basis of 226, *242–249*
Steady states 30 *see also* Stable steady state
  and "adaptation" to inputs 41
  assumed, in most compartmental models 120, 132
  biological 26, 30, 45
  concentrations of reproductive hormones at 219–220
  difficulties in attaining 41
  and equifinality 43
  in feedback systems 49
    magnification or gain at 50–52
  using Laplace transforms 37
  linearity and non-linearity of 32
  measurement of, in endocrinology 53
  not attained for drug 120
  of ovulatory cycle model 221–222
  several in non-linear systems 43–44
  stability of 37, 42–43, 56–58
Steepest descent method 254
Stepwise regression 87
Steroid hormones *see also* Hormone; Oestradiol; Progesterone; Testosterone
  competitive protein-binding assays 155–170
  estimated 99
  metabolism 54
  ovarian follicle production of, characterized by multivariate analysis 234–240
  in pregnancy 110, 146, 150
  SBG 110–114, 146–150

Stewart-Hamilton equation *116*–117, 119
Stiff differential equations 29, 88
  AUX subprograms define 279–281
  initial conditions 88
  integration requires special methods 88, 253
  models involving 253, 279–282, 290
STIFF (D02AEF) subprogram 253, 279–282, 290
  input to 281
Stimuli
  acting on
    linear systems 33, 37, 39
    non-linear systems 33
  adaptation to 53
  controlling biological responses 174
  effects
    recede with time 39
    on rhythms 175–188
    at sensitive phases of biological rhythms 176–180
  previous and current, in feedback 52
  pulse, causing phase changes in rhythms 181–186
  and responses, identifying appropriate 53, 221
Stimulus *see also* Input
  levels of, organism adapted to 49
  and response 7–8, 34
  in endocrine systems 53, 221
Stochastic
  behaviour *11*
    and instability 55
    producing deterministic results 29
  description of deterministic outcome 57
  models 76, 226–240
  systems 29–30
    biological 26
    and hierarchy 11
  variation in input tests stability 45
  in ovulatory cycle model 220–222
Stochiometric binding constants 154
Stress effects on ovulatory cycle 220, 224
Structural
  organization, models of 66
  stability *42*, 64
    in non-linear models 45
  of ovulatory cycle model 220–221
Subjectivity in modelling 2, 17, 19
Subprogram *see* Computer subprograms
Subsystems
  characteristics distinguished 40
  combining 39–40
    in compartmental analysis 31
    in feedback loops 47
    in large system modelling 201–225
    in linear and non-linear systems 33, 40
    by transfer functions 37
  removed by ablation or drugs 44

Superposition, principle of 33
Surgery, opening feedback loops by 51
Synchronizing biological function 186
Systems *see also* Biological, Closed, Dynamic, Endocrine, Isolated systems
   analysis in biology 201
   components of 6
   distinguishing 6

t-Test for comparing two parameters 98, 228, *246–248*
   bias tested by 92
   comparison of two estimates only 195, 248
   competitive protein-binding assays 160, 168–169
   empirical parameters 98
   F-test as preliminary to 247
   one- or two-tailed 247
   non-linear models, precautions 247
   rhythm analysis 191, 195
T-values *106*–109, 111, 132
   directing experimental design 113–114
   DESIGN program 276
   influence on parameter precision 106
   TCALC subprogram 268, *275–276*
Target cell organ response 53–54, 189–190, 221
   energy and 190
   in feedback 48
Taylor series 44, 81
TCALC subprogram 268, 275–276
Technological
   development compared to biological research 19
   interference 24
Technology, mathematics developed for 26
Temperature
   body, during menstrual cycle 172, 192–197
   variations and diapause control 178
Termination criteria 84, 107–108
Testes
   annual rhythm in function of 176–178
   feedback from 206–207
Testing
   classes of individuals modelled 12
   hypotheses 2, 19, 25
   models 3–5, 14, 17, 19, 24, 224
      outside physiological conditions 23, 224
      of ovulatory cycle 211, 216, 220–222
      sensitivity to assumptions 224
      using computers 20
Testosterone
   assay for 157–160, 167–168
      confidence intervals in 169
      precision of 156, 169
      sensitivity of 156, 168–169
   simulation of 164–165
   equilibrim dialysis 110, 146–150
   feedback model 206
   ovarian follicle production of 234–237, 239–240
   pregnancy and 110, 146–150
   sex steroid binding globulin 110–114, 146–150
Theca cells
   mass of 99
   production of cAMP by 228–229
Theoretical
   modelling 26–31
      assumptions in, of enzyme kinetics 31
      biological systems to which applied 31
      compartmental analysis not 31
      in endocrinology 31
   of feedback systems 47, 49, 52
   of rhythms 176
   models 3–4, 74, 103
      of biological cycles 191
      conflict with metaphoric models 5, 13
      derivation of, example 100–102
      of growth 96, 98
      of instability 55
      interpretation of parameters in 8, 74, 87
      ligand-macromolecule binding 111–114, 143, 147–150, 156–160, 168, 284–286, 288
      many are non-linear in their parameters 78
      necessary for understanding biology 23
      of ovulation 223
      prediction from 3, 202
      in self-modelling 36
      testing of feedback 52
      of thickness of ovarian follicle wall 100–102
Thermal convection, organization in 55
Thermodynamic metaphor 64
Thermodynamics
   classical and stability 42
   explaining evolution 54
Thermoregulation model 52
Three-dimensional drawing of cortisol molecule 21
Thresholds 65 *see also* Bifurcation; Catastrophe theory; Decision functions; Discontinuities; Instability
   biological 26
   in clocks 184, 188
   of instability 55
   in models of the ovulatory cycle 208, 210–213, 219, 222
Thyroid
   control uncoupling 52
   stimulating hormone 54
Thyroxine 292
Ties *228*

Subject Index

Time
  constants see also Rate constants
    modelling systems with a wide range of 69
    of target cell response 53, 223
    in differentials 27
    discrete in biology 29, 69
    domain analysis 191, 194–195
    frame, selection simplifies 9, 220
    importance in biological systems 27, 69, 212
    of influence of previous events 216, 223
Time-series see also Circadian rhythms; Cycles; Oscillations; Rhythms
  aliasing 196
  amplitude 173, 191–192, 195
  auto-correlation function 191, 194–196
    coefficient 194
    correlogram 195, 197
    lag 194–195, 197
  auto-regression 195
  baseline 191–192
  bivariate process 198–200
    Bode diagrams 40–41, 49–51, 199
    coherency squared 199
    cross-correlation 198
    cross-spectra 199
    examples 200
    gain spectrum 199
    limitations 199
    relationship between time-series 199
  central mean 191–192, 290
  continuous and discrete 196
  empirical characterization of rhythms 191–200
  Fourier analysis 195–197
  frequency 28, 191–192, 195
    domain analysis 40–41, 49, 191, 195–197
    limitations in biology 196
  harmonic analysis 191, 195–197
  intuitive search for rhythm in 179, 192
  LIMIT FUNCTN subprogram 290
  observations, frequency required 196
  period 173, 191–192, 194, 290
  periodically varying rate constant 121
  phase 173, 191–192, 195, 290
  random 192, 195
  resting value 191–192, 290
  sampling rate 196
  SIN FUNCTN subprogram 290
  sine wave model 173–174, 191–194
  spectral analysis 191, 195–197
  stationary 192
  time domain analysis 191, 194–196
  trend 191, 195, 197
  window 191, 196
Tissue culture
  ovarian follicles 228–231, 234–240
  simplex method optimizes conditions of 81

Topology and biological metaphors 64
Tracers 120
  binding of 156–157
  dynamic systems analysis and 115–142
  iodine-labelled albumin 137–138
  radioactive, effect of contaminants 150, 156
  specific activity of 122
  testosterone 157
  writing differential equations of compartmental model 122–123, 131–132
  zinc transport in rabbit tissues 123–130
Trajectories 42, 56
  aperiodic 57
  in catastrophes 64–65
  in difference equations 56–58
  in instability 65
  near limit cycles 59–60, 181, 183
  oscillatory 44
  on perturbing non-linear systems 44
  near stable and unstable steady states 42–43
  thermodynamic 64
Transformation of data 99
  competitive protein-binding assays 157, 161
  linear 99, 232–233
  Lineweaver-Burke plot 70–72, 244
  logarithmic 73, 227, 234, 239
  logit-log 162
  multivariate analysis 232–240
  normalization 102, 232, 244
  spline functions 167
  statistical properties of 232
  weighting required 168
  z-score 232–233, 244
Transfer functions 37–39
  calculated by computer 39
  and characteristic equations 44
  in combining subsystems 39–40
  of components in frequency analysis 40
  difficulties in biology 41
  in feedback modelling 47, 50–51
    stability 49
  in ovulatory cycle model 215–216, 218
Transient states 30
  in endocrinology 53
  in frequency analysis 40–41
  linearity in response of 32–33
Transport
  effect of hormone dependent on 180
  lags in feedback systems 49
  properties and steady states 43
  rates, through membranes, rhythmic 189
Trend
  residuals 84, 91, 116, 138
  rhythm characterization 191, 195, 197
  runs test 192
Tukey's smoothing function 196

Turnover time *121*
  calcium 131
  carnitine 131
  corpus luteum zinc 128
  endometrial zinc 126
  zinc 126, 129, 130

Uncertainty *243 see also* Coefficient of variation; Error; Standard deviation; Variance
  analogue computer 75
  competitive protein-binding assay 167–168
  estimation
    before experimentation 104
    essential need 70
  experimental
    in biological experiments 12
    caused by unrecognized cycles 12
    in description of models 22
    effects of, shown by simulation 14
    estimated from replication 82–83, 97, 147, 165–166
    in finite level modelling 10
    and individual variation 12
    Monte Carlo simulation 72, 91–95, 111–113
    poor estimates of 99
    relationship to parameter uncertainty 95, 104
  independent variable, assumed free of 82
  parameter 90, 92
  random 91–95, 111, 112
  reduced chi-square 246
  reduction by matching pairs 104
  SIMUL program analyses 92
  total, in parameters 276
Uniqueness in compartmental models 121
UNIT 1 265, 268, 275
UNIT 2
  CA1, CA2, CA2A FUNCTN subprograms 125–128, 132–135, 278–281
  GENBIND FUNCTN subprogram 153, 155, 287
  RIA FUNCTN subprogram 158, 288
UNIT 5 253, 268, 278
UNIT 6 268
UNIT 16 268, 275–276
Unstable *see also* Instability
  behaviour in feedback 48
  steady state *42,* 57–58
  systems and magnification 50
Uterine fluid, transport of zinc in 123
Uterus in ovulatory cycle 203

Variables 7–9, 22 *see also* Dependent, Independent variables
  behaviour near a steady state 42
  constraints on values 30
    found by simulation 14
  decisive, in biological behaviour 26

discrete 75
extraneous (uncontrolled) 103
in finite level modelling 67–68, 213
interdependent 8
lumping of 9
and operators 32
postulated in theoretical modelling 31
quantized 66–67, 213–214
require manipulation 224
significance to model behaviour required 22
state *31*
unidentified in modelling instabilities 64
used in studying the ovulatory cycle 203
values altered at thresholds 208
Variance *242*
  in any function 243
  auto-correlation coefficient *195*
  analysis of *247*–248
    Bartlett's test 248
    between, as against within, samples 248
    comparing parameter estimates 248
    F-test 105, 227, *248*
    factorial experiments 105
    Friedman two-way, by ranks 230–231
    rhythms 191
  competitive protein-binding assays 167–168
  discriminant analysis 238
  experimental, estimation 147
  factor analysis 233
  heterogeneity of 99
  homogeneity 246, 248
  multivariate analysis 233
  pooling 167–168
  propagation of 243
  ratio test *248* see also *F*-Test
  reduction of, by
    clustering individuals 238
    normalization 99
    pairing data 229
    rotation of axes in multivariate analyses 234–235
  reliability measure 82
  residual 109, 111–112
  transmission of 243
Variance-covariance matrix 257
Variety of behaviour 67
Vasopressin feedback 48

Wasp, diapause control in 178
Waves 61–63
Weight of elephants 95–99
Weighted mean 267
Weighting 99, 227, *243,* 253, 265
  competitive protein-binding assays 157–158, 163, 167–168
  Lineweaver-Burke plot 70–72, 243
  MODE *253*

Weighting
  most likely model given most 276
  percent coefficient of variation 167–168
  POLYNOM FUNCTN subprogram 267
  by reciprocal of data variance 82–83, 147
  RIA FUNCTN subprogram 157
  T-weighted differences in model response 276
Wilcoxon
  matched-pairs signed-ranks test 229
  (Mann-Whitney) two-sample randomization test 228
Wilks' lambda 238–239
"World" model 1, 22

X 250

YFIT 250, 257, 281

z-Score 90, 92, 94, 111, 135, 165, 244, 258
  analysis of residuals 84
  detecting outliers 84
  discriminant analysis 238–240
  factor analysis 234, 236–237
  multivariate analysis 232–240
  principal component analysis 233
Zhabotinski-Zaikin reaction 61
Zilversmit criterion 125
Zinc
  radioactive tracer 123, 125, 278
  transport in tissues 123–130

Other Volumes in This Series:

Volume 15: A. T. Cowie, I. A. Forsyth, I. C. Hart
Hormonal Control of Lactation
1980. 64 figures, 7 tables. Approx. 320 pages
ISBN 3-540-09680-9

Volume 14: J. H. Clark, E. J. Peck, Jr.
Female Sex Steroids
Receptors and Function
1979. 116 figures, 18 tables. XII, 245 pages
ISBN 3-540-09375-3

Volume 13: H. F. DeLuca
Vitamin D – Metabolism and Function
1979. 14 figures. VIII, 80 pages
ISBN 3-540-09182-3

Volume 12
Glucocorticoid Hormone Action
Editors: J. D. Baxter, G. G. Rousseau
1979. 176 figures, 58 tables. XIX, 638 pages
ISBN 3-540-08973-X

Volume 11: S. Ohno
Major Sex-Determining Genes
1979. 34 figures, 6 tables. XIII, 140 pages
ISBN 3-540-08965-9

Volume 10: W. I. P. Mainwaring
The Mechanism of Action of Androgens
1977. 12 figures, 17 tables. XI, 178 pages
ISBN 3-540-07941-6

Volume 9: R. E. Mancini
Immunologic Aspects of Testicular Functions
1976. 36 figures, 8 tables. IX, 114 pages
ISBN 3-540-07496-1

Volume 8: E. Gurpide
Tracer Methods in Hormone Research
1975. 35 figures. XI, 188 pages
ISBN 3-540-07039-7

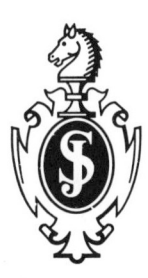

Springer-Verlag
Berlin
Heidelberg
New York

Volume 7: E. W. Horton
Prostaglandins
1972. 97 figures. XI, 197 pages
ISBN 3-540-05571-1

Volume 6: K. Federlin
Immunopathology of Insulin
Clinical and Experimental Studies
1971. 53 figures. XIII, 185 pages
ISBN 3-540-05408-1

Volume 5: J. Müller
Regulation of Aldosterone Biosynthesis
1971. 19 figures. VII, 137 pages
ISBN 3-540-05213-5

Volume 4: U. Westphal
Steroid-Protein Interactions
1971. 144 figures. XIII, 567 pages
ISBN 3-540-05312-3

Volume 3: F. G. Sulman
Hypothalamic Control of Lactation
In collaboration with M. Ben-David, A. Danon, S. Dikstein, Y. Givant, K. Khazen, J. Mishkinsky-Shani, I. Nir, C. P. Weller

1970. 58 figures. XII, 235 pages
ISBN 3-540-04973-8

Volume 2: K. B. Eik-Nes, E. C. Horning
Gas Phase Chromatography of Steroids
1968. 85 figures. XV, 382 pages
ISBN 3-540-04277-6

Springer-Verlag
Berlin
Heidelberg
New York

Volume 1: S. Ohno
Sex Chromosomes and Sex-Linked Genes
1967. 33 figures. X, 192 pages
ISBN 3-540-03934-1

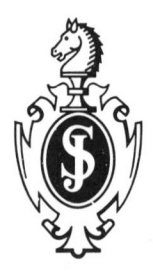

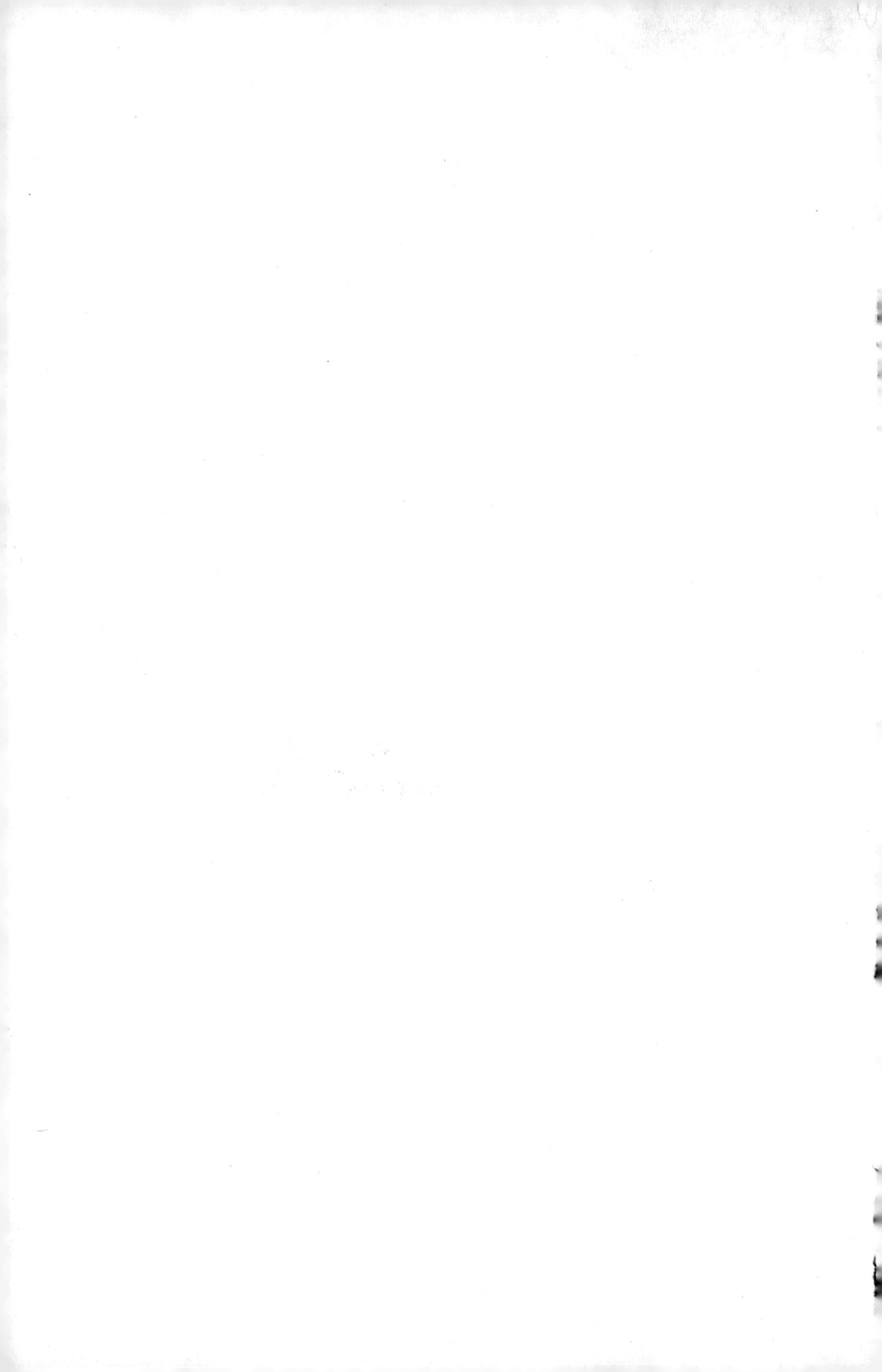